20 Years of Guided Bone Regeneration in Implant Dentistry

Second Edition

SECOND EDITION

20 Years of GUIDED BONE REGENERATION in Implant Dentistry

Edited by

Daniel Buser, DDS, PROF DR MED DENT

Professor and Chairman

Department of Oral Surgery and Stomatology

School of Dental Medicine

University of Bern

Bern, Switzerland

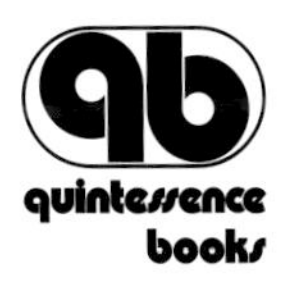

Quintessence Publishing Co, Inc

Chicago, Berlin, Tokyo, London, Paris, Milan, Barcelona, Istanbul, São Paulo, New Delhi, Moscow, Prague, and Warsaw

Library of Congress Cataloging-in-Publication Data

20 years of guided bone regeneration in implant dentistry / edited by Daniel Buser. —
2nd ed.
p. ; cm.
Rev. ed. of: Guided bone regeneration in implant dentistry / edited by Daniel Buser,
Christer Dahlin, Robert K. Schenk. c1994.
Includes bibliographical references and index.
ISBN 978-0-86715-401-6 (hardcover)
1. Endosseous dental implants. 2. Guided bone regeneration. I. Buser, Daniel. II.
Guided bone regeneration in implant dentistry. III. Title: Twenty years of guided bone
regeneration in implant dentistry. IV. Title: Guided bone regeneration in implant
dentistry.
[DNLM: 1. Guided Tissue Regeneration, Periodontal. 2. Bone Regeneration. 3. Dental
Implantation, Endosseous—methods. WU 240 Z999 2009]
RK667.I45G84 2009
617.6'92—dc22
2009024243

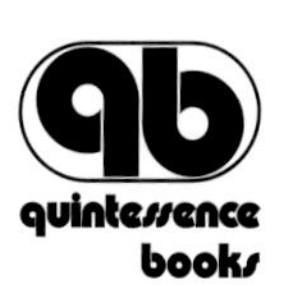

Quintessence Publishing Co Inc
4350 Chandler Drive
Hanover Park, IL 60133
www.quintpub.com

Editor: Kathryn Funk
Design: Gina Ruffolo
Production: Angelina Sanchez

Printed in Singapore

Contents

To the pioneers of
guided bone regeneration

L. A. Hurley
C. A. L. Bassett
P. J. Boyne
T. P. Rüedi
T. Karring
S. Nyman
C. Dahlin
R. K. Schenk

Foreword

To be provided with the opportunity to write a foreword for a significant new textbook represents both a true honor and privilege, but certainly also a genuine responsibility toward the authors. The work at hand not only represents a definite landmark in clinical dentistry but also has been carefully edited and in part written by my close friend of many years. The text comprehensively surveys 20 years of a fundamental and ever-growing field in implant dentistry and defines the current state of the art in guided bone regeneration. At the end of the first decade of the new millennium, guided bone regeneration and peri-implant contour augmentation are well established and inseparably connected to successful clinical implant dentistry. In fact, the knowledge of what techniques, procedures, and associated biomaterials are available today, linked to indispensable scientific documentation, provide the clinician with the basis for appropriate clinical decision making and—according to the practitioner's education and competence—subsequent treatment. In this context, the SAC concept, which objectively differentiates between straightforward (S), advanced (A), and complex (C) clinical situations, has particular importance and therefore has been strongly promoted by the author. Furthermore, as the title of this textbook suggests, guided bone regeneration, although an independent discipline, is strongly and primarily connected to implant dentistry, which now promotes prosthetically driven implant placement, rather than the antiquated bone-driven approach. The authors, all of them highly qualified and considered experts in the field, guarantee both the impressive quality of this work and its completeness in covering all the various aspects involved. Oral surgeons, periodontists, prosthodontists, general practitioners, and dental students are certain to find information that is relevant to their unique goals and perspectives. This textbook is destined to quickly reach the level of a true standard and long-standing reference.

Urs C. Belser, DDS, Prof Dr Med Dent
Professor
Department of Prosthodontics
School of Dental Medicine
University of Geneva
Geneva, Switzerland

Preface

The use of barrier membranes for the regeneration of bone defects has significantly changed implant dentistry in the past 20 years. This principle, often called *guided bone regeneration* (*GBR* or *GBR technique*), was first described in 1959 by Hurley and colleagues for experimental spinal fusion treatment. In the 1960s, the research teams of Bassett and Boyne tested microporous cellulose acetate laboratory filters (Millipore) for the healing of cortical defects in long bones and for osseous facial reconstruction, respectively. The authors used these filters to establish a suitable environment for osteogenesis by excluding fibrous connective tissue cells from bone defects. However, these pioneering studies did not immediately lead to a broad clinical application of barrier membranes in patients. The clinical potential of the membrane technique was not recognized until the early 1980s, when the research team of Karring and Nyman systematically examined barrier membranes in various experimental and clinical studies for periodontal regeneration. A few years later, barrier membrane techniques were tested in experimental studies on bone regeneration. Based on promising results in these studies, clinical testing of membranes began in implant patients in the late 1980s.

In 1994, after 5 years of intensive experimental and clinical work, the first edition of this textbook, *Guided Bone Regeneration in Implant Dentistry*, was published and generated a high level of interest among those in the field of implant dentistry. Since that time, the GBR technique has continued to evolve, necessitating an updated analysis of its scientific basis and clinical applications. The result is in your hands—the second edition of the GBR book, *20 Years of Guided Bone Regeneration in Implant Dentistry*.

This book is again written for the clinician with interest and experience in implant dentistry. The first four chapters focus on the basic science of GBR in implant dentistry. These chapters help the reader to understand the biologic and biomaterial background of this well-documented and well-established surgical technique in implant dentistry—essential knowledge for the use of barrier membranes in patients. As an introduction to the topic of the book, chapter 1 discusses the development of the GBR technique over the past 20 years. In this chapter, the four factors important for a successful regenerative outcome are described. Chapter 2 covers the biologic basis of bone regeneration and presents a scientific update on bone formation and remodeling. It features excellent histologic images obtained using undecalcified sections over the course of more than 30 years of experimental orthopedic research. Chapter 3 describes the characteristics, advantages, and disadvantages of nonresorbable and bioresorbable barrier membranes used in implant dentistry. Chapter 4 contains information about the various types of bone grafts and bone substitutes routinely used in combination with barrier membranes. These bone fillers not only provide support and thus help prevent membrane collapse but also influence new bone formation and bone remodeling in the defect area. The various characteristics of bone fillers, such as their osteogenetic and osteoconductive potential and substitution rates, are presented based on various experimental studies.

Chapters 5 through 9 focus on the clinical applications of GBR. Each chapter presents specific indications and describes the criteria for patient selection, the step-by-step surgical procedure, and aspects of postoperative treatment. Emphasis is placed on incision technique, flap design, the handling and placement of barrier membranes, the combination of membranes with autogenous bone grafts and low-substitution bone fillers, and approaches to wound closure. These five clinical chapters reflect the immense progress of GBR in the past 10 to 15 years and the current clinical status of GBR in implant dentistry.

As editor, I cordially thank all the authors and coauthors for the great amount of time and effort they contributed to the realization of this textbook. It has been a very intensive but satisfying experience to collaborate with colleagues of such quality. I also thank Ms Jeannie Wurz for her excellent work in editing and checking all manuscripts prior to submission to the publisher. Last but not least, I thank the staff of Quintessence Publishing for their excellent collaboration in completing this book and again providing superb quality in their work and printing.

Contributors

Michael M. Bornstein, Dr Med Dent
Assistant Professor and Head
Section of Dental Radiology and Stomatology
Department of Oral Surgery and Stomatology
University of Bern
Bern, Switzerland

Dieter D. Bosshardt, PhD, Dr Sc Nat
Senior Scientist and Head
Laboratory of Oral Histology
School of Dental Medicine
University of Bern
Bern, Switzerland

Daniel Buser, DDS, Prof Dr Med Dent
Professor and Chairman
Department of Oral Surgery and Stomatology
School of Dental Medicine
University of Bern
Bern, Switzerland

Stephen T. Chen, BDS, MDSc, PhD
Senior Fellow in Periodontics
School of Dental Science
University of Melbourne
Victoria, Australia

Simon Storgård Jensen, DDS
Consulting Oral and Maxillofacial Surgeon
Department of Oral and Maxillofacial Surgery
Copenhagen University Hospital
Glostrup, Denmark
Research Fellow
Department of Oral Surgery and Stomatology
School of Dental Medicine
University of Bern
Bern, Switzerland

Isabella Rocchietta, DDS
Research Fellow
Department of Periodontology
School of Dentistry
University of Milan
Milan, Italy

Robert K. Schenk, MD, Prof Dr Med
Professor Emeritus of Anatomy
Department of Oral Surgery and Stomatology
School of Dental Medicine
University of Bern
Bern, Switzerland

Massimo Simion, MD, DDS
Professor and Chairman
Department of Periodontology
School of Dentistry
University of Milan
Milan, Italy

Thomas von Arx, DDS, Prof Dr Med Dent
Associate Professor
Department of Oral Surgery and Stomatology
School of Dental Medicine
University of Bern
Bern, Switzerland

CHAPTER 1

Guided Bone Regeneration over the Past 20 Years

Daniel Buser

Based on fundamental experimental studies performed by the research teams of Per-Ingvar Brånemark from the University of Gothenburg (Sweden) and André Schroeder from the University of Bern (Switzerland), the use of dental implants has become a scientifically accepted treatment for the replacement of lost or missing teeth in fully and partially edentulous patients. In landmark papers published in the late 1960s and 1970s, both research teams described the phenomenon of osseointegrated titanium implants.[1–3] An osseointegrated implant is characterized by direct apposition of living bone to the titanium surface.[4,5]

Several prerequisites have been defined for achieving osseointegration of titanium implants with high predictability.[1,2] Some of these have been revised over the past 30 years; others are still considered important. To achieve osseointegration, the implant must be inserted with a low-trauma surgical technique to avoid overheating of the bone during preparation of a precise recipient site, and the implant should be placed with sufficient primary stability.[6] When these clinical guidelines are followed, successful osseointegration will predictably occur for nonsubmerged titanium implants (single-stage procedure) as well as for submerged titanium implants (two-stage procedure), as demonstrated in comparative, experimental studies.[7,8]

When clinical testing of osseointegrated implants first began, the majority of treated patients were fully edentulous. Promising results were reported in various retrospective studies.[9–13] Encouraged by these good treatment outcomes, clinicians started to utilize osseointegrated implants in partially edentulous patients, and the first reports of promising short-term results were published in the late 1980s and early 1990s.[14–18] As a consequence, single-tooth gaps and distal-extension situations have become more and more common indications for implant therapy in daily practice, and today these applications dominate in many clinical centers.[19]

One of the most important prerequisites for achieving and maintaining successful osseointegration is the presence of a sufficient volume of healthy bone at the recipient site. This includes not only bone of sufficient height to allow the insertion of an implant of appropriate length but also a ridge of sufficient crest width. Clinical studies have shown that implants placed in a site with a missing buccal bone wall have a greater rate of soft tissue complications[20] and/or a compromised long-term prognosis.[21,22] To avoid increased rates of implant complications and failures, these studies suggested that sites with inadequate bone volume either should be considered local contraindications to implant placement or should be locally augmented with an appropriate surgical procedure to regenerate the bone and allow implant placement.

In the 1980s and early 1990s, several attempts were made to develop new surgical techniques to augment bony defects in the alveolar ridge to overcome these local contraindications to implant-borne prostheses. The proposed techniques included vertical ridge augmentation with autogenous bone grafts from the iliac crest in extremely atrophic mandibles or maxillae,[23,24] sinus floor elevation procedures in partially or fully edentulous maxillae,[25–27] the application of autogenous onlay grafts for lateral ridge augmentation,[28–30] or split-crest techniques, such as alveolar extension plasty.[31–33]

During the same period, in addition to these new surgical techniques, the concept of guided bone regeneration (GBR) utilizing barrier membranes was introduced. Based on case reports and short-term clinical studies, various authors reported first results with this membrane technique for the regeneration of localized bone defects in implant patients.[34–39]

This textbook provides an update on the biologic basis of the GBR technique and its clinical applications, predominantly in partially edentulous patients. Clinical experience with GBR in implant patients now spans 20 years. These 20 years can be divided into a development phase and a phase of routine application.

Development Phase

The utilization of barrier membranes for implant patients was certainly triggered by the clinical application of barrier membranes for periodontal regeneration, called *guided tissue regeneration* (GTR). GTR was first developed in the early 1980s by Nyman et al.[40,41] The initial studies were made with Millipore filters (Millipore), which had already been used in the late 1950s and 1960s for the regeneration of bone defects in experimental studies.[42–44] However, these studies had no impact on the development of new surgical techniques to regenerate localized defects in the jaws because the potential of this membrane application probably was not recognized.

The articles by Nyman et al[40,41] in the field of GTR, both of which demonstrated successful treatment outcomes of GTR procedures, created a great deal of interest and led to much research activity in the mid- to late 1980s.[45–48] These studies were performed with expanded polytetrafluoroethylene (ePTFE), which is a bioinert membrane and became the standard membrane for GTR and GBR procedures during the development phase of both techniques. The use of ePTFE membranes for bone regeneration was initiated in the mid-1980s by the group led by Nyman and Dahlin, who performed a series of experimental studies.[49–51] These studies confirmed the concept that the application of an ePTFE membrane creates a physical barrier that separates the tissues and cells that could potentially participate in the wound healing events. The barrier membrane creates a secluded space and facilitates the proliferation of angiogenic and osteogenic cells from the marrow space into that defect without interference by fibroblasts. These events were nicely demonstrated by Schenk et al[52] in a landmark experimental study in foxhounds. The current understanding of wound healing events in membrane-protected bone defects are presented in chapter 2.

The utilization of ePTFE membranes for GBR procedures in patients started in the late 1980s. The main objective was to regenerate peri-implant bone defects in implant sites with local bone deficiencies. The GBR technique has been used with a simultaneous or a staged approach.[35] Implant placement with simultaneous GBR was predominantly used for immediate implant placement in postextraction sites to regenerate peri-implant bone defects[34,37] or for implants with crestal dehiscence defects.[39] The staged approach was used in clinical situations with healed implant sites but an insufficient crest width. The membrane technique was utilized to enlarge the crest width with a first surgery, and implant placement took place in a second surgical procedure performed after 6 to 9 months of healing.[36]

Early on, several complications were noted with both approaches, and modifications of the surgical techniques were proposed to improve the predictability for successful treatment outcomes. One frequently seen complication was the collapse of ePTFE membranes, which reduced the volume of the regenerated tissue underneath the membrane. In addition, some of the regenerated sites demonstrated insufficient bone formation and the formation of a periosteum-like tissue underneath the membrane.[36,39] Therefore, bone fillers such as autografts or allografts were recommended by various groups, not only to support the membrane and eliminate membrane collapse but also to enhance new bone formation through the osteogenic potential of autogenous bone grafts.[53–55] The combination of ePTFE membranes and autogenous bone grafts provided good clinical outcomes with both approaches (Figs 1-1 and 1-2).

In the mid-1990s, several expert meetings took place to discuss the potential and limitations of the GBR technique used in daily practice at that time. These meetings clearly showed that an improvement of the GBR technique was necessary to allow its widespread use in implant dentistry. The experts agreed that the GBR technique—based on the utilization of ePTFE membranes in combination with bone grafts or bone substitutes—had the following weaknesses: *(1)* a significant rate of membrane exposures arising from soft tissue dehiscences, often leading to local infection underneath the membrane and subsequently to a compromised treatment outcome of the GBR procedure[56–59]; *(2)* difficult handling of the membrane during surgery because of its hydrophobic properties, requiring stabilization of the membrane with miniscrews and tacks[54,60]; and *(3)* the need for a second surgical procedure to remove the bioinert, nonresorbable membrane.

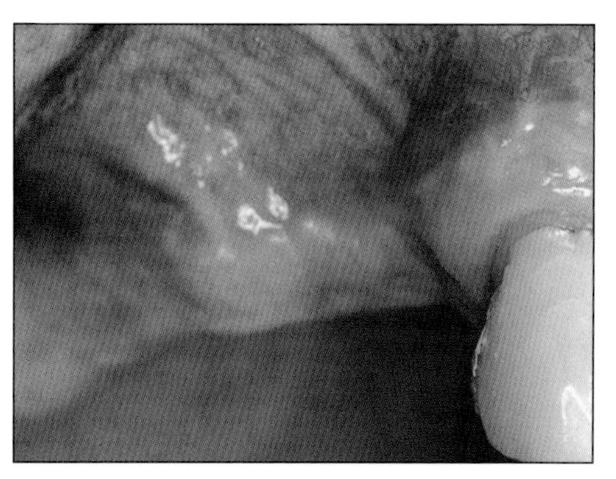

Fig 1-1a Distal-extension situation in the right maxilla. Two titanium implants are planned to allow placement of a fixed dental prosthesis.

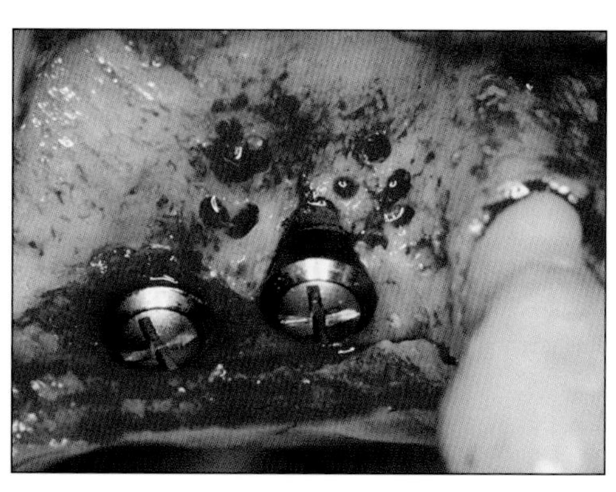

Fig 1-1b The insertion of both implants has resulted in a crestal dehiscence defect at the mesial implant. The corticalized bone surface has been perforated with a small round bur to open the marrow cavity and stimulate bleeding in the defect area.

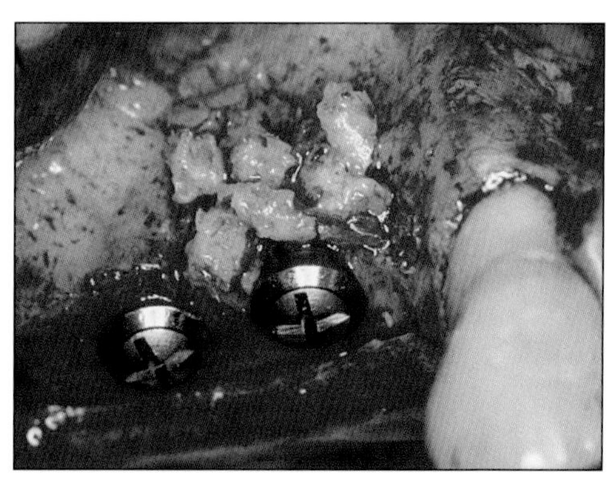

Fig 1-1c Locally harvested bone chips are applied to support the ePTFE membrane and to stimulate new bone formation in the defect area.

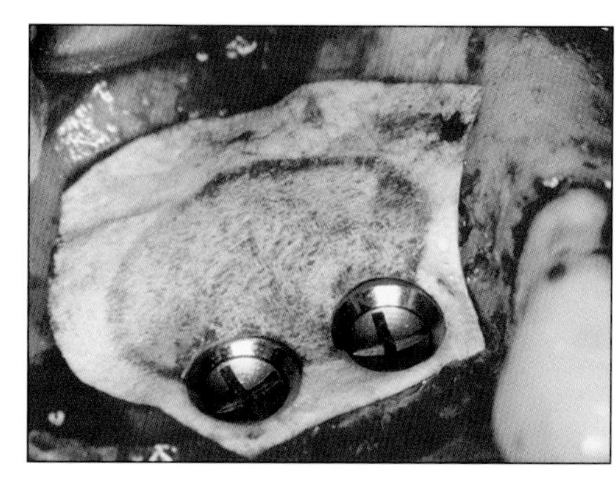

Fig 1-1d A nonresorbable ePTFE membrane is applied to function as a physical barrier. The punched membrane is stabilized around the neck of both implants.

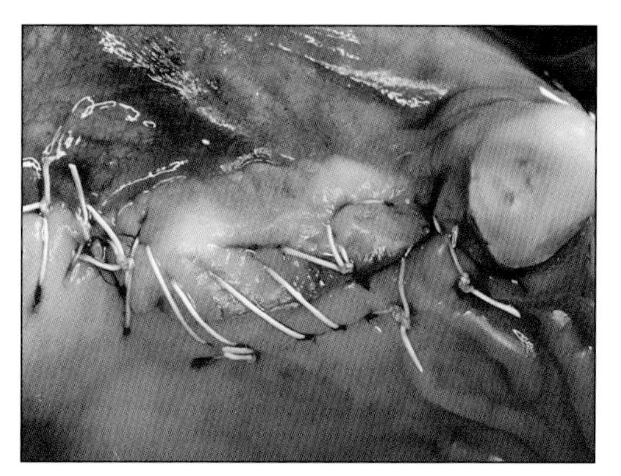

Fig 1-1e Following incision of the periosteum, the surgery is completed with a tension-free primary wound closure.

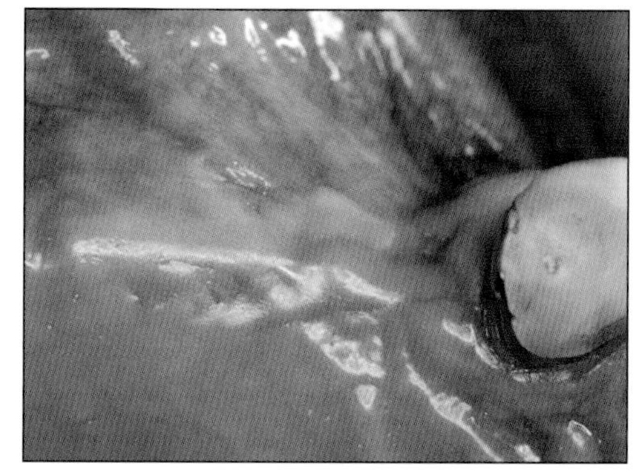

Fig 1-1f The clinical status is satisfactory 4 months following implant surgery. Wound healing was uneventful and without complication.

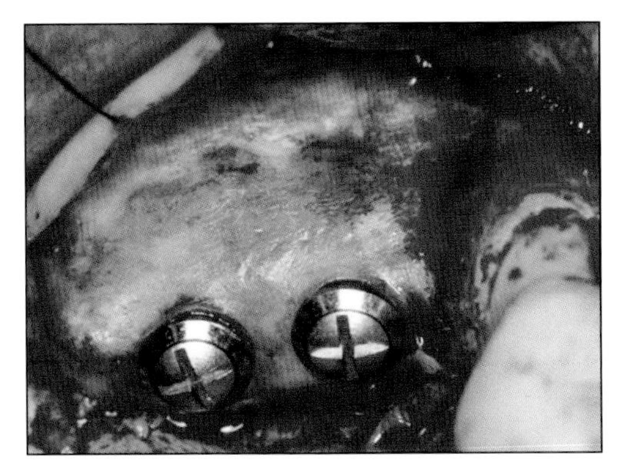

Fig 1-1g The site is reopened after 4 months of healing. A second surgery is necessary to remove the nonresorbable membrane.

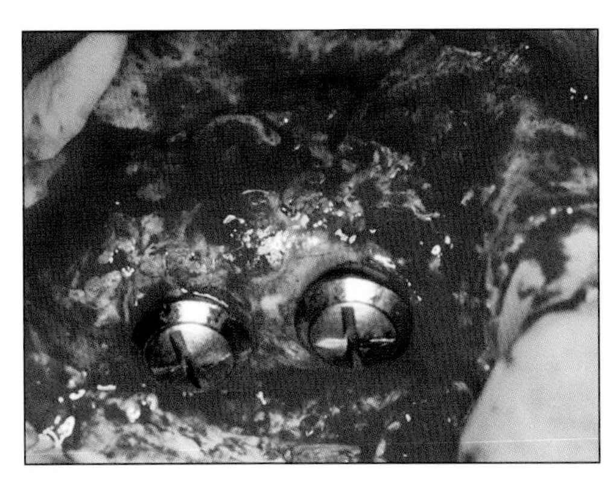

Fig 1-1h The clinical status following membrane removal shows successful bone regeneration in the defect area.

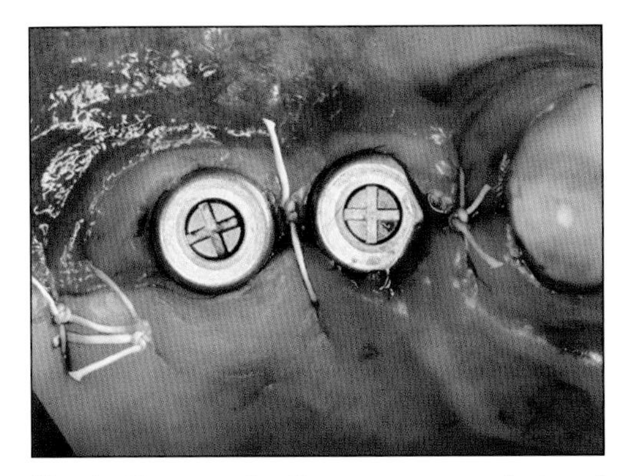

Fig 1-1i Longer healing caps are applied, and the soft tissue margin is adapted and secured in place with interrupted sutures.

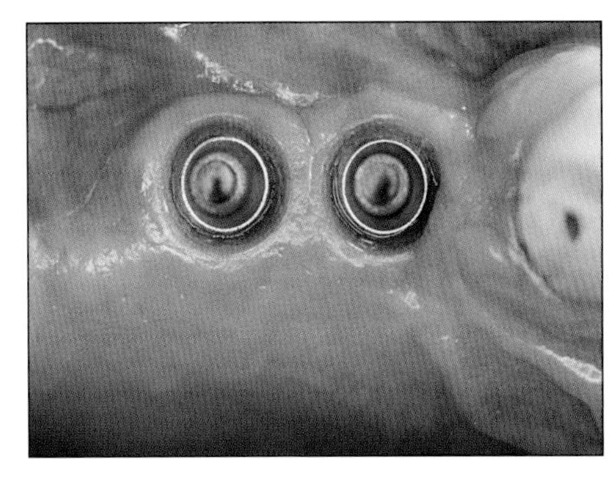

Fig 1-1j Two weeks later, the soft tissues have healed and both implants can be restored with a single crown.

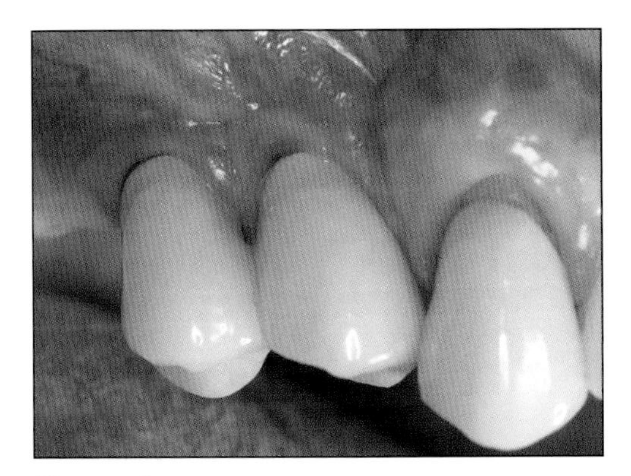

Fig 1-1k A satisfactory treatment outcome is evident at the 15-year follow-up examination.

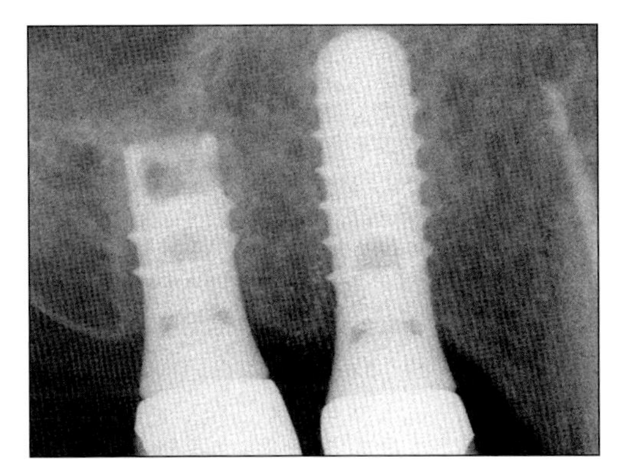

Fig 1-1l The radiographic follow-up at 15 years reveals that the bone crest levels are stable around both implants.

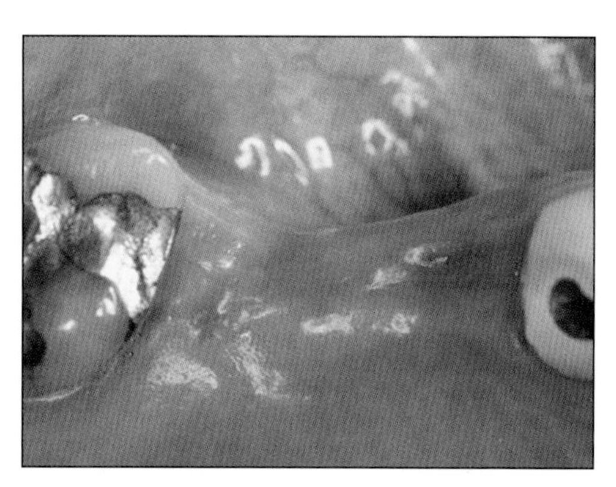

Fig 1-2a Preoperative occlusal view of the right maxilla with two missing premolars. The facial mucosa is flattened.

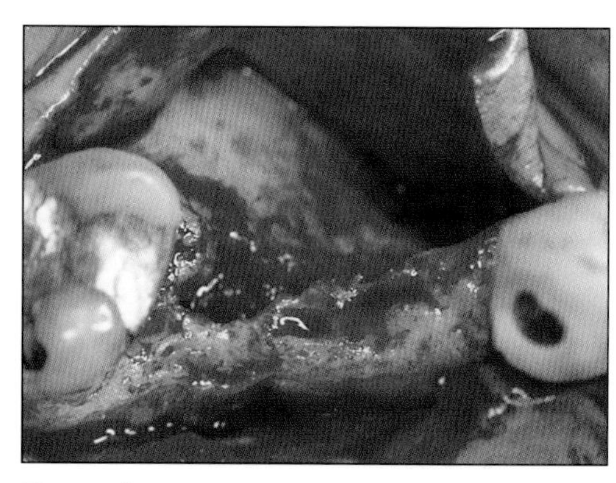

Fig 1-2b Elevation of a mucoperiosteal flap reveals an insufficient crest width of less than 4 mm. The clinical situation requires a staged approach.

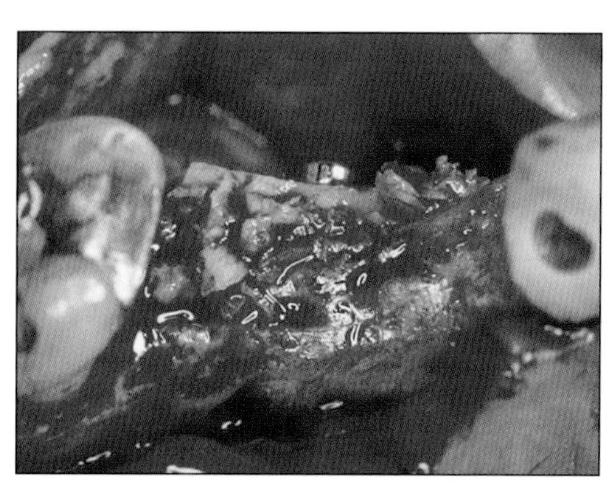

Fig 1-2c A block graft is applied to increase the width of the alveolar crest.

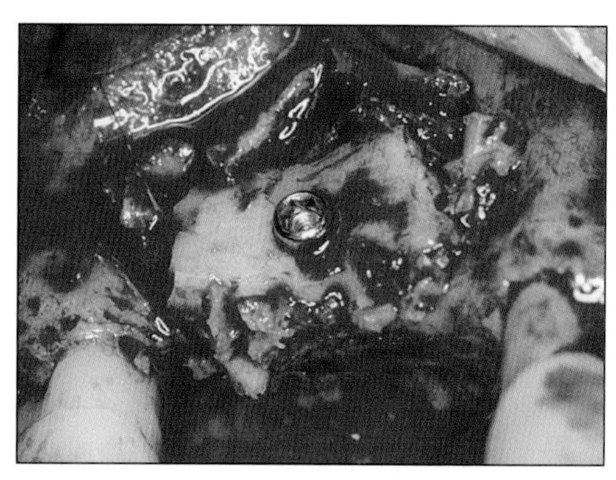

Fig 1-2d The facial view shows the applied block graft stabilized with a titanium screw.

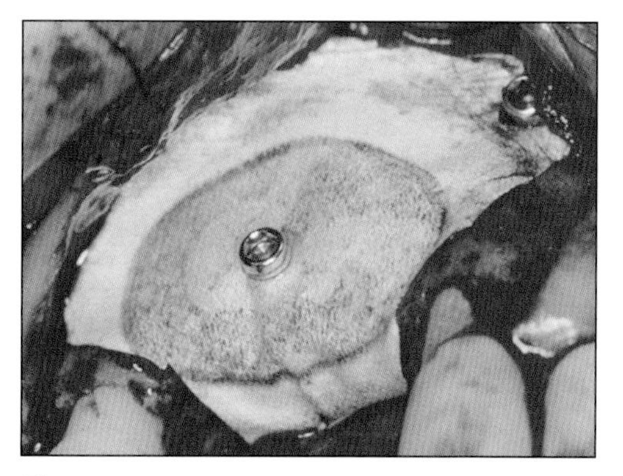

Fig 1-2e Following application of an ePTFE membrane, miniscrews are used to stabilize the hydrophobic membrane.

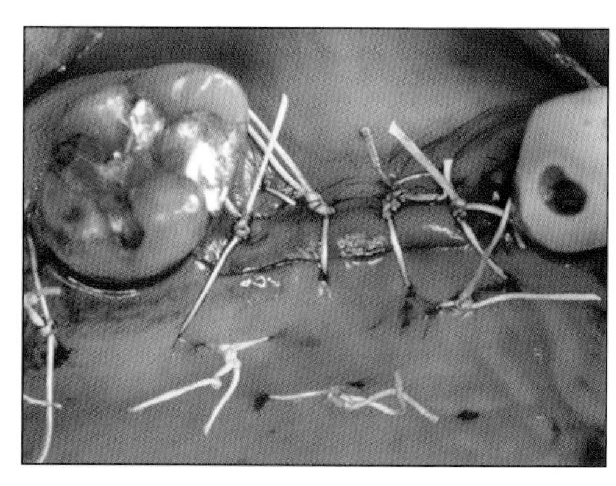

Fig 1-2f Primary wound closure is achieved with mattress and interrupted single sutures using 4-0 ePTFE sutures.

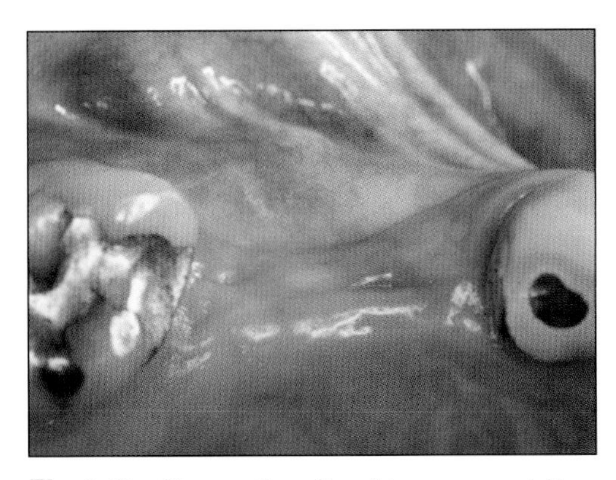

Fig 1-2g Six months after ridge augmentation, healthy soft tissues are found following a healing period that was free of complications.

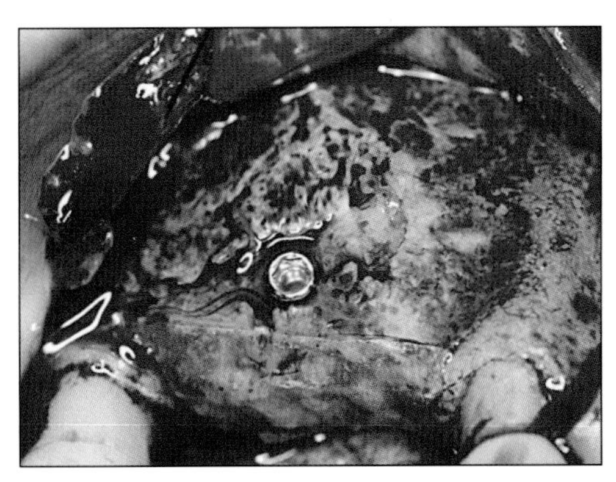

Fig 1-2h Following flap elevation and membrane removal, the facial view shows regenerated tissue. The block graft can still be recognized but is covered in some areas with newly formed bone.

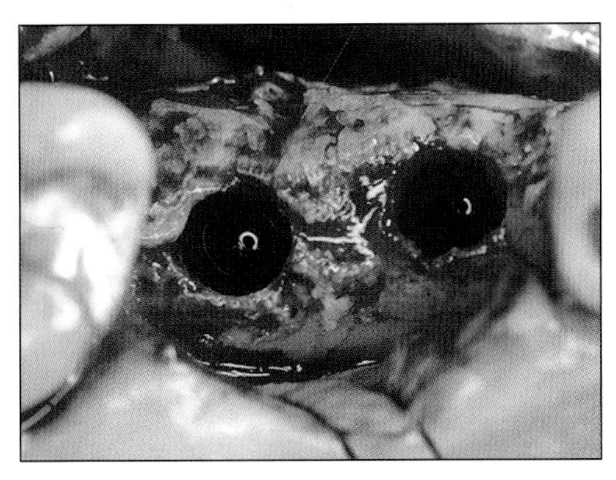

Fig 1-2i The occlusal view confirms successful ridge augmentation. The crest width measures more than 6 mm, allowing the placement of two implants.

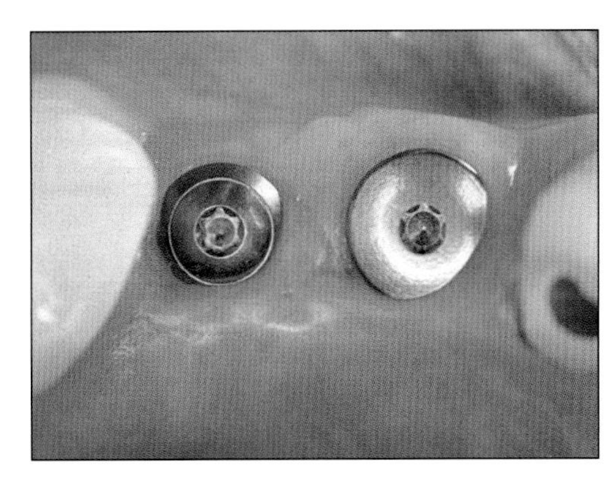

Fig 1-2j Following 3 months of nonsubmerged healing of both implants, the peri-implant mucosa is healthy.

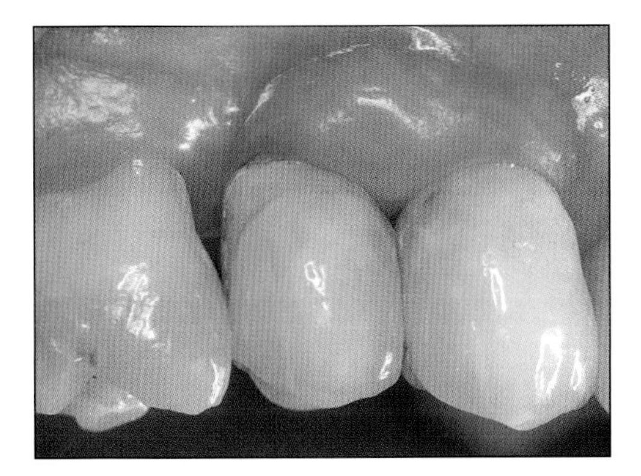

Fig 1-2k Fourteen years after implant placement, the peri-implant mucosa is healthy and stable.

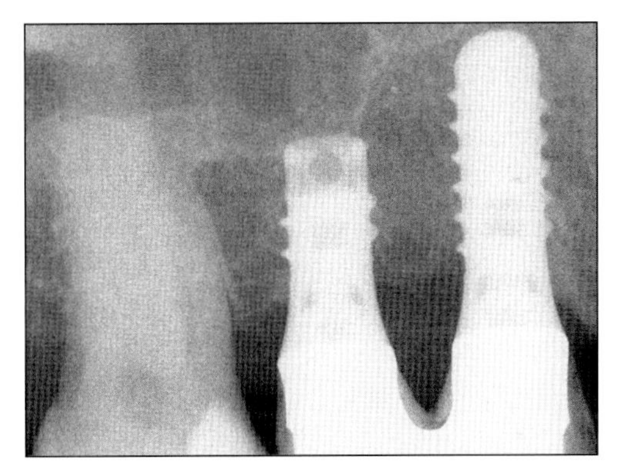

Fig 1-2l The periapical radiograph at the 14-year examination confirms the stable bone crest levels around both implants.

Box 1-1	Objectives for improvements of the GBR technique

- To make successful outcomes more predictable and reduce the rate of complications with membrane exposure and membrane infection
- To make the technique more user friendly, with easier membrane application during surgery
- To make the technique more patient friendly by eliminating a second surgical procedure for membrane removal whenever possible and by reducing healing periods as much as possible

During these meetings, the participants defined objectives to improve the predictability and attractiveness of GBR procedures in implant patients for both the patient and the clinician (Box 1-1). It was clear to the participants at these expert meetings that these objectives could only be achieved with the utilization of a bioresorbable membrane. This trend was again initiated in the field of GTR, with the introduction of the first bioresorbable membranes in the early 1990s.[61,62] Subsequently, numerous studies in animals examined different bioresorbable membranes for GBR procedures as well.[63–74] In general, two different groups of bioresorbable membranes were evaluated: *(1)* polymeric membranes made of polylactic or polyglycolic acid and *(2)* collagen membranes produced from various animal sources.[75] The characteristics of different barrier membranes used for GBR procedures are discussed in detail in chapter 3.

Compared with the selection of an appropriate barrier membrane, the selection of appropriate bone fillers to support membranes is at least as important for the treatment outcome. The various bone grafts and bone substitutes that can be used as bone fillers underneath membranes are discussed in detail in chapter 4.

Routine Application

Parallel to these experimental studies, clinicians started to use bioresorbable membranes in patients. The first published clinical reports were predominantly studies with collagen membranes.[76–81] Today, collagen membranes are routinely used in daily practice for GBR procedures.

In the past 10 years, the GBR technique has become the standard of care for the regeneration of localized bone defects in implant patients. A systematic review by Aghaloo and Moy[82] demonstrated that implants placed with the GBR procedure have favorable survival rates and that the GBR procedure is the only well-documented surgical technique among various surgical techniques used for localized ridge augmentation. The only other scientifically well-documented surgical technique at present is sinus grafting (sinus floor elevation). Today, clinicians performing GBR procedures are in the favorable situation of selecting their surgical approach and biomaterials from a

Box 1-2 Objectives for GBR procedures

Primary objectives
- Successful bone regeneration of the defect with high predictability to provide long-lasting function and esthetics
- Low risk of complications

Secondary objectives
- The least number of surgical interventions
- Low morbidity for the patient
- Reduced healing periods

variety of options. The chosen GBR procedure should always attempt to fulfill the primary and secondary objectives in a given clinical situation (Box 1-2).

The primary objectives of a GBR procedure are the achievement of successful bone regeneration in the defect area with high predictability and a low risk of complications. The secondary objectives are to obtain a successful outcome with the least number of surgical interventions, a low morbidity for the patient, and a shortened healing period. As already discussed, these secondary objectives have been very important in the past 10 to 15 years because clinicians around the globe have tried to improve these clinical aspects in an attempt to make GBR procedures less stressful and/or more attractive for patients in daily practice. These secondary objectives should not compromise the primary objectives of GBR procedures, however. In other words, a therapeutic approach that promises a low number of surgical procedures, a low morbidity for the patient, or a short treatment time should neither reduce the predictability of successful treatment outcomes nor increase the risk of complications. Therefore, all aspects are important, but the primary objectives have a clear priority.

The anticipated treatment outcome is influenced by four factors that have recently been described in detail by Buser and Chen[83] for implant placement in postextraction sites (Fig 1-3). These factors are valid for GBR procedures in general. The key factor is the clinician, who makes all decisions based on a proper assessment of the clinical situation. The clinician evaluates the patient, selects appropriate biomaterials, and decides on the most suitable treatment approach to provide the anticipated treatment outcome.

A comprehensive analysis of the patient enables the clinician to determine whether the situation can be classified as low, medium, or high risk. In addition to determining if the patient has a smoking habit, the clinician should evaluate medical, dental, and anatomical risk factors in detail, in particular the morphology of the bone defect to be regenerated. The defect morphology plays an important role in the selection of the appropriate surgical technique and particularly in determining whether a simultaneous or a staged approach is more appropriate. These aspects are discussed in detail in chapter 6.

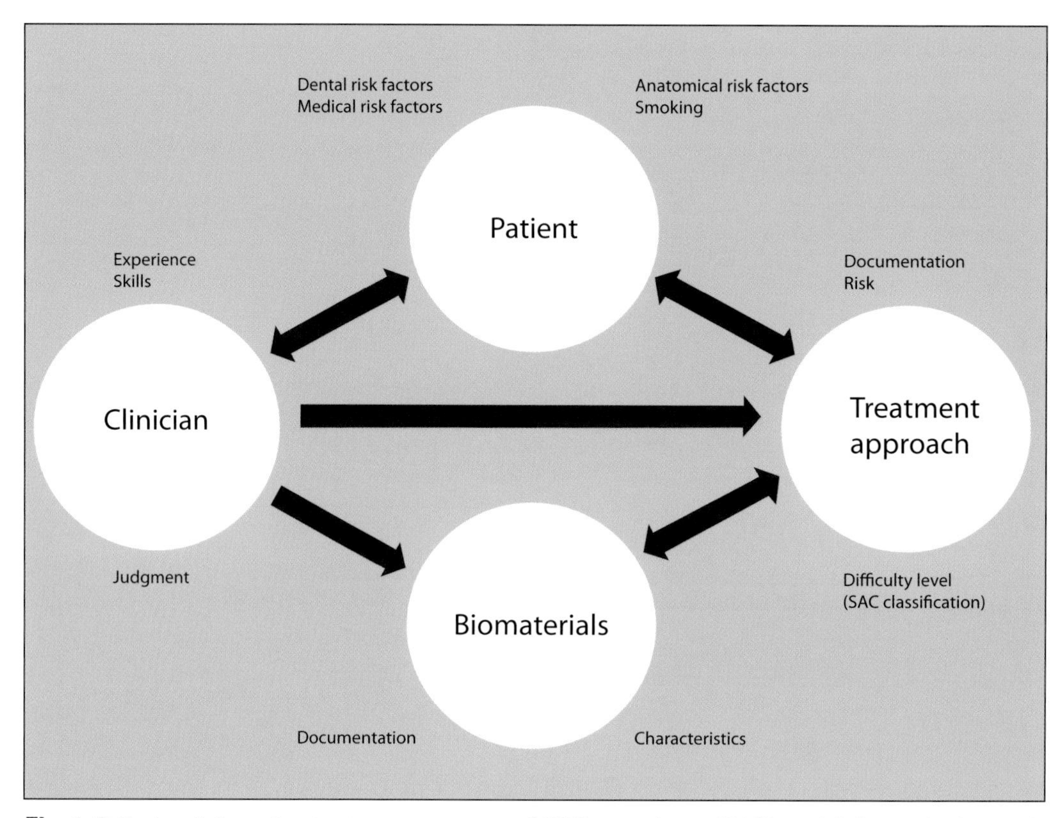

Fig 1-3 Factors influencing treatment outcomes of GBR procedures. (SAC) straightforward-advanced-complex. (Reprinted from Buser and Chen[83] with permission.)

Conclusion

Over the past 20 years, significant progress has been made in developing GBR procedures in implant dentistry. GBR has become a standard of care for the regeneration of localized bone defects in the alveolar ridge of potential implant patients. This progress has been an important contributing factor in the rapid expansion of implant therapy in the past 10 to 15 years.

The recommended step-by-step procedures in various clinical situations are presented in chapters 6 through 9. The reader of this textbook will quickly realize that the recommended surgical techniques are rather conservative. This conservative approach offers the best level of predictability in attaining a successful treatment outcome with a low risk of complications. Hence, this conservative approach offers the best chance to be a successful clinician who is able to satisfy patients' high expectations.

References

1. Brånemark PI, Breine U, Adell R, Hansson BO, Lindström J, Ohlsson A. Intra-osseous anchorage of dental prostheses. 1. Experimental studies. Scand J Plast Reconstr Surg 1969;3:81–100.
2. Schroeder A, Pohler O, Sutter F. Gewebsreaktion auf ein Titan-Hohlzylinderimplantat mit Titan-Spritzschichtoberfläche. Schweiz Monatsschr Zahnmed 1976;86:713–727.
3. Schroeder A, van der Zypen E, Stich H, Sutter F. The reactions of bone, connective tissue, and epithelium to endosteal implants with titanium-sprayed surfaces. J Maxillofac Surg 1981;9:15–25.
4. Albrektsson T, Brånemark PI, Hansson HA, Lindström J. Osseointegrated titianium implants. Requirements for ensuring a long-lasting direct bone anchorage in man. Acta Orthop Scand 1981;52: 155–170.
5. Schenk RK, Buser D. Osseointegration: A reality. Periodontol 2000 1998;17:22–35.
6. Buser D, von Arx T, ten Bruggenkate C, Weingart D. Basic surgical principles with ITI implants. Clin Oral Implants Res 2000;11(suppl 1):59–68.
7. Gotfredsen K, Rostrup E, Hjørting-Hansen E, Stoltze K, Budtz-Jörgensen E. Histological and histomorphometrical evaluation of tissue reactions adjacent to endosteal implants in monkeys. Clin Oral Implants Res 1991;2:30–37.
8. Weber HP, Buser D, Donath K, et al. Comparison of healed tissues adjacent to submerged and non-submerged unloaded titanium dental implants. A histometric study in beagle dogs. Clin Oral Implants Res 1996;7:11–19.
9. Brånemark PI, Hansson BO, Adell R, et al. Osseointegrated implants in the treatment of the edentulous jaw. Experience from a 10-year period. Scand J Plast Reconstr Surg 1977;16(suppl):1–132.
10. Adell R, Lekholm U, Rockler B, Brånemark PI. A 15-year study of osseointegrated implants in the treatment of the edentulous jaw. Int J Oral Surgery 1981; 10:387–416.
11. Cox JF, Zarb GA. The longitudinal clinical efficacy of osseointegrated dental implants: A 3-year report. Int J Oral Maxillofac Implants 1987;2:91–100.
12. Albrektsson T, Dahl E, Enbom L, et al. Osseointegrated oral implants. A Swedish multicenter study of 8139 consecutively inserted Nobelpharma implants. J Periodontol 1988;59:287–296.
13. Babbush CA, Kent JN, Misiek DJ. Titanium plasma-sprayed (TPS) screw implants for the reconstruction of the edentulous mandible. J Oral Maxillofac Surg 1986;44:274–282.
14. Jemt T, Lekholm U, Adell R. Osseointegrated implants in the treatment of partially edentulous patients: A preliminary study on 876 consecutively placed fixtures. Int J Oral Maxillofac Implants 1989; 4:211–217.
15. Buser D, Weber HP, Lang NP. Tissue integration of non-submerged implants. 1-year results of a prospective study with 100 ITI hollow-cylinder and hollow-screw implants. Clin Oral Implants Res 1990;1:33–40.
16. Buser D, Weber HP, Bragger U, Balsiger C. Tissue integration of one-stage ITI implants: 3-year results of a longitudinal study with hollow-cylinder and hollow-screw implants. Int J Oral Maxillofac Implants 1991;6:405–412.
17. Zarb GA, Schmitt A. The longitudinal clinical effectiveness of osseointegrated dental implants in anterior partially edentulous patients. Int J Prosthodont 1993;6:180–188.
18. Zarb GA, Schmitt A. The longitudinal clinical effectiveness of osseointegrated dental implants in posterior partially edentulous patients. Int J Prosthodont 1993;6:189–196.
19. Bornstein MM, Halbritter S, Harnisch H, Weber HP, Buser D. A retrospective analysis of patients referred for implant placement to a specialty clinic: Indications, surgical procedures, and early failures. Int J Oral Maxillofac Implants 2008;23:1109–1116.
20. Lekholm U, Adell R, Lindhe J, et al. Marginal tissue reactions at osseointegrated titanium fixtures. 2. A cross-sectional retrospective study. Int J Oral Maxillofac Surg 1986;15:53–61.
21. d'Hoedt B. 10 Jahre Tübinger Implantat aus Frialit - Eine Zwischenauswertung der Implantatdatei. Z Zahnärztl Implantol 1986;2:6–10.
22. Dietrich U, Lippold R, Dirmeier T, Behneke W, Wagner W. Statistische Ergebnisse zur Implantatprognose am Beispiel von 2017 IMZ-Implantaten unterschiedlicher Indikationen der letzten 13 Jahre. Z Zahnärztl Implantol 1993;9:9–18.
23. Lindstrom J, Brånemark PI, Albrektsson T. Mandibular reconstruction using the preformed autologous bone graft. Scand J Plastic Reconstr Surg 1981;15: 29–38.
24. Jensen J, Sindet-Pedersen S. Autogenous mandibular bone grafts and osseointegrated implants for reconstruction of the severely atrophic maxilla: A preliminary report. J Oral Maxillofac Surg 1991;49: 1277–1287.
25. Boyne PJ, James RA. Grafting of the maxillary sinus floor with autogenous bone and marrow. J Oral Surg 1980;38:613–616.
26. Wood RM, Moore DL. Grafting of the maxillary sinus with intraorally harvested autogenous bone prior to implant placement. Int J Oral Maxillofac Implants 1988;3:209–214.
27. Kent JN, Block MS. Simultaneous maxillary sinus floor bone grafting and placement of hydroxylapatite-coated implants. J Oral Maxillofac Surg 1989;47:238–242.
28. ten Bruggenkate CM, Kraaijenhagen HA, van der Kwast WAM, Krekeler G, Oosterbeek HS. Autogenous maxillary bone grafts in conjunction with placement of ITI endosseous implants: A preliminary report. Int J Oral Maxillofac Surg 1992;21:81–84.

29. Triplett RG, Schow SR. Autologous bone grafts and endosseous implants: Complementary techniques. J Oral Maxillofac Surg 1996;54:486–494.
30. Widmark G, Andersson B, Ivanoff CJ. Mandibular bone graft in the anterior maxilla for single-tooth implants. Presentation of surgical method. Int J Oral Maxillofac Surg 1997;26:106–109.
31. Osborn JF. Extension alveoloplasty (I). New surgical procedures for the treatment of alveolar collapse and residual ridge atrophy [in German]. Quintessenz 1985;36:9–16.
32. Khoury F. Die modifizierte Alveolar-Extensionsplastik. Z Zahnärztl Implantol 1987;3:174–178.
33. Simion M, Baldoni M, Zaffe D. Jawbone enlargement using immediate implant placement associated with a split-crest technique and guided tissue regeneration. Int J Periodontics Restorative Dent 1992;12:463–473.
34. Lazzara RJ. Immediate implant placement into extraction sites: Surgical and restorative advantages. Int J Periodontics Restorative Dent 1989;9:332–343.
35. Nyman S, Lang NP, Buser D, Bragger U. Bone regeneration adjacent to titanium dental implants using guided tissue regeneration: A report of two cases. Int J Oral Maxillofac Implants 1990;5:9–14.
36. Buser D, Bragger U, Lang NP, Nyman S. Regeneration and enlargement of jaw bone using guided tissue regeneration. Clin Oral Implants Res 1990;1: 22–32.
37. Becker W, Becker BE. Guided tissue regeneration for implants placed into extraction sockets and for implant dehiscences: Surgical techniques and case reports. Int J Periodontics Restorative Dent 1990;10: 376–391.
38. Dahlin C, Andersson L, Linde A. Bone augmentation at fenestrated implants by an osteopromotive membrane technique. A controlled clinical study. Clin Oral Implants Res 1991;2:159–165.
39. Jovanovic SA, Spiekermann H, Richter EJ. Bone regeneration around titanium dental implants in dehisced defect sites: A clinical study. Int J Oral Maxillofac Implants 1992;7:233–245.
40. Nyman S, Lindhe J, Karring T, Rylander H. New attachment following surgical treatment of human periodontal disease. J Clin Periodontol 1982;9: 290–296.
41. Nyman S, Gottlow J, Karring T, Lindhe J. The regenerative potential of the periodontal ligament. An experimental study in the monkey. J Clin Periodontol 1982;9:257–265.
42. Hurley LA, Stinchfield FE, Bassett CAL, Lyon WH. The role of soft tissues in osteogenesis. J Bone Joint Surg 1959;41a:1243.
43. Bassett CAL, Creighton DK, Stinchfield FE. Contribution of endosteum, cortex and soft tissues to osteogenesis. Surg Gynecol Obstet 1961;112:145.
44. Boyne PJ. Regeneration of alveolar bone beneath cellulose acetate filter implants [abstract]. J Dent Res 1964;43:827.
45. Gottlow J, Nyman S, Karring T, Lindhe J. New attachment formation as the result of controlled tissue regeneration. J Clin Periodontol 1984;11:494–503.
46. Gottlow J, Nyman S, Lindhe J, Karring T, Wennstrom J. New attachment formation in the human periodontium by guided tissue regeneration. Case reports. J Clin Periodontol 1986;13:604–616.
47. Pontoriero R, Nyman S, Lindhe J, Rosenberg E, Sanavi F. Guided tissue regeneration in the treatment of furcation defects in man. J Clin Periodontol 1987;14:618–620.
48. Pontoriero R, Lindhe J, Nyman S, Karring T, Rosenberg E, Sanavi F. Guided tissue regeneration in the treatment of furcation defects in mandibular molars. A clinical study of degree III involvements. J Clin Periodontol 1989;16:170–174.
49. Dahlin C, Linde A, Gottlow J, Nyman S. Healing of bone defects by guided tissue regeneration. Plastic Reconstr Surg 1988;81:672–676.
50. Dahlin C, Sennerby L, Lekholm U, Linde A, Nyman S. Generation of new bone around titanium implants using a membrane technique: An experimental study in rabbits. Int J Oral Maxillofac Implants 1989;4:19–25.
51. Dahlin C, Gottlow J, Linde A, Nyman S. Healing of maxillary and mandibular bone defects using a membrane technique. An experimental study in monkeys. Scand J Plast Reconstr Surg Hand Surg 1990;24:13–19.
52. Schenk RK, Buser D, Hardwick WR, Dahlin C. Healing pattern of bone regeneration in membrane-protected defects: A histologic study in the canine mandible. Int J Oral Maxillofac Implants 1994;9: 13–29.
53. Nevins M, Mellonig JT. Enhancement of the damaged edentulous ridge to receive dental implants: A combination of allograft and the Gore-Tex membrane. Int J Periodontics Restorative Dent 1992;12: 97–111.
54. Buser D, Dula K, Belser U, Hirt HP, Berthold H. Localized ridge augmentation using guided bone regeneration. 1. Surgical procedure in the maxilla. Int J Periodontics Restorative Dent 1993;13:29–45.
55. Buser D, Dula K, Belser UC, Hirt HP, Berthold H. Localized ridge augmentation using guided bone regeneration. 2. Surgical procedure in the mandible. Int J Periodontics Restorative Dent 1995;15:10–29.
56. Becker W, Dahlin C, Becker BE, et al. The use of e-PTFE barrier membranes for bone promotion around titanium implants placed into extraction sockets: A prospective multicenter study. Int J Oral Maxillofac Implants 1994;9:31–40.
57. Gotfredsen K, Nimb L, Buser D, Hjørting-Hansen E. Evaluation of guided bone generation around implants placed into fresh extraction sockets: An experimental study in dogs. J Oral Maxillofac Surg 1993;51:879–884; discussion 885–886.
58. Augthun M, Yildirim M, Spiekermann H, Biesterfeld S. Healing of bone defects in combination with immediate implants using the membrane technique. Int J Oral Maxillofac Implants 1995;10:421–428.
59. Rosenquist B, Grenthe B. Immediate placement of implants into extraction sockets: Implant survival. Int J Oral Maxillofac Implants 1996;11:205–209.

60. Becker W, Becker BE, McGuire MK. Localized ridge augmentation using absorbable pins and ePTFE barrier membranes: A new surgical approach. Int J Periodontics Restorative Dent 1994;14:48–61.
61. Gottlow J. Guided tissue regeneration using bioresorbable and non-resorbable devices: Initial healing and long-term results. J Periodontol 1993;64:1157–1165.
62. Gottlow J, Laurell L, Lundgren D, et al. Periodontal tissue response to a new bioresorbable guided tissue regeneration device: A longitudinal study in monkeys. Int J Periodontics Restorative Dent 1994;14:436–449.
63. Becker J, Neukam FW, Schliephake H. Restoration of the lateral sinus wall using a collagen type I membrane for guided tissue regeneration. Int J Oral Maxillofac Surg 1992;21:243–246.
64. Aaboe M, Pinholt EM, Hjørting-Hansen E, Solheim E, Praetorius F. Guided tissue regeneration using degradable and non-degradable membranes in rabbit tibia. Clin Oral Implants Res 1993;4:172–176.
65. Gotfredsen K, Nimb L, Hjørting-Hansen E. Immediate implant placement using a biodegradable barrier, polyhydroxybutyrate-hydroxyvalerate reinforced with polyglactin 910. An experimental study in dogs. Clin Oral Implants Res 1994;5:83–91.
66. Schliephake H, Neukam FW, Hutmacher D, Becker J. Enhancement of bone ingrowth into a porous hydroxylapatite-matrix using a resorbable polylactic membrane: An experimental pilot study. J Oral Maxillofac Surg 1994;52:57–63.
67. Hurzeler MB, Quinones CR, Schupbach P. Guided bone regeneration around dental implants in the atrophic alveolar ridge using a bioresorbable barrier. An experimental study in the monkey. Clin Oral Implants Res 1997;8:323–331.
68. Schliephake H, Kracht D. Vertical ridge augmentation using polylactic membranes in conjunction with immediate implants in periodontally compromised extraction sites: An experimental study in dogs. Int J Oral Maxillofac Implants 1997;12:325–334.
69. Hurzeler MB, Kohal RJ, Naghshbandi J, et al. Evaluation of a new bioresorbable barrier to facilitate guided bone regeneration around exposed implant threads. An experimental study in the monkey. Int J Oral Maxillofac Surg 1998;27:315–320.
70. Hockers T, Abensur D, Valentini P, Legrand R, Hammerle CH. The combined use of bioresorbable membranes and xenografts or autografts in the treatment of bone defects around implants. A study in beagle dogs. Clin Oral Implants Res 1999;10:487–498.
71. Alliot B, Piotrowski B, Marin P, Zahedi S, Brunel G. Regeneration procedures in immediate transmucosal implants: An animal study. Int J Oral Maxillofac Implants 1999;14:841–848.
72. von Arx T, Cochran DL, Schenk RK, Buser D. Evaluation of a prototype trilayer membrane (PTLM) for lateral ridge augmentation: An experimental study in the canine mandible. Int J Oral Maxillofac Surg 2002;31:190–199.
73. Donos N, Kostopoulos L, Karring T. Alveolar ridge augmentation using a resorbable copolymer membrane and autogenous bone grafts. An experimental study in the rat. Clin Oral Implants Res 2002;13:203–213.
74. Oh TJ, Meraw SJ, Lee EJ, Giannobile WV, Wang HL. Comparative analysis of collagen membranes for the treatment of implant dehiscence defects. Clin Oral Implants Res 2003;14:80–90.
75. Hutmacher D, Hurzeler MB, Schliephake H. A review of material properties of biodegradable and bioresorbable polymers and devices for GTR and GBR applications. Int J Oral Maxillofac Implants 1996;11:667–678.
76. Hurzeler MB, Strub JR. Guided bone regeneration around exposed implants: A new bioresorbable device and bioresorbable membrane pins. Pract Periodontics Aesthet Dent 1995;7:37–47.
77. Zitzmann NU, Naef R, Schärer P. Resorbable versus nonresorbable membranes in combination with Bio-Oss for guided bone regeneration. Int J Oral Maxillofac Implants 1997;12:844–852.
78. Zitzmann NU, Schärer P, Marinello CP. Factors influencing the success of GBR. Smoking, timing of implant placement, implant location, bone quality and provisional restoration. J Clin Periodontol 1999;26:673–682.
79. Nemcovsky CE, Artzi Z, Moses O. Rotated split palatal flap for soft tissue primary coverage over extraction sites with immediate implant placement. Description of the surgical procedure and clinical results. J Periodontol 1999;70:926–934.
80. Nemcovsky CE, Artzi Z, Moses O, Gelernter I. Healing of dehiscence defects at delayed-immediate implant sites primarily closed by a rotated palatal flap following extraction. Int J Oral Maxillofac Implants 2000;15:550–558.
81. Hammerle CH, Lang NP. Single stage surgery combining transmucosal implant placement with guided bone regeneration and bioresorbable materials. Clin Oral Implants Res 2001;12:9–18.
82. Aghaloo TL, Moy PK. Which hard tissue augmentation techniques are the most successful in furnishing bony support for implant placement? Int J Oral Maxillofac Implants 2007;22(suppl):49–70.
83. Buser D, Chen ST. Factors influencing treatment outcomes in post-extraction implants. In: Buser D, Wismeijer D, Belser UC (eds). ITI Treatment Guide. Vol 3: Implant placement in post-extraction sites: Treatment options. Berlin: Quintessence, 2009:18–28.

CHAPTER 2

Biologic Basis of Bone Regeneration

Dieter D. Bosshardt
Robert K. Schenk

For both the esthetic outcome and long-term success, a sufficient amount of living bone is required to place an endosseous dental implant in jawbone. In about 50% of implant sites, however, there is a need for a procedure that predictably generates enough bone volume for the placement of a dental implant. There are several options for the enhancement of bone formation, including *(1)* osteoinduction by bone grafts or growth factors; *(2)* osteoconduction by bone grafts or substitute materials that serve as a scaffold for new bone formation; *(3)* transfer of stem cells or progenitor cells that differentiate into osteoblasts; *(4)* distraction osteogenesis; and *(5)* guided bone regeneration (GBR) using barrier membranes. Regardless of the method used, there is always an underlying basic mechanism of bone healing.

Bone reveals a unique potential for regeneration, which is probably best illustrated by fracture repair. Bone is able to heal fractures or local defects with regenerated tissue, or regenerate, of equally high structural organization without leaving a scar. The mechanism of this healing pattern is often considered to be a recapitulation of embryonic osteogenesis and growth. Because bone has a unique spontaneous healing capacity, the trick in reconstructive surgery is to harness this great regenerative potential to enhance bone formation for clinical applications. Thus, adequate bone augmentation or treatment of any bone defect requires a profound understanding of bone development and morphogenesis at the cellular and molecular levels. This chapter will summarize the development, structure, function, biochemistry, and cell biology of bone to provide the biologic basis for discussion of the GBR healing pattern.

Development and Structure of Bone

Functions

Bone is certainly a high achievement in the evolution of supporting tissues. However, it has functions that go beyond mere body support. Functions of bone include *(1)* mechanical body support, motion, and locomotion; *(2)* support of teeth for biting and crushing of food; *(3)* support and protection of the brain, spinal cord, and internal organs; *(4)* housing of bone marrow, which is the source of hematopoietic cells; and *(5)* calcium homeostasis.

It is probably because these functions are of vital importance that bone possesses an exceptional capacity for self-healing, repair, and regeneration.

Skeletogenesis

From the tip of the toe to the crown of the head, bone is present throughout the body at various anatomical sites. Its structure is not homogenous because bone is structurally adapted to meet its specific functional requirements. The mammalian skeleton consists of so-called long bones and flat bones and develops from two embryonic sources—the mesoderm in the somites and the branchial arches. Bone formation depends on two prerequisites: ample blood supply and mechanical support.

There are two different modes of ossification: intramembranous and chondral (endochondral). In the case of direct or intramembranous ossification, connective tissue serves as a template for bone matrix deposition. During indirect or chondral ossification, cartilage forms a model and, after its calcification, serves as a solid base that is first covered with and then substituted by bone. Endochondral ossification takes place in growth cartilage.

During embryonic development, the shape of the individual bone is elaborated either directly or indirectly. In the following fetal and postnatal growth periods, the bones undergo three changes: *(1)* growth in length and diameter, *(2)* refinement of the shape by periosteal and endosteal modeling, and *(3)* remodeling. (The terms *modeling* and *remodeling* often cause confusion. Modeling indicates a change in shape, whereas remodeling refers to tissue replacement or substitution without a change in architecture.) Thus, modeling and remodeling are important processes not only in the mature skeleton but also during development and growth of bone. Basically, the diaphysis of a long bone grows in diameter by periosteal apposition and endosteal resorption. In addition, modeling of the shape is also regulated by changes in the rate of matrix apposition.

Types and structural organization

Based on the orientation of the collagen fibrils, three types of bone tissue can be identified: woven bone, lamellar bone, and an intermediate type—the primary parallel-fibered bone.

Woven bone is formed predominantly in embryos and growing children and later is replaced by lamellar bone. In the adult, woven bone reappears when accelerated bone formation is required, as in the bony callus during fracture repair, and in pathologic conditions such as Paget disease, renal osteodystrophy, hyperparathyroidism, or fluorosis. In woven bone, the collagen fibrils are oriented in a random manner. The interfibrillar spaces are comparatively wide.[1] Besides having intertwined collagen fibrils, woven bone is characterized by a high number of large osteocytes and a high mineral density (Fig 2-1).

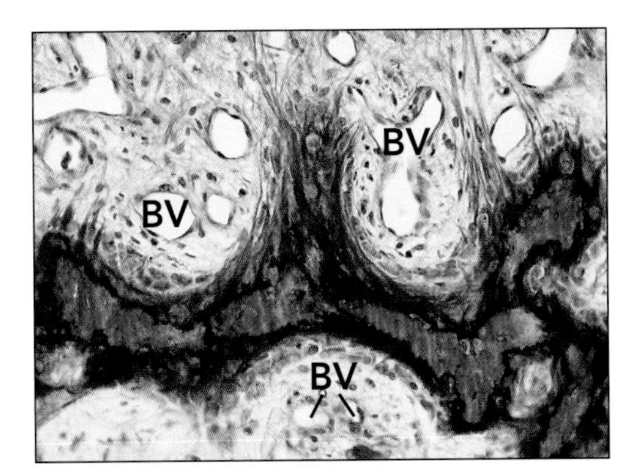

Fig 2-1 Light microscopic view of woven bone. This type of bone is able to form struts and ridges, which are always closely associated with blood vessels (BV) (Goldner trichrome stain).

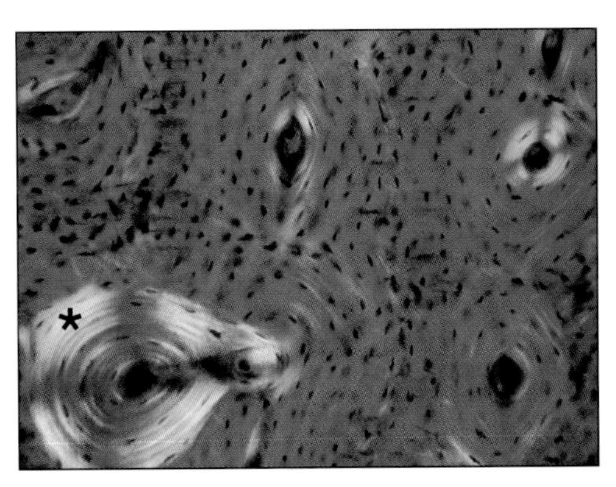

Fig 2-2 Primary and secondary osteons in equine cortical bone. In polarized light, secondary osteons *(asterisk)* reveal a clear lamellar pattern. The wall of primary osteons consists of primary parallel-fibered bone, which is less birefringent.

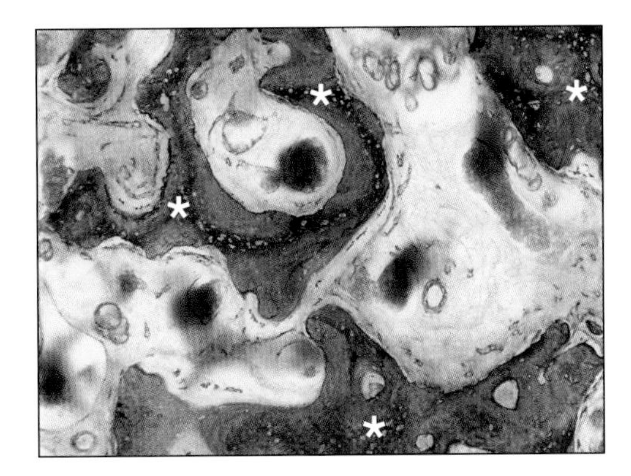

Fig 2-3 Light microscopic micrograph showing reinforcement of woven bone *(asterisks)* by parallel-fibered bone (toluidine blue surface stain).

Lamellar bone possesses a much more complex structure, characterized by matrix layers that consist of a parallel collagen fibril arrangement. One lamellar unit is about 3 to 5 μm wide, and the orientation of the fibrils changes from one lamella to another (Fig 2-2). Thus, lamellar bone may be regarded as a complex, plywood-like structure.[2]

Primary parallel-fibered bone is deposited during early stages of bone formation as well as during periosteal and endosteal bone apposition. Its collagen fibrils run parallel to the bone surface but lack a lamellar organization (Fig 2-3). Primary parallel-fibered bone shares most physiologic properties with woven bone.

Mature bone consists of cortical (compact) and cancellous (trabecular or spongy) bone. Based on the orientation of the lamellae, cortical bone matrix is subdivided into different compartments. The basic structural units are the osteons (or haversian systems), longitudinally oriented cylindric structures with vascular (haversian) canals in the center. In secondary osteons, the wall consists of concentric lamellae, whereas primary osteons are characterized by a more primitive parallel-fibered bone matrix

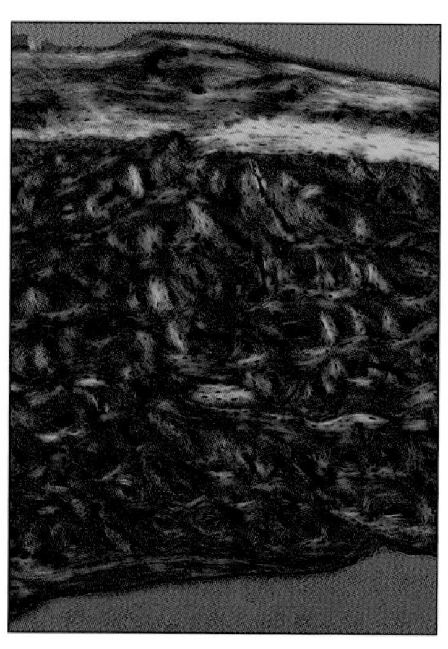

Fig 2-4 Polarized light micrograph of cortical bone from a rabbit tibia. Osteons built around haversian canals are sandwiched between circumferential lamellae at the periosteal *(top)* and endosteal *(bottom)* surfaces.

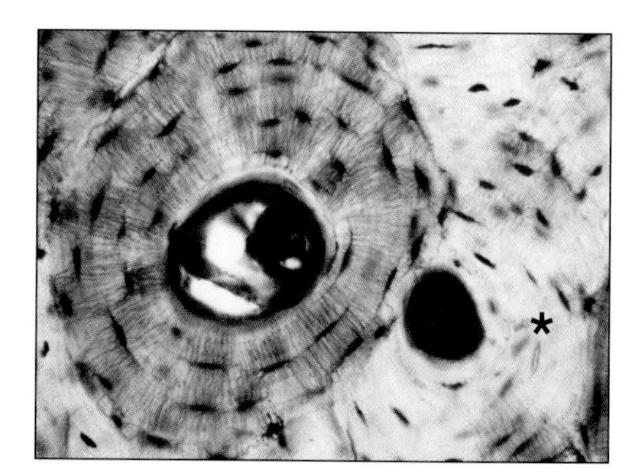

Fig 2-5 Osteons are metabolic units. Staining of osteocytes demonstrates the canaliculolacunar system. *(asterisk)* Necrotic fragment of an osteon after obliteration of the haversian canal (undecalcified ground section; basic fuchsin stain).

(see Fig 2-2). Along the periosteal and endosteal surfaces, appositional growth often results in packets of circumferential lamellae (Fig 2-4). Remnants of circumferential lamellae and of earlier generations of osteons occupy the remaining space as interstitial lamellae. The osteocytes within these remnants of cortical remodeling activity are often cut off from their vascular supply and die (Fig 2-5).[3]

The trabeculae of cancellous bone are also composed of bone structural units, ie, packets or walls, separated (or glued together) by cement lines. They also reflect local remodeling in earlier periods of growth and cancellous bone turnover[4] (see the discussion of cancellous bone modeling and remodeling later in this chapter).

Bone cells

Bone formation, maintenance, and repair are regulated by four different types of cells. Osteoblasts, bone-lining cells, and osteoclasts cover bone surfaces, whereas osteocytes are found in the interior of the bone matrix. A prerequisite for bone formation and survival is sufficient blood supply. Thus, angiogenesis is a necessary prerequisite not only for bone development but also for maintenance and repair.

Osteoblasts are large cuboidal cells that form a single layer covering all periosteal or endosteal surfaces where bone formation is active.[5] They are polarized cells that secrete osteoid unidirectionally toward the bone surface. The osteoblast's nucleus is ovoid, and its cytoplasm is filled with abundant rough endoplasmic reticulum and a prominent Golgi complex (Fig 2-6). Heterogeneity among osteoblasts seems to exist and may reflect differences between types of bone and/or anatomical sites.[6] The osteoblast is responsible for synthesis, assembly, and mineralization of the bone matrix.

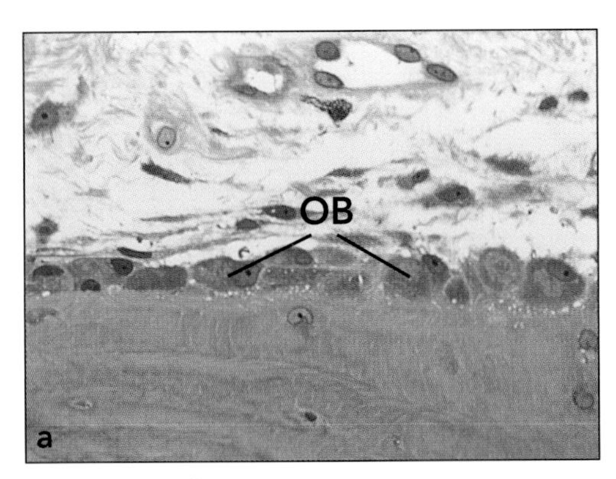

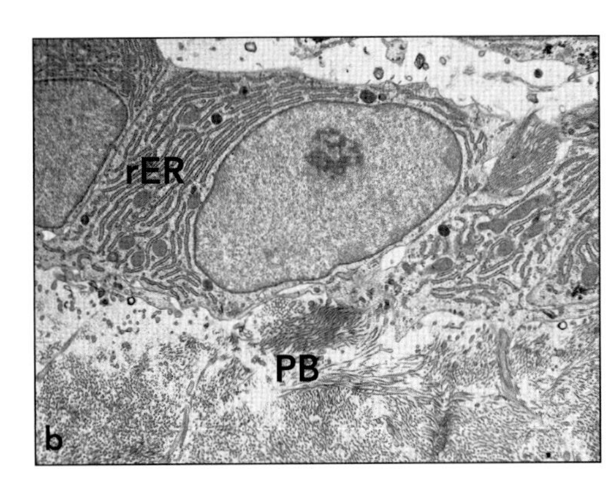

Fig 2-6 *(a)* Light micrograph showing a single layer of osteoblasts (OB) lining the bone matrix (toluidine blue stain). *(b)* Transmission electron micrograph illustrating osteoblasts with abundant rough endoplasmic reticulum (rER) lining the osteoid or prebone (PB).

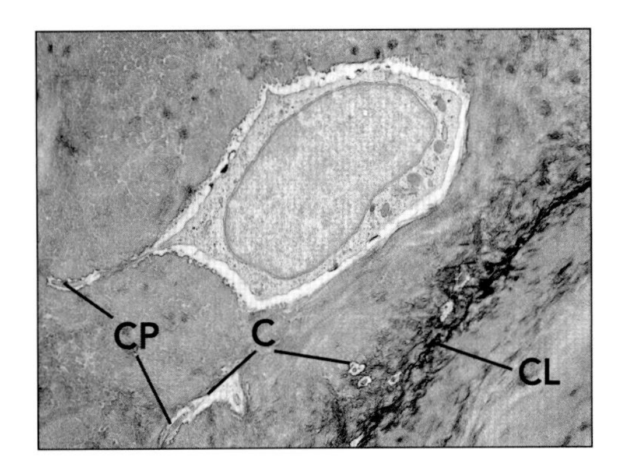

Fig 2-7 Transmission electron micrograph showing an osteocyte embedded in its lacuna next to a cement line (CL). Longitudinally and transversely cut canaliculi (C) containing cytoplasmic processes (CP) are visible close to the osteocyte.

Some osteoblasts become osteocytes by inversion of matrix secretion or by entrapment through neighboring osteoblasts.[5] The speed of matrix deposition may determine the number of embedded osteocytes.[7] This is exemplified in woven bone, which is formed much more quickly than any other type of bone and possesses a high number of embedded osteocytes.[8]

The osteocyte is trapped in the bone matrix in a lacuna (Fig 2-7), and neighboring osteocytes are interconnected by tiny cytoplasmic processes extending through a dense canalicular system. This canaliculolacunar system allows for diffusion of metabolites and signaling molecules for cell communication with neighboring osteocytes, osteoblasts, and bone-lining cells. It is indispensable for osteocyte survival because diffusion of nutrients and waste products through the heavily mineralized bone matrix is almost impossible. However, the transport capacity of this system also has limitations. In mammals, the critical transport distance to keep the osteocytes alive is approximately 100 µm.[9] This explains why the wall thickness of both osteons and packets in trabecular bone rarely exceeds 100 µm. Osteocytes may actively participate in bone homeostasis through their involvement in bone turnover, ion exchange, and sensing of mechanical signals.[10]

The bone-lining cell is the third cell type that belongs to the osteoblast family. It is regarded as an inactive osteoblast covering the bone surface. Bone-lining cells are flat and have a reduced armamentarium of cytoplasmic organelles, which is indicative of

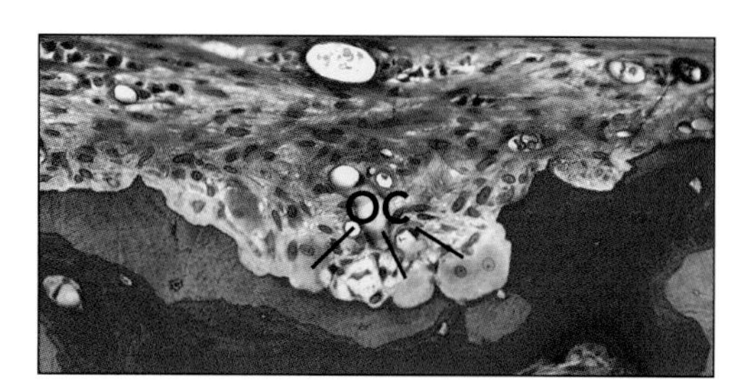

Fig 2-8 Light micrograph showing osteoclasts (OC) in Howship lacunae formed in the alveolar bone (fuchsin and toluidine blue stain).

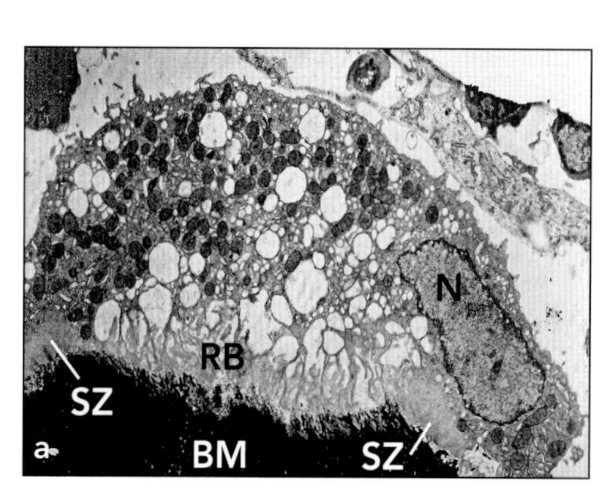

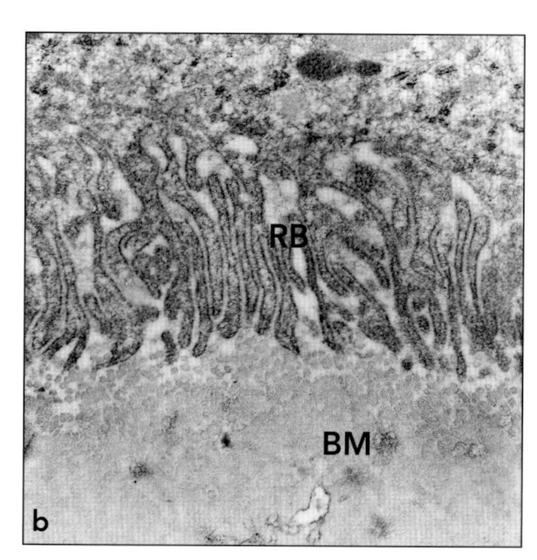

Fig 2-9 *(a)* Transmission electron micrograph showing an osteoclast with the ruffled border (RB), the sealing zone (SZ), and numerous mitochondria, vesicles, and vacuoles, but with only a single nuclear profile (N). The ruffled border represents the site of bone matrix (BM) dissolution and degradation (undecalcified ultrathin section). *(b)* Enlarged transmission electron micrograph of the ruffled border (RB) and bone matrix (BM) (decalcified ultrathin section).

low activity of both cell metabolism and protein synthesis. They are, therefore, also called *inactive* or *resting osteoblasts*. Bone-lining cells may participate in the initiation of resorption by release of osteoclast activation factors and by active contraction, which is thought to expose the bone surface for the attachment of osteoclasts.[11]

Osteoclasts are cells of the monocyte-macrophage hematopoietic cell lineage.[12] Their primary function is to degrade bone matrix in various physiologic and pathologic contexts. They differ from other giant cells, especially from foreign-body giant cells, and are conventionally identified by their location in a resorption cavity, the Howship lacuna (Fig 2-8). Furthermore, they are large and multinucleated and stain positive for tartrate-resistant acid phosphatase.[13] Other characteristic features are the presence of a number of cell surface receptors, including those for receptor activator for nuclear factor κB (RANK), macrophage colony-stimulating factor, vitronectin, and calcitonin. Their size varies from 30 to 100 μm, and the number of nuclei ranges roughly from 3 to 30.

The cytoplasm is acidophilic and often contains vacuoles (Fig 2-9a). The marginal area of the osteoclast adheres to the mineralized surface and seals off the actual resorption chamber with the so-called sealing zone (clear zone). In the central part of this

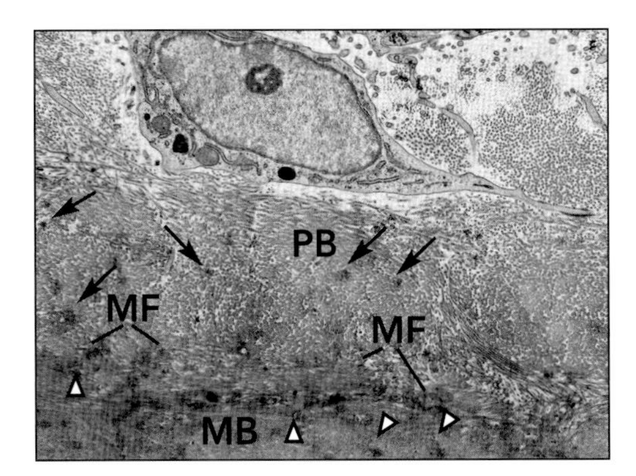

Fig 2-10 Transmission electron micrograph illustrating an osteoblast, the osteoid or prebone (PB), the mineralization front (MF), and the mineralized bone matrix (MB). Mineralization foci *(arrows)* and "gray patches" *(arrowheads)* are visible in the osteoid and the mineralized bone matrix, respectively.

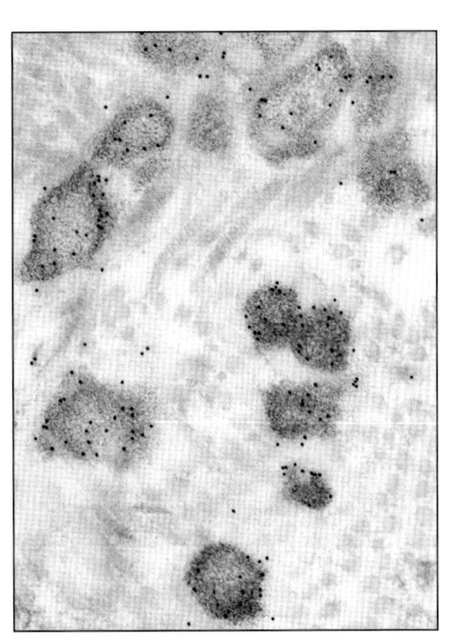

Fig 2-11 High-resolution immunocytochemistry showing an association between gold particle labeling for osteopontin and mineralization foci in the osteoid.

chamber, the cell surface is enlarged by numerous cytoplasmic foldings that form the ruffled border (Fig 2-9b). Through the enlarged cell membrane, hydrogen ions and proteolytic enzymes are released to dissolve the mineral crystals and to degrade the organic bone matrix.

Bone matrix

Deposition and mineralization

The osteoblast synthesizes a mixture of macromolecules that are secreted into the extracellular milieu to form the bone matrix—the osteoid or prebone—which consists of a matrix seam made up of collagens and noncollagenous proteins. At a certain distance from the osteoblast, at the mineralization front, the osteoid converts into mineralized bone. The mineralization of woven bone is initiated by matrix vesicles. In contrast, matrix vesicles are rarely seen in the osteoid of mineralizing lamellar bone. However, the first mineral to appear among the collagen fibrils may be found at small discrete foci that are distributed within the osteoid and accumulate at the mineralization front (Fig 2-10). The co-localization of noncollagenous bone proteins such as osteopontin (Fig 2-11) and bone sialoprotein with these small mineralization foci and with amorphous gray or reticular patches of mineralized bone indicates the association of these proteins with the mineralization process. Bone acidic glycoprotein 75 and osteocalcin, on the other hand, show a diffuse distribution pattern throughout the mineralized bone matrix.[14]

Constituents

The bone matrix is a biologic composite consisting of water, mineral, collagens, and noncollagenous macromolecules, the latter usually referred to as *noncollagenous proteins.* The biochemical composition of bone has recently been reviewed.[15–19] The collagens play structural and morphogenetic roles.[20] In mineralized tissues, they interact with various noncollagenous proteins and provide a scaffold for the accommodation of the mineral crystals.[21] The noncollagenous proteins of bone can roughly be classified into glycoproteins, proteoglycans, plasma-derived proteins, growth factors, and other macromolecules. Besides having a structural function, the bone matrix harbors molecules that play roles in biomineralization and matrix-cell interactions, and it serves as a reservoir for growth factors and cytokines.

During tissue repair, growth and differentiation factors not only may be produced by the local cells but also can be released from the mineralized matrix. The prevailing opinion is that growth factors released from the mineralized bone matrix during the resorption process of osteoclasts exert their functions on local cells. Growth factors present in the bone matrix include insulin-like growth factors, fibroblast growth factors, transforming growth factor β (TGF-β), and platelet-derived growth factors.

Of great interest with regard to bone regeneration, but also for heterotopic (de novo) bone formation, is the TGF-β superfamily. Members of this family are soluble factors that regulate embryonic development, morphogenesis, and a variety of functional responses, including cell proliferation, differentiation, apoptosis, and the cell cycle. Their action depends not only on the cell type but also on the cytokines and other growth factors present in the local milieu.

Osteoblasts

Osteoblasts originate from mesenchymal stem cells in bone marrow.[22] Differentiation of cells of the osteoblastic lineage is controlled by multiple transcription factors at various stages of their development. Core-binding factor α1 (Cbfa1), also known as *runt-related transcription factor 2 (Runx2),* and osterix (Osx), downstream from Cbfa1, are master switches for osteoblast differentiation.[23] The expression of Cbfa1 is not restricted to cells of the osteogenic and chondrogenic lineage,[24,25] and the expression of Cbfa1 in fully differentiated cells suggests additional roles in osteoblast function.

Throughout life, the skeleton undergoes continuous remodeling, which serves the purpose of repair and mechanical adaptation. The consequences of an imbalance in the expression of signaling molecules are metabolic bone disorders or diseases such as Paget disease, osteopetrosis, osteoporosis, arthritis, or bone loss in periodontitis.[26,27] Regulation of bone remodeling is under both systemic and local control. Local factors are operative in a paracrine and autocrine fashion, and osteoblasts, osteoclasts, and inflammatory and immune cells function as both sources and targets of signaling molecules. Numerous cytokines and growth factors have anabolic and/or catabolic effects on bone formation.[28,29] Among these bone-regulatory molecules are parathyroid hormone, parathyroid hormone–related peptide, calcitonin, calcitriol (the active form of vitamin D), prostaglandin E_2, growth hormone, thyroid hormone, sex

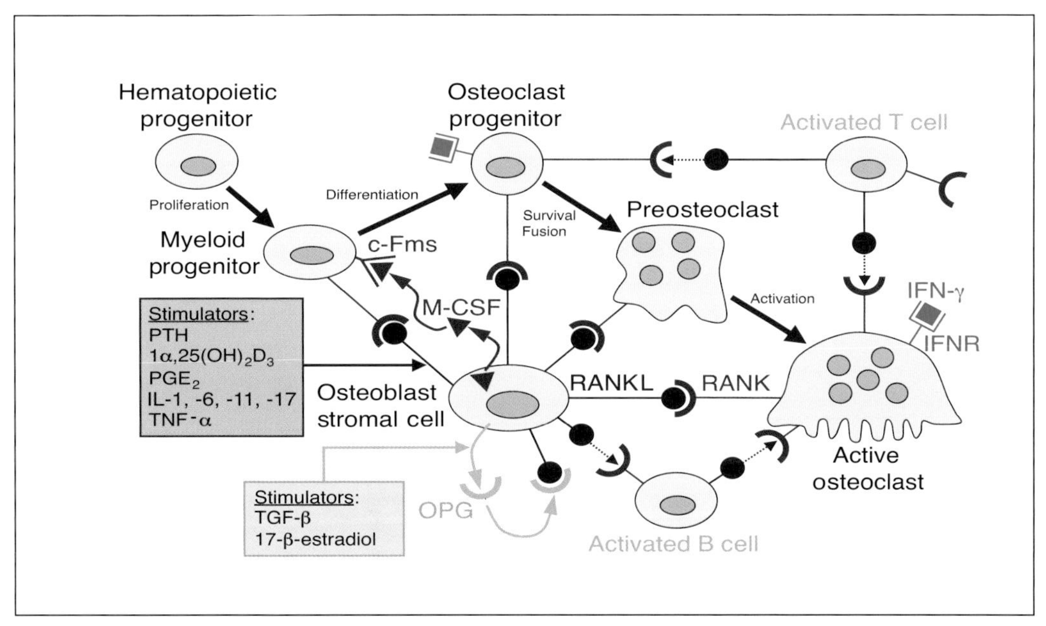

Fig 2-12 RANK-RANKL-OPG system. (PTH) parathyroid hormone; ($1\alpha,25[OH]_2D_3$) 1α,25-dihydroxyvitamin D_3; (PGE_2) prostaglandin E_2; (IL-1) interleukin 1; (IL-6) interleukin 6; (IL-11) interleukin 11; (IL-17) interleukin 17; (TNF-α) tumor necrosis factor α; (M-CSF) macrophage colony-stimulating factor; (c-Fms) M-CSF receptor; (RANK) receptor activator for nuclear factor κB; (RANKL) RANK ligand; (IFN-γ) interferon γ; (IFNR) IFN-γ receptor; (TGF-β) transforming growth factor β; (OPG) osteoprotegerin.

steroids (estrogen and testosterone), leptin, statins, interferon γ, tumor necrosis factor α, transforming growth factor α (TGF-α), TGF-β, bone morphogenetic proteins (BMPs), fibroblast growth factor, insulin-like growth factor 1, platelet-derived growth factors, and interleukins 1, 6, 11, and 17.

Osteoclasts

Unlike osteoblasts, osteoclasts originate from hematopoietic stem cells.[12] It is therefore not surprising that many growth factors and transcription factors that are involved in hematopoietic differentiation of other cells also affect osteoclast differentiation.[23]

Normal bone remodeling depends on a delicate balance between bone formation and resorption. Bone resorption is regulated by a system consisting of RANK and its ligand (RANKL), which are members of the tumor necrosis factor ligand and receptor families, and osteoprotegerin (OPG) (Fig 2-12). RANKL is expressed by bone marrow stromal cells, osteoblasts, and certain fibroblasts, whereas RANK is expressed by osteoclast precursors and mature osteoclasts. The binding of RANK to RANKL induces osteoclast differentiation and activity and regulates osteoclast survival. OPG, however, which is produced by bone marrow stromal cells, osteoblasts, and certain fibroblasts, is a soluble decoy receptor for RANKL that competes for this binding. Thus, OPG is a natural inhibitor of osteoclast differentiation and activation.

Any interference with this system can shift the balance between bone apposition and resorption. The expression of macrophage colony-stimulating factor plays an essential role in this regulatory system. Furthermore, a number of pro-inflammatory cytokines and growth factors, in particular interleukin 1 and tumor necrosis factor α, regulate the expression of RANKL and OPG. The immune system modifies the balance between bone formation and resorption in a complex process involving T and B lymphocytes, dendritic cells, and cytokines. By the expression of RANKL on B cells, T cells, and marrow stromal cells and the expression of RANK on osteoclast precursors, mature osteoclasts, T lymphocytes, B lymphocytes, and dendritic cells, these cells can directly influence bone resorption.[30–32]

The discovery of this important regulatory system, which links bone biology with immune cell biology, has created the possibility of new therapeutic strategies. Attempts using recombinant OPG were successful in preventing bone resorption and loss. However, production of significant antibody titers in a patient given OPG brought this development to an early end. Another way of blocking RANK signaling is through the use of denosumab, a fully human monoclonal antibody against RANKL. Clinical trials are currently exploring its effects on bone loss in patients with osteoporosis, bone metastasis, myeloma, and rheumatoid arthritis.[33]

Maintenance of Bone

Bone modeling and remodeling continue after cessation of growth. The signaling molecules involved in regulation of cell differentiation and activity already have been discussed. The aim of this section is to discuss the morphologic aspects of bone modeling and remodeling after completion of development and growth. Cortical bone remodeling may be distinguished from trabecular bone remodeling. Both types of bone undergo physiologic remodeling.

Cortical bone

Primary osteons are formed during appositional growth, whereas secondary osteons are the result of matrix substitution. The fundamental structural unit of cortical bone remodeling is the osteon (see Fig 2-2). The remodeling sequence is illustrated in transverse sections in Fig 2-13. First, a resorption canal is formed by osteoclasts. Later, osteoblasts appear and start refilling the canal with concentric lamellae. In compact human bone, completed secondary osteons have an outer diameter of 200 to 250 µm, with the central vascular canal—the haversian canal—measuring 50 to 80 µm.[34] As a coherent cylindric structure, secondary osteons rarely measure more than 2.0 to 3.0 mm in length. They are interconnected at intervals of 0.5 to 1.0 mm by transverse vascular channels, the Volkmann canals.

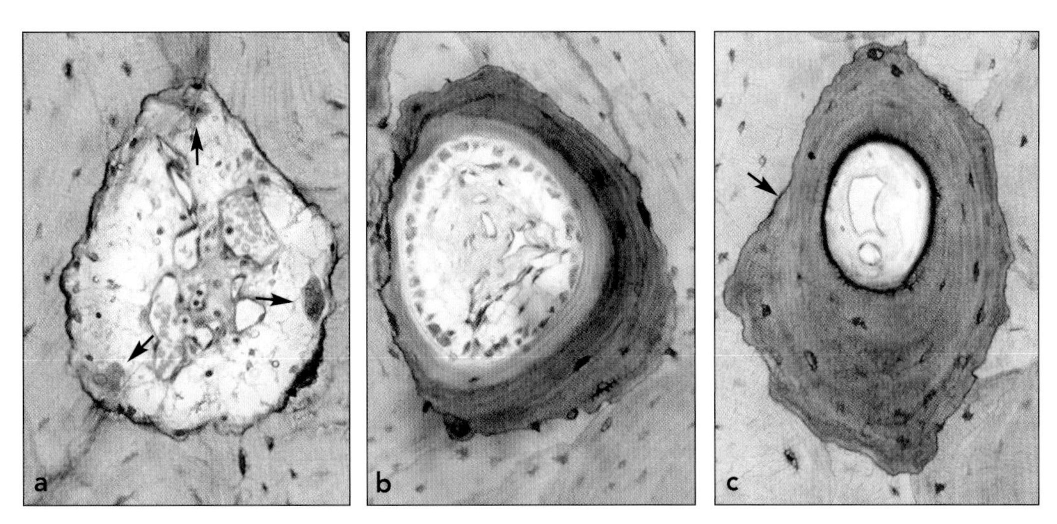

Fig 2-13 Cortical bone remodeling in the humerus of an adult man. *(a)* Resorption canal with osteoclasts *(arrows)*. *(b)* Concentric lamellae deposited by osteoblasts. *(c)* Completed secondary osteon, bound by a cement line *(arrow)* (transverse sections through evolving secondary osteons; toluidine blue surface stain).

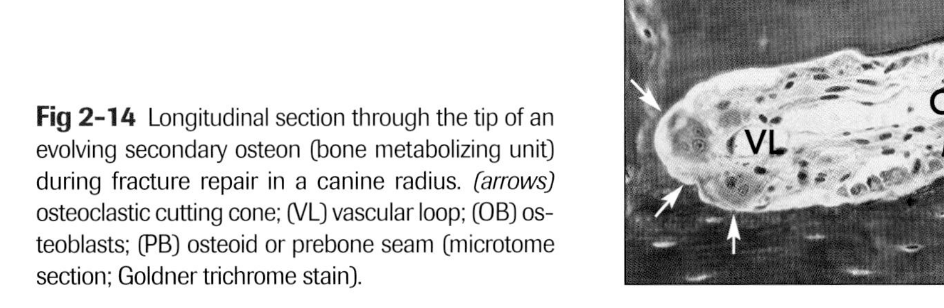

Fig 2-14 Longitudinal section through the tip of an evolving secondary osteon (bone metabolizing unit) during fracture repair in a canine radius. *(arrows)* osteoclastic cutting cone; (VL) vascular loop; (OB) osteoblasts; (PB) osteoid or prebone seam (microtome section; Goldner trichrome stain).

Longitudinal sections of newly formed osteons have shown that bone resorption and deposition are coupled in time and space and occur in discrete remodeling sites called *bone metabolizing units*. At the advancing front of a resorption canal, osteoclasts are assembled in a cutting cone (Fig 2-14). While the osteoclasts advance longitudinally, they widen the resorption canal up to its final diameter. The tip of a vessel loop follows immediately behind the osteoclasts. This loop lies in the center of the canal and is surrounded by perivascular cells thought to include osteoclast and osteoblast precursor cells. In the reversal phase, ie, between bone resorption and bone matrix deposition, the wall of the canal is lined by mononuclear cells. Further in the back of the cutting cone, osteoblasts appear and deposit the lamellar bone matrix, which will later mineralize. Depending on the species, completion of the osteon requires 2 to 4 months.

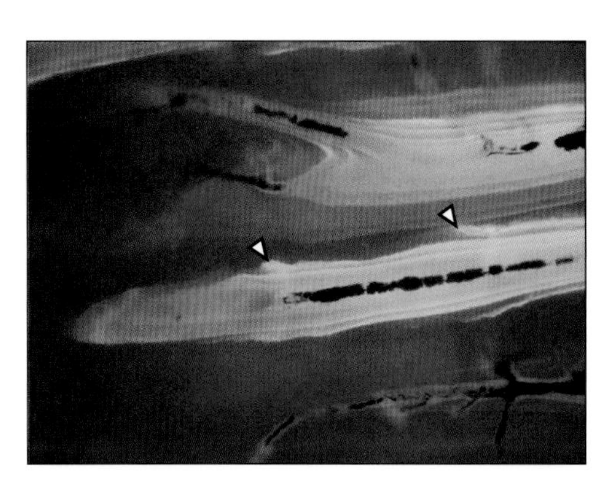

Fig 2-15 Sequential polychrome labeling of a bone metabolizing unit at weekly intervals *(arrowheads)* to measure the daily osteoclastic resorption rate.

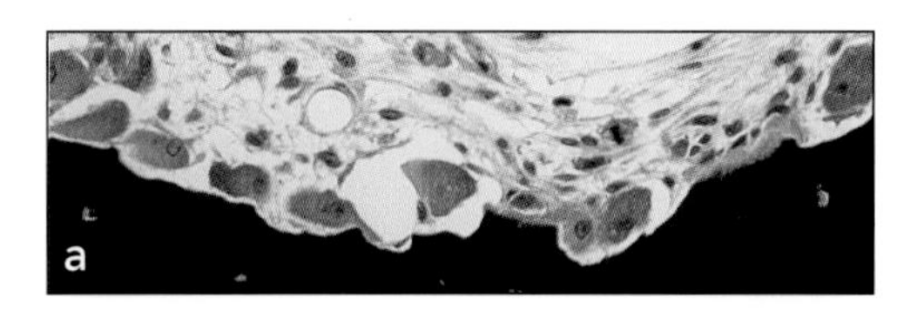

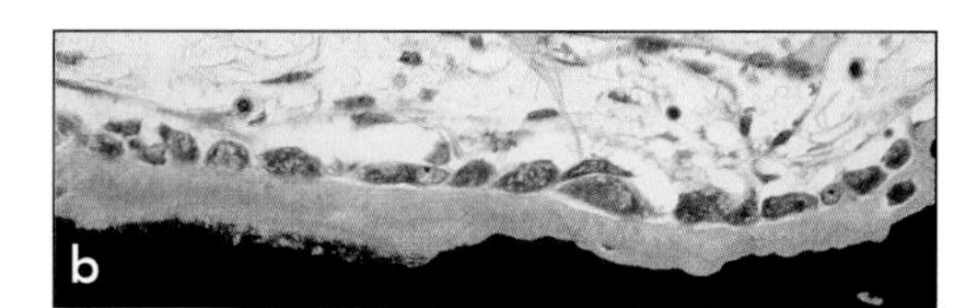

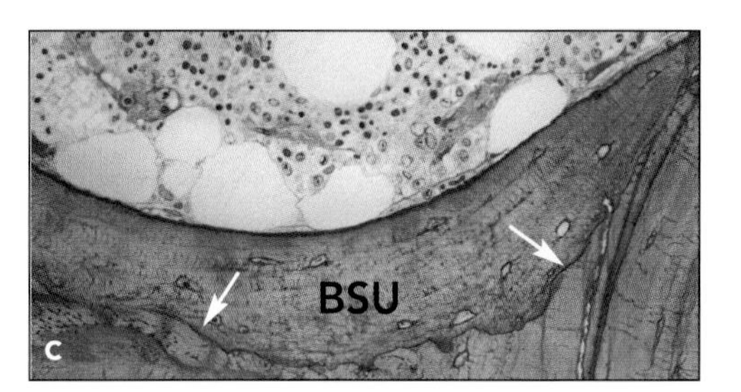

Fig 2-16 Trabecular bone remodeling in a human iliac crest biopsy. *(a)* Resorptive phase. *(b)* Early formative phase. *(c)* Newly formed packet (bone structural unit [BSU]), clearly delineated by a reversal or cement line *(arrows)* (*[a and b]* Von Kossa–McNeal stain; *[c]* toluidine blue surface stain).

These measurements and calculations are based on sequential fluorochrome labelings (Fig 2-15) and also allow an accurate determination of the osteoclast's resorption rate in longitudinal sections, which amounts to 50 to 60 µm per day in dogs.[35–37]

Cancellous bone

While the original architecture of the trabecular framework is determined by the growth pattern, modeling in the spongiosa specifically changes the architecture of cancellous bone throughout life. The trabecular network undergoes profound changes that result in a structural adaptation to the prevailing functional load, or, as often stated, "according to Wolff's law."[38] This adaptation enables bone to withstand a given stress with a minimum amount of material. The mechanism of functional adaptation is not fully understood, and at present, Wolff's law just offers a convenient way to accept it as a fact without looking for other explanations.

Bone remodeling improves the quality of the tissue, with regard to both its mechanical and metabolic properties. Remodeling of trabecular bone replaces discrete portions (or packets) with new lamellar bone (Fig 2-16). Formation of a new packet begins with local recruitment of osteoclasts that form a cavity on the trabecular surface.

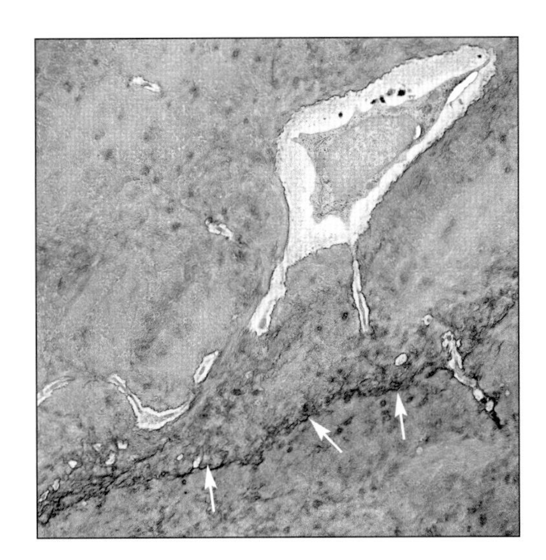

Fig 2-17 Transmission electron micrograph showing a cement line *(arrows)* at the interface between old and new bone.

The mean depth of these cavities is around 50 μm and rarely exceeds 70 μm. At the end of this resorptive phase, and after a short intermission or reversal phase, osteoblasts start depositing new bone matrix during the formative phase. In analogy to the osteons, the new packet is considered a bone structural unit, and the cell populations involved in its formation are considered a bone metabolizing unit.

Considering the extent of the trabecular surface in the human skeleton, the control and dynamics of cancellous bone remodeling play an important role in the pathogenesis of metabolic bone disorders, particularly in osteoporosis.

Cement line

The cement line is a very characteristic structural entity of bone. It delineates (demarcates) the interface between new and old bone. Two types of cement lines are distinguished: resting lines and reversal lines. Resting lines are smooth and strictly parallel to the lamellae. They are formed when bone formation is arrested and, after a resting period, resumes again. Reversal lines are formed during the reversal phase, ie, they constitute the matrix that is deposited directly against a bone surface previously resorbed by osteoclasts (Fig 2-17). Resting lines, which are produced by osteoblasts at sites not exposed to osteoclastic resorption, show structure and composition similar to those of reversal lines.

Secondary osteons are always separated from (or connected to) the surrounding older bone matrix by a cement line. Likewise, the new packet formed after the completion of the trabecular bone remodeling is separated from the older bone matrix by a cement line. Howship lacunae left behind by the osteoclasts give the cement line a crenated appearance (see Figs 2-13c and 2-16c). The number of cement lines—both resting and reversal—indicates the intensity of matrix turnover.

Biology of Bone Regeneration

Physiologic versus reparative regeneration

Regeneration is commonly understood as replacement of vanishing or lost components in the body by elements of equally high structural organization so that structure and function are completely restored. Physiologic regeneration is distinguished from reparative regeneration.

Many tissues or organ systems undergo physiologic regeneration, ie, continuous replacement of cells or tissue elements. Remodeling of cortical and trabecular bone also represents regeneration; both cells and matrix are replaced.

Reparative regeneration takes place when tissues are lost because of injury or disease. Bone has the unique potential to completely restore its original architecture, but there are certain limitations. The reconstruction of the original level of tissue organization occurs sequentially and closely repeats the pattern of bone formation occurring during development and growth. Likewise, some basic conditions have to be fulfilled, such as ample blood supply and mechanical stability provided by a solid base. This pattern of bone regeneration and some possibilities for promoting and protecting the repair process will be demonstrated by histologic observations in selected experimental studies.

Activation of bone regeneration

Any bone lesion (fracture, defect, insertion of an implant, or interruption of blood supply) activates local bone regeneration by the release and local production of growth factors and other signaling molecules. Bone is one of the richest sources of growth factors. Osteoinduction in its classic concept implies initiation of heterotopic (ectopic) bone formation, that is, bone formation at sites where bone physiologically does not normally exist. The term *osteoinduction* is, however, just as frequently applied if ossification is activated in contact with existing bones, that is, in the case of orthotopic bone induction. To avoid confusion, the term *bone activation* is preferred for orthotopic bone formation.

In heterotopic bone formation, inducible osteoprogenitor cells are found far from bone. These mesenchymal cells are abundant in subcutaneous connective tissue, skeletal muscles, and the spleen and kidney capsule. Their response to inductive stimuli, such as BMPs, is more complex than in orthotopic bone formation and, in fact, mimics endochondral bone formation.[39] After subcutaneous implantation of BMPs in rats, proliferation of mesenchymal cells starts after 3 to 4 days. From days 5 to 8 onward, cartilage develops and, within 1 day, starts to mineralize. Vascular invasion and bony substitution of the calcifying cartilage follows from days 10 to 11 and onward. Intermediate cartilage differentiation seems to be mandatory if induction acts on inducible osteoprogenitor cells. Importantly, the response is always indirect bone formation.

In orthotopic bone formation, osteoprogenitor cells are found in tissues in direct proximity to bone, such as in bone marrow stroma, periosteum, endosteum, and intracortical canals. These cells respond to inductive signals with proliferation and differentiation directly into osteoblasts. Thus, in orthotopic bone induction, the inducing agents act on determined osteoprogenitor cells, and the cellular response is direct bone formation. The lag phase is short—seldom longer than 1 to 3 days—and the newly formed bone is laid down on preexisting bone surfaces.

Repair of bone defects

The repair of bone defects is a good model for the study of bone regeneration. In contrast to fractures, defects are less subject to mechanical factors and to obstructions of the blood supply. Therefore, defect healing has been used in many classic experiments dealing with the influence of surgical and pharmacologic measures on bone regeneration. The basic pattern of defect healing with regard to physiologic ossification and growth is discussed in the next sections.

Small cortical bone defects

Johner[40] examined the healing of bore holes with diameters of 0.1 to 1.0 mm in the tibias of rabbits. Bone formation within these holes starts within a couple of days, without preceding osteoclastic resorption, and reveals a clear-cut size dependency. Holes with a diameter in the range of osteons (0.2 mm) are concentrically filled with lamellar bone (Fig 2-18). In larger holes, a scaffold of woven bone is formed first, and then lamellar bone is deposited in the newly formed intertrabecular spaces, which have a corresponding diameter of 150 to 200 µm (Fig 2-19). As in appositional growth, the matrix deposition rate of lamellar bone is restricted to a couple of microns per day, whereas woven bone rapidly bridges larger defects. After 4 weeks, both the small and the larger defects are filled with compact bone. There is, however, a threshold for this rapid bridging by woven bone. This threshold lies around 1 mm for bore holes in rabbit cortical bone.[41]

Experimental studies on bony ingrowth into porous acetabular components for total hips in dogs demonstrate similar results,[42] summarized in the often-quoted phrase *osteogenic jumping distance*. This term indicates that bone is not able to cross gaps wider than 1 mm in one single jump. In the case of implants, the situation becomes even more difficult because bridging the defects starts from the bony side only. This does not mean that larger holes or gaps will stay open indefinitely, but filling takes longer, and there is no doubt that bore holes of 3 to 5 mm persist for several weeks, if not months, until repair is completed. The bone healing around dental implants has recently been analyzed in relation to the distance between the implant surface and the surrounding bone[43] and in relation to the implant surface characteristics.[44,45]

Completion of filling does not mean that healing is complete, however. Although the bony regenerate appears compact, its structure is still far from that of the osteonal cortical bone. The latter must be formed by haversian remodeling. Bone remodeling starts in the cortex immediately surrounding the margin of the original bore

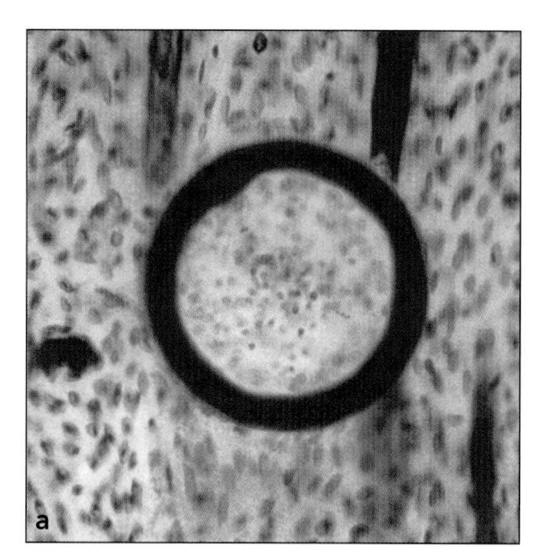

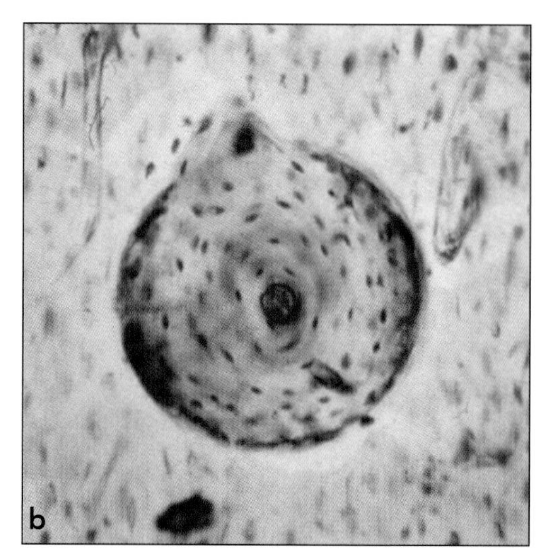

Fig 2-18 Repair of very small cortical bone defects. Bur holes with a diameter of 0.2 mm in the cortex of rabbit's tibia after 1 week *(a)* and after 4 weeks *(b)* (basic fuchsin stain).

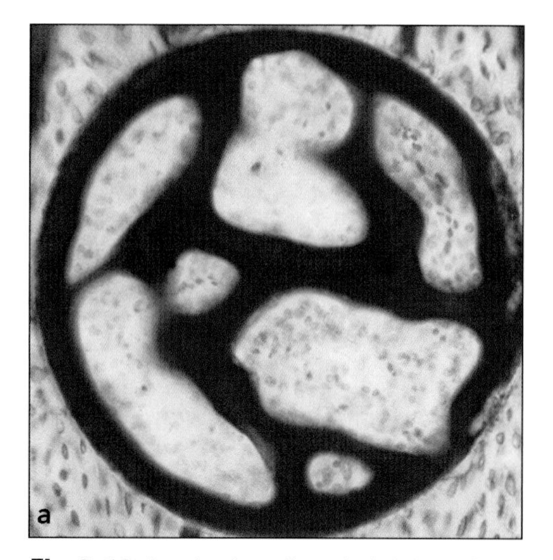

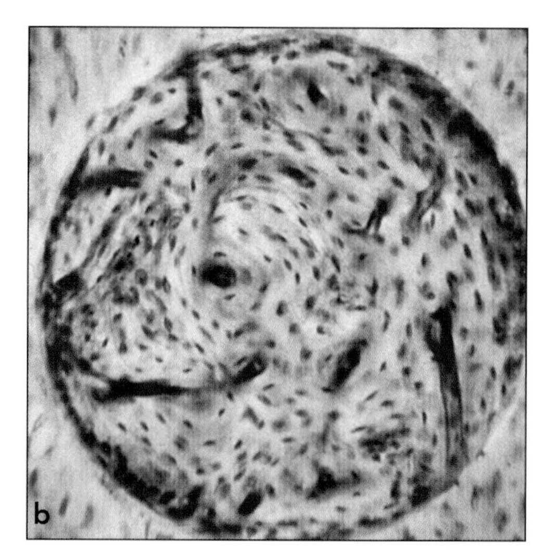

Fig 2-19 Repair of small cortical defects. Bur holes with a diameter of 0.4 mm in the cortex of rabbit's tibia after 1 week *(a)* and after 4 weeks *(b)* (basic fuchsin stain).

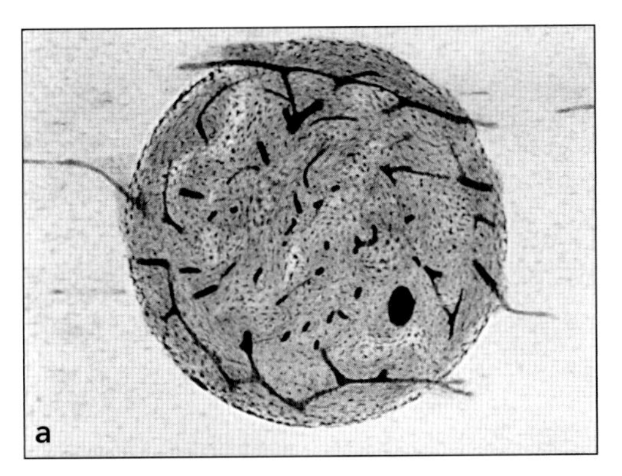

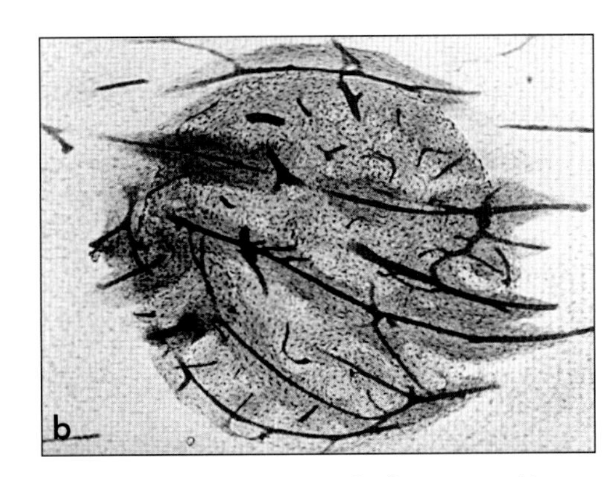

Fig 2-20 Microradiographs showing repair of small cortical defects, measuring 0.6 mm in diameter, and haversian remodeling after 6 weeks *(a)* and after 6 months *(b)*. The original compact filling is partially substituted by newly formed osteons.

hole about 3 weeks after defect creation. Remodeling is activated by the local tissue environment, including vascular damage that was produced during drilling. From the margin of the defect, remodeling progresses into the newly formed bone and replaces it with longitudinally oriented, secondary osteons (Fig 2-20). Within a couple of months, the small cortical defects are fully reconstructed and can only be identified by detailed microscopic evaluation.

In summary, repair of small cortical defects can be divided into two phases that closely resemble the formation of compact bone during development and growth. The simple lesion produced by drilling a hole seems to activate a programmed sequence of events, starting with the filling of the defect by appositional bone formation and then leading to a structural integration of the defect area by haversian remodeling.

Small cancellous bone defects

Small cancellous bone defects reveal a similar healing pattern. Healing also occurs in two phases, starting with woven bone formation across the defect and within the adjacent intertrabecular spaces. This primary scaffold is then reinforced by concentric filling of the spongework lattice with primary parallel-fibered bone, which considerably increases the density in the former defect area. In a second phase, remodeling restores the trabecular architecture.

Promotion of Bone Regeneration

As outlined before, bone tissue exhibits a remarkable regenerative potential and perfectly restores its original structure and mechanical properties. This capacity has limitations, however, and may even fail if certain conditions are not fulfilled. Factors that impede or even prevent bone repair are, among others, *(1)* failure of vascular supply,

(2) mechanical instability, *(3)* oversized defects, and *(4)* competing tissues of high proliferative activity. However, several options, alone or in combination, are available to promote and to support bone formation, including *(1)* osteoinduction by growth factors, *(2)* osteoconduction by bone grafts or substitutes, *(3)* transfer of stem cells or progenitor cells that differentiate into osteoblasts, *(4)* distraction osteogenesis, and *(5)* GBR using barrier membranes. In the following section, the principles and experimental observations of some of these methods are discussed.

Therapeutic use of growth and differentiation factors

The induction of bone formation requires three elements: *(1)* soluble osteoinductive signals, *(2)* cells that are able to respond to these and other signals, and *(3)* a supporting matrix or scaffold to carry and deliver cells and/or molecular factors. Growth factors such as fibroblast growth factors, platelet-derived growth factors, vascular endothelial growth factor, insulin-like growth factors, and growth hormone are undergoing experimental investigation to clarify their potential roles in enhancing skeletal repair. However, these growth factors do not have true osteoinductive properties. Therefore, researchers and clinicians invest hope in the therapeutic use of BMPs in dentistry to enhance bone formation.

The osteoinductive capacity of demineralized bone[46] and dentin matrix[47] has been known for many years and was attributed to the activity of molecules that were later referred to as *bone morphogenetic proteins*.[48] To date, at least 20 members of the BMP family have been identified. Two of them, BMP-2 and BMP-7, have attracted considerable attention and appear to be most promising as therapeutic tools for the enhancement of bone repair. In the United States and Europe, recombinant human BMP-2 (rhBMP-2) and BMP-7 (rhBMP-7) are currently in clinical use for problematic cases. Non-union, open tibial fractures, and spinal fusions are the three conditions for which there is clinical approval.

Although rhBMPs have been experimentally tested, their use in implant dentistry and periodontology is not yet routine. In a study by Jung and coworkers,[49] the effect of rhBMP-2 in conjunction with deproteinized bovine bone mineral as a bone substitute material was evaluated in bone regeneration in humans. Histomorphometric analysis showed that there was no statistically significant difference in the relative amount of newly formed bone. However, the addition of rhBMP-2 increased the graft-to-bone contact and enhanced the maturation process of the newly formed bone. Nevertheless, hopes should not be set too high when it comes to the routine therapeutic use of rhBMPs for relatively small bone defects or deficiencies in periodontics and implant dentistry.

rhBMP-2 and rhBMP-7 are currently predominantly used in orthopedic patients for whom all other treatment options have been exhausted. In the oral cavity, an extraordinary reconstruction was achieved by Warnke and coworkers[50] in a patient who had undergone a subtotal mandibulectomy. Mandibular reconstruction was achieved with a de novo mandibular segment that developed in a titanium mesh cage filled with mineral blocks, the patient's bone marrow, and 7 mg of rhBMP-7 after implantation into the latissimus dorsi muscle on the vascular pedicle of the thoracodorsal artery. Seven weeks later, a free vascularized bone-muscle flap was transferred and anastomosed to repair the mandibular defect.

There are several reasons why routine application of rhBMPs is not yet possible, including the need for very high dosages to be effective in humans, decreasing responsiveness with increasing patient age, rapid clearance, and high costs. The use of an appropriate carrier to deliver and release rhBMPs may prolong their resident time in the wound environment. However, the search for the perfect carrier system is still ongoing. An unexpected issue that emerged in recent years is the observation that rhBMPs applied at a bone defect or injury initiate the release of factors that promote osteoclastogenesis and activation of osteoclasts, which leads to bone resorption.[51]

Advances in gene transfer technology provide an opportunity to deliver complementary DNAs that can encode osteogenic proteins. This strategy, which is currently being tested under experimental conditions, enables a sustained local presence of the growth or differentiation factor with minimal exposure of nontarget sites. Whether gene transfer technology will find its way into routine reconstructive dentistry, which does not treat life-threatening diseases, remains to be seen.

Bone grafting and bone graft substitutes

Bone grafting materials are used in reconstructive surgery to fill voids, replace portions of bone, augment bone, facilitate or enhance repair of bone defects through osteoconduction, provide mechanical membrane support, stabilize the blood clot, and serve as vehicles for antibiotics or growth factors. A bone filler should at least be safe, nontoxic, and biocompatible; provide mechanical support and an osteoconductive scaffold; become osseointegrated or replaced; allow ingrowth of blood vessels; and be easy to use and cost-effective. Several options for a grafting material currently exist, including autologous or allogeneic bone and xenogeneic or alloplastic bone graft substitutes. These materials may display one or more of the properties that are commonly described as *(1)* osteoconductive, *(2)* osteoinductive, and *(3)* osteogenic. Chapter 4 discusses the current status of bone fillers in implant dentistry.

Osteoconductive materials possess a matrix that serves as a scaffold or framework that is used as a template and enlarged solid base for bone deposition. Materials with *osteoinductive* properties contain proteins that stimulate and support proliferation and differentiation of progenitor cells to become osteoblasts. *Osteogenic* means that the material contains osteogenic cells (osteoblasts or osteoblast precursors) that are capable of forming bone if placed in the proper environment.

Autologous bone is a preferred bone graft material because it possesses osteoinductive, osteogenic, and osteoconductive properties. However, the harvesting of autologous bone may require an additional surgical intervention, which increases the operative time, costs, intraoperative blood loss, pain, and recovery time. Moreover, it is associated with an increased risk of donor site morbidity (eg, increased postoperative pain, nerve injury, blood vessel injury, hematoma, infection, hernia formation, and cosmetic disadvantages). Finally, the supply of autologous bone graft may be limited.

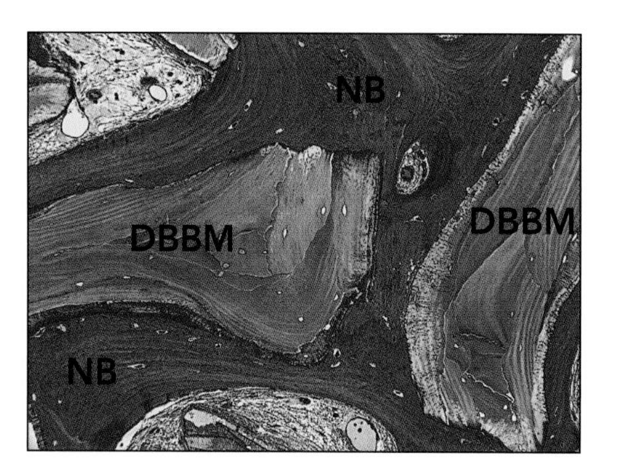

Fig 2-21 Semithin section illustrating the osteoconductive property of deproteinized bovine bone mineral (DBBM). The newly formed bone (NB) stains more intensely than does the DBBM. However, note the differential staining of the DBBM particles (decalcified tissue embedded in acrylic resin; basic fuchsin and toluidine blue stain).

Allogeneic bone and certain bone-derived or synthetic bone graft substitutes may have similar osteoconductive properties. Allografts have been used alone or in combination with autologous bone to manage bone defects. However, their efficacy is less than that of autologous bone alone.[52] When human demineralized bone matrix, which is commercially available, was used alone, it failed to demonstrate efficacy equivalent to that of autologous bone.[52] In cases of non-union bone fractures treated with Allomatrix (demineralized bone matrix with calcium sulfate, Wright Medical), a high incidence of wound drainage, infection, and treatment failure was reported.[53]

Xenogeneic and alloplastic bone graft substitutes are increasingly appearing on the market and are becoming more and more popular. They have osteoconductive properties, albeit to varying degrees (Fig 2-21). Bony filling of larger defects is greatly facilitated by osteoconduction. Two important conditions must be fulfilled for successful osteoconduction: *(1)* the scaffold must consist of a bioinert or bioactive material and *(2)* the shape and dimensions of its external and internal structure should favor tissue ingrowth and bone deposition. With regard to shape and dimension, a material resembling spongeous bone provides the ideal conditions for bony ingrowth, which always also depends on vascular ingrowth by angiogenesis.[54]

Guided bone regeneration

Principles

GBR, usually in combination with a grafting material, is the method most widely used to augment bone in routine dental practice. Because bone is a relatively slow-growing tissue, both fibroblasts and epithelial cells have the opportunity to occupy available space more efficiently and to build up a soft connective tissue much faster than bone is able to grow. Thus, the biologic mechanism behind GBR is the exclusion of undesirable cells from the wound environment to enable cells from the bone tissue to proliferate into the coagulum-filled space under the barrier membrane. If the occlusive barrier function lasts long enough and if the barrier membrane is not exposed to the oral cavity, optimal conditions exist for the stem cells and osteoprogenitor cells

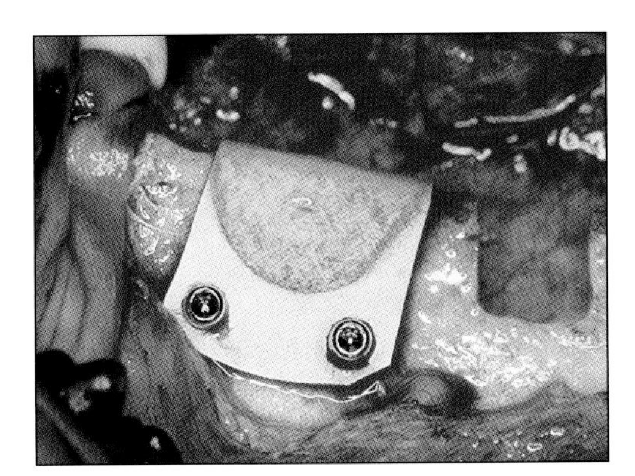

Fig 2-22 Surgical procedure of GBR. Exposure of the alveolar crest and defect creation in a canine mandible 2 months after extraction of the premolars. The distal defect is open, but the mesial one is covered with a barrier membrane. Miniscrews fix the membrane and mark the corners of the defect for radiography.

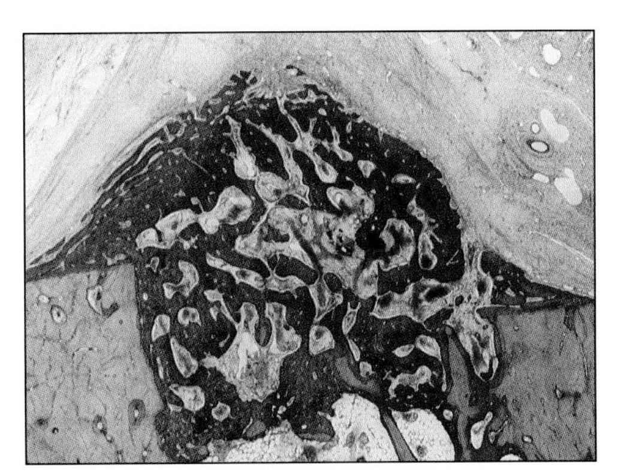

Fig 2-23 Ground section through the central portion of a control defect without a barrier membrane after 2 months. A bony cover seals the marrow space in the bottom of the defect (toluidine blue and basic fuchsin surface stain).

to differentiate into osteoblasts, which deposit the bone matrix. In other words, the barrier membrane creates a secluded space that allows bone to use its great, natural healing capacity in an undisturbed or protected manner. Both resorbable and nonresorbable membranes are available on the market.

Bone healing pattern

In the following sections, the histologic healing pattern of bone regeneration in membrane-protected defects is illustrated and discussed using data from an experimental study in the canine mandible.[55] In this study, saddle-type defects measuring approximately 8 × 12 × 10 mm were created 2 months after premolar extraction. The defects were covered with or without a barrier membrane (Fig 2-22). A standard expanded polytetrafluoroethylene (ePTFE) membrane and two different prototype ePTFE membranes reinforced by polypropylene mesh were used. The position of the membranes was secured by two miniscrews. No bone filler was used. However, intravenously aspirated blood was injected under each membrane. Histologic analysis was performed after healing periods of 2 and 4 months.

Healing without a barrier membrane. The control defects, which did not receive a barrier membrane, showed a consistent repair pattern in which bone formation was restricted to the defect margins, ie, mesial and distal walls of the defect and at the defect bottom (Fig 2-23). Closure of the marrow space was completed after 2 months, but bone formation made no further progress. At 4 months, bone had slightly increased in density.

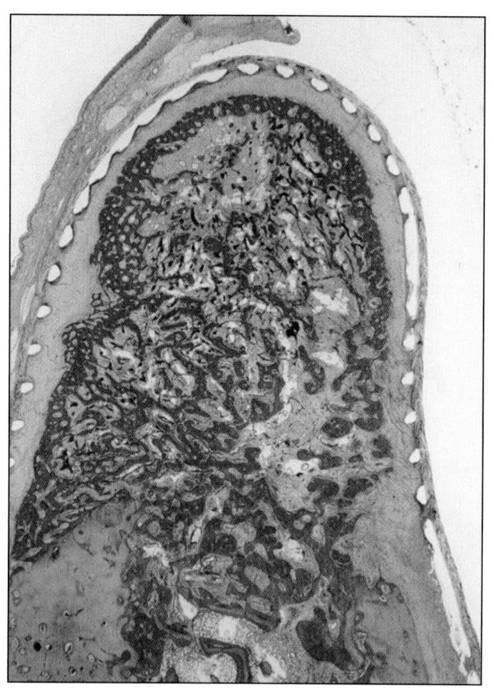

Fig 2-24 Buccolingual ground section of a membrane-covered defect after 2 months, revealing the bony filling of the secluded volume beneath the barrier membrane (toluidine blue and basic fuchsin surface stain).

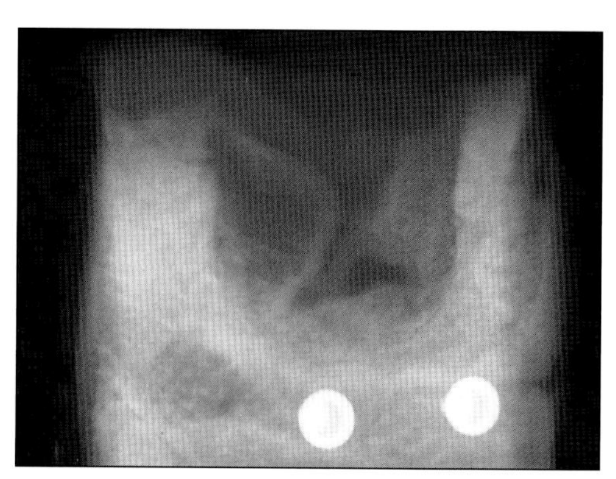

Fig 2-25 Radiograph of a membrane-covered defect after 2 months revealing bony ingrowth from the mesial and distal walls as well as from the bottom of the defect. (Reprinted from Schenk et al[55] with permission.)

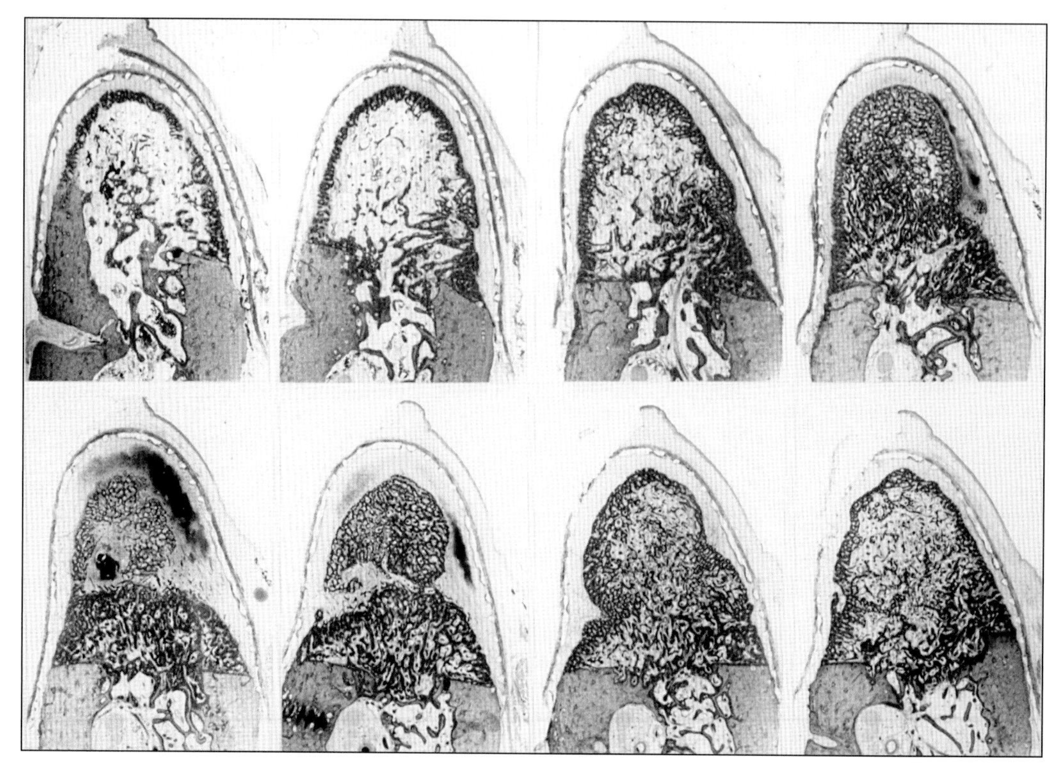

Fig 2-26 Selected serial buccolingual sections, arranged in a mesiodistal sequence, of a membrane-covered defect after 2 months (original magnification ×2.5). (Reprinted from Schenk et al[55] with permission.)

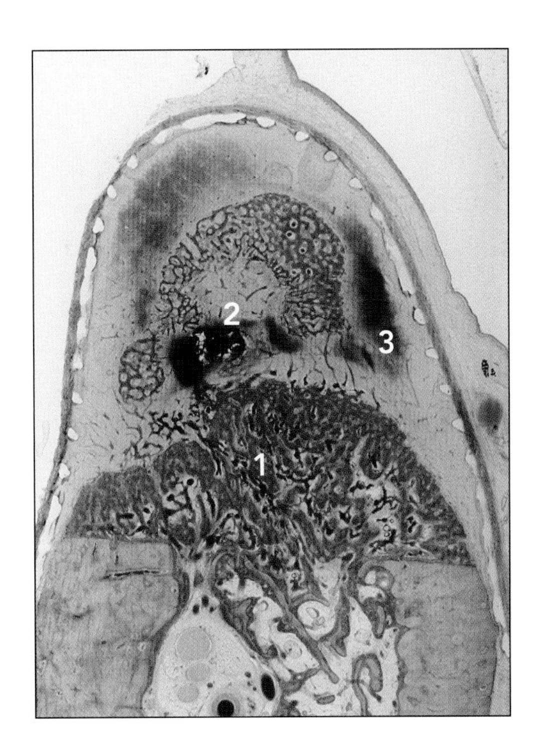

Fig 2-27 Section adjacent to section 5 of the series (*bottom left* in Fig 2-26) revealing the bony cover of the bottom marrow space (1) and a tangential section through the top of the bony hill originating from the mesial wall of the defect (2), as well as the associated hematoma (3).

Healing under a barrier membrane. Membrane protection resulted in a dramatic change in bone and tissue regeneration. The membrane maintained the space created during surgery and clearly separated the outer compartment, constituting the oral mucosa, from the inner space, which is mainly accessible from the marrow cavity (Fig 2-24).

This inner compartment was initially filled with a blood clot, and at 2 months, remnants of the coagulum could still be recognized in the middle portion of the defect (Figs 2-25 to 2-27). However, the hematoma was completely penetrated by granulation tissue and blood vessels. The majority of the secluded volume now consisted of a spongeous bony regenerate that enclosed, between its trabeculae, a labyrinth of tiny, interdigitating marrow spaces filled with hypervascularized, loose soft connective tissue. Both the vessels and the fibrous tissue were in continuity with the original bone marrow. Bone formation started, as in the controls, from the margins of the defects, where it spread over the openings of the marrow cavity (Fig 2-27).

Thus, there were basically three centers of bone formation, which formed a dome-shaped seal over the openings of the marrow cavity. From these bony covers, bone further expanded into the center of the membrane-bound space. Both radiographs (see Fig 2-25) and serial ground sections (see Fig 2-26) demonstrated this characteristic pattern of bone healing. Figure 2-27 illustrates the third center of bone formation at the bottom of the defect.

Formation of the primary spongeous scaffold. The histology of bone formation in the membrane-protected space exhibited a remarkable similarity to that found during bone development and growth (Fig 2-28). The infiltration of the hematoma by granulation tissue followed the basic pattern of wound healing. The invading vascular sprouts were accompanied by cells originating from the bone marrow at the periphery

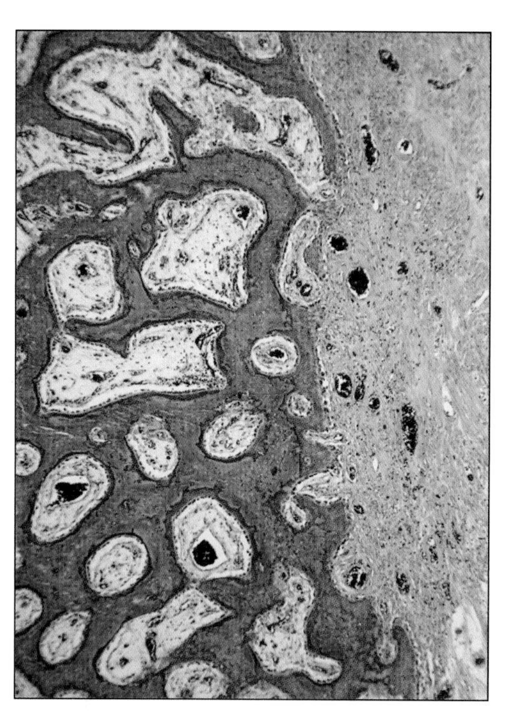

Fig 2-28 Organization of the hematoma and woven bone formation. Blood vessels and bone-forming cells invade the former hematoma *(right)* and construct a scaffold of woven bone (Goldner trichrome stain).

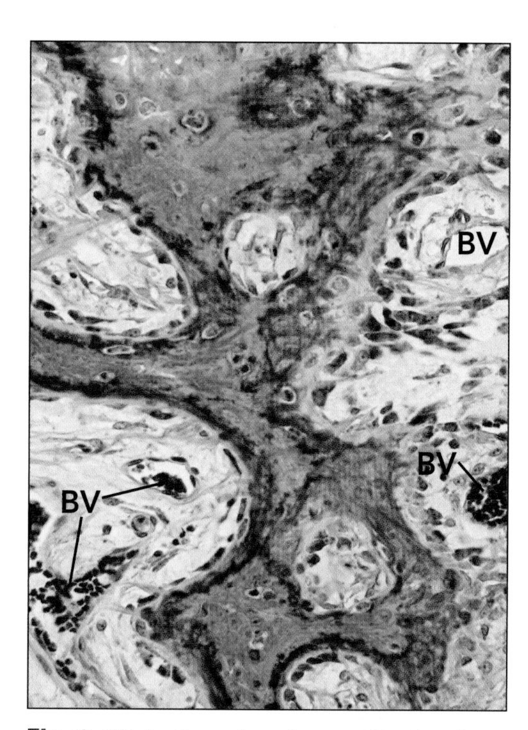

Fig 2-29 In the advancing ossification front, blood vessels (BV) and outgrowing trabeculae are tightly interconnected. Osteoid seams are stained in red, and mineralized bone matrix is in green (Goldner trichrome stain).

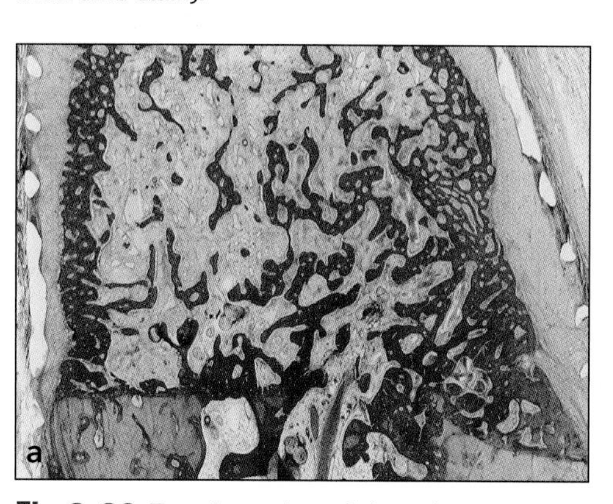

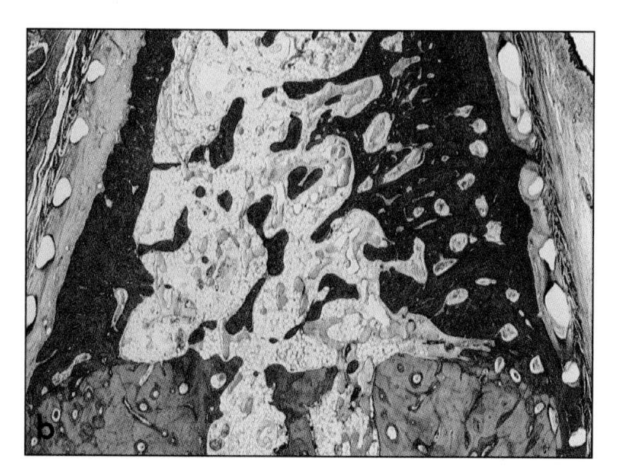

Fig 2-30 Transformation of the primary spongiosa spongework into cortical bone and cancellous bone. *(a)* After 2 months, the spongiosa is denser at the periphery than in the center of the bony regenerate. *(b)* Cortical bone and secondary spongiosa after 4 months. A compact bone layer in the periphery confines a cancellous bone in the center with well-defined trabeculae and regular bone marrow (toluidine blue and basic fuchsin surface stain).

of the defect. The bone marrow contained adult mesenchymal stem cells capable of adipogenic, chondrogenic, and osteogenic differentiation.[56] From the cut cortical and trabecular surfaces, woven bone sprouted out, mostly in the shape of thin, bifurcating plates (Fig 2-29). A particular characteristic of this primary spongeous scaffold is the perfect interdigitation with the vascular plexus. As already mentioned, angiogenesis and ample blood supply are mandatory for bone development and maintenance.

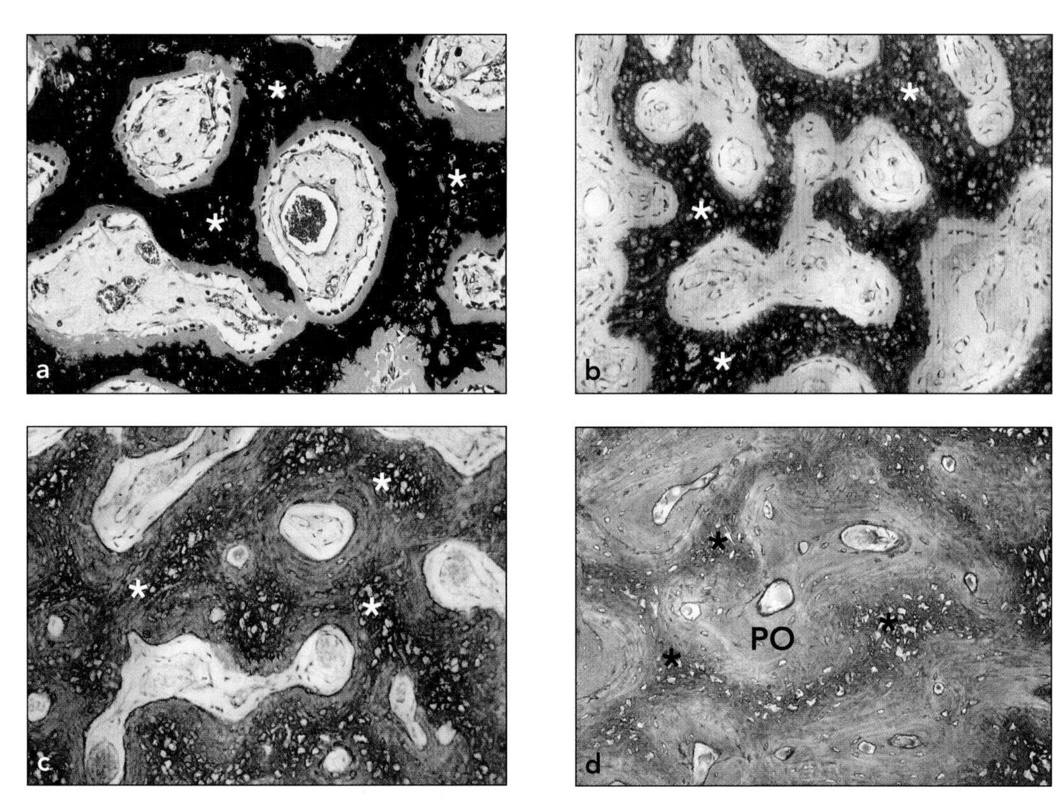

Fig 2-31 Transformation of a scaffold of woven bone into cortical bone. Microtome section *(a)* and ground section *(b)* showing newly formed woven bone *(asterisks)* covered by a contiguous layer of osteoblasts and surrounded by well-vascularized intertrabecular spaces. Reinforcement of woven bone *(asterisks)* by parallel-fibered bone 2 months after surgery *(c)* and transformation into primary osteons (PO) by continuous filling of the intertrabecular spaces 4 months after surgery *(d)*. Woven bone *(asterisks)* is still clearly recognizable (*[a]* von Kossa–McNeal stain; *[b to d]* toluidine blue surface stain). (Reprinted from Schenk et al[55] with permission.)

Transformation into compact bone and a regular spongiosa. While the original primary spongework exclusively consisted of woven bone, it later served as a template for the apposition of lamellar bone, which eventually would constitute both compact bone and a regular spongiosa with mature bone marrow. These events occurred 3 to 4 months after surgery (Fig 2-30).

The formation of a peripheral cortical bone layer started in the vicinity of the mesial and distal walls of the defect as a continuation of the original cortex. The surface of the trabeculae in the primary spongework was lined by a coherent layer of osteoblasts (Fig 2-31a). Continuous bone deposition increased the diameter of the trabeculae and narrowed the intertrabecular spaces (Figs 2-31b and 2-31c). The structure of the newly formed bone changed gradually from woven to lamellar bone, parallel-fibered bone being an intermediate stage of this maturation process. The endpoint of this process was reached when the former intertrabecular spaces attained the size of regular cortical canals and, together with the surrounding concentric lamellae, constituted primary osteons (Fig 2-31d).

The formation of a secondary or regular spongiosa started in the central portion of the defect space, where the marrow space was expanded by resorption of the primary

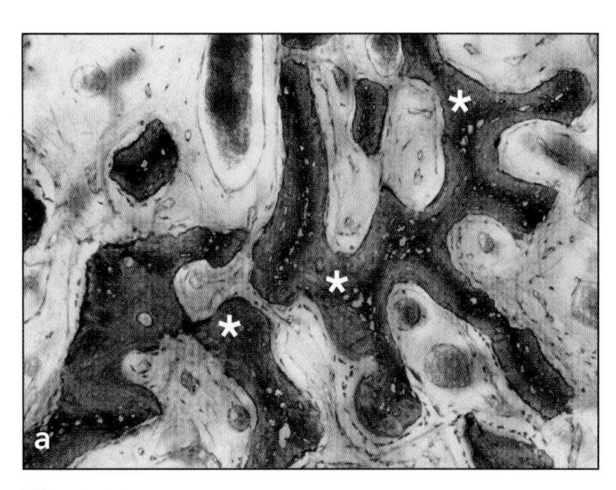

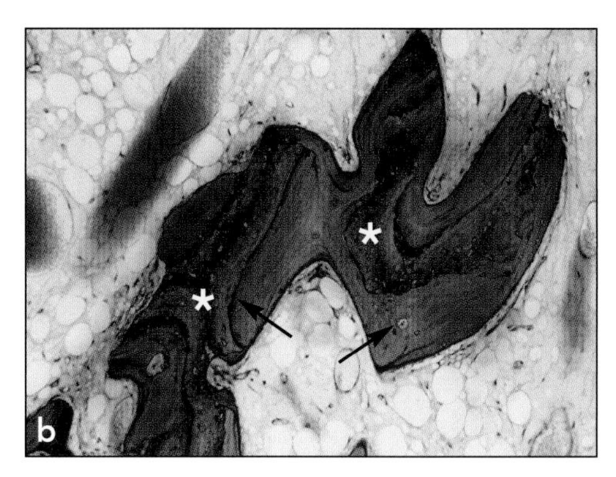

Fig 2-32 Formation of a secondary spongiosa. *(a)* After 2 months, the trabeculae of the primary spongework consist of woven bone *(asterisks)* reinforced by a layer of parallel-fibered bone. *(b)* After 4 months, remodeling results in bone trabeculae that are composed of remnants of the original scaffold *(asterisks)* covered by packets of lamellar bone *(arrows)* (toluidine blue surface stain).

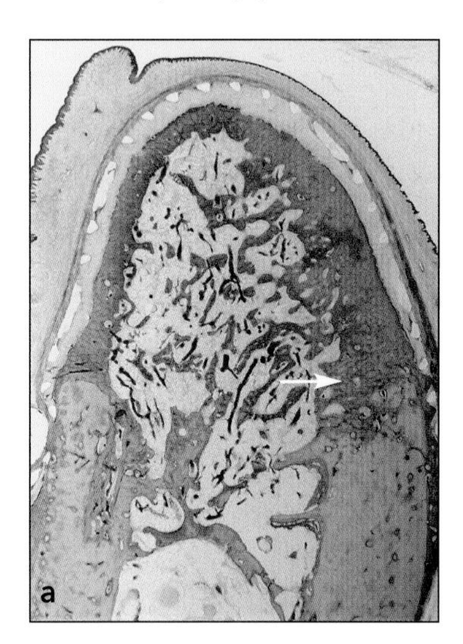

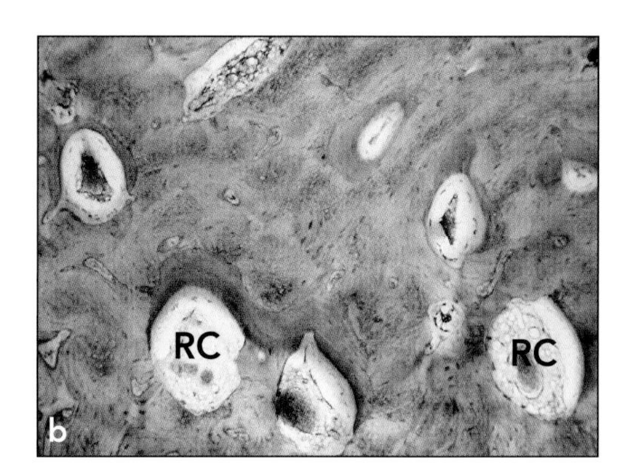

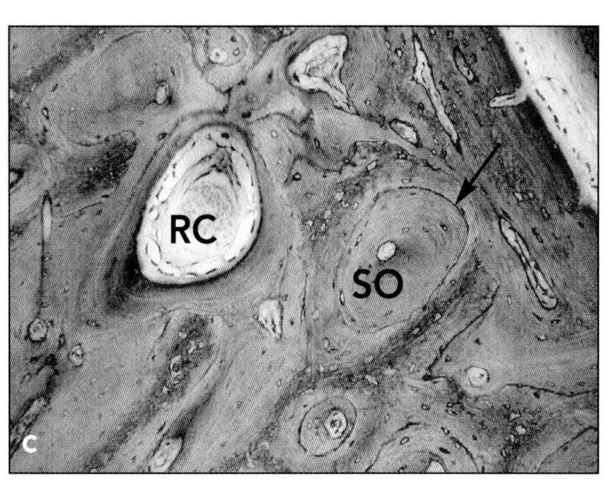

Fig 2-33 Cortical bone remodeling at 4 months (ground sections; toluidine blue surface stain). *(a)* Haversian remodeling starts within the compact cortical layer, preferentially in close proximity to the original cortex *(arrow)*. *(b)* Initially formed resorption canals (RC) will be filled with mature lamellar bone. *(c)* Higher magnification shows a resorption canal (RC) with beginning bone deposition and a completed secondary osteon (SO) confined by a cement line *(arrow)*.

spongework (Fig 2-32a). The spared trabeculae underwent profound remodeling, and the remnants of woven and parallel-fibered bone were gradually replaced by packets of lamellar bone (Fig 2-32b). This process also started mesially and distally and proceeded into the central defect portion. The resulting cancellous bone was contiguous with preexisting trabeculae in the walls of the defect.

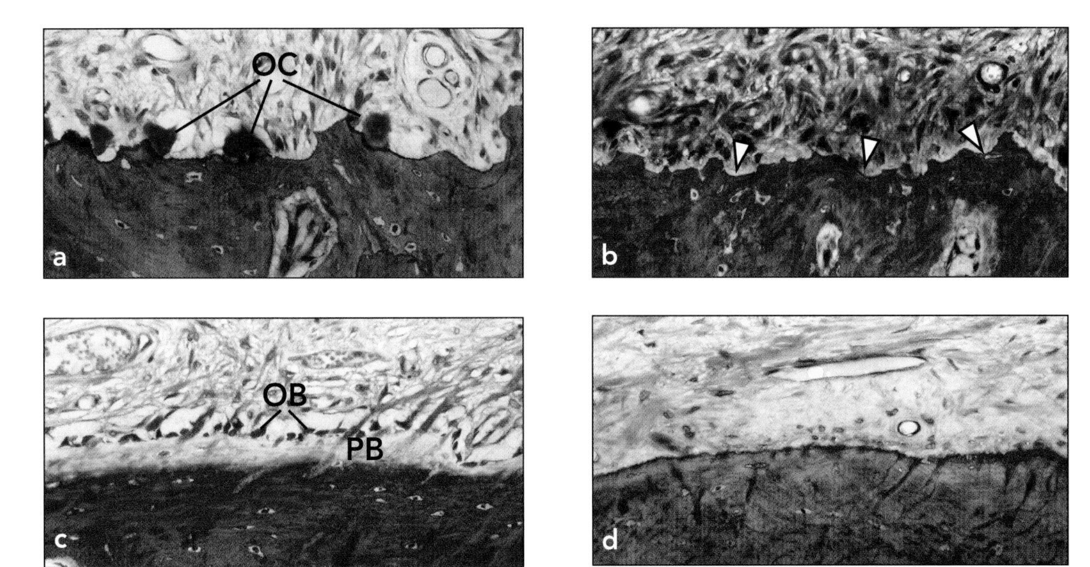

Fig 2-34 Modeling of cortical bone. *(a)* Active, ongoing resorption is indicated by the presence of osteoclasts (OC). *(b)* Howship lacunae *(arrowheads)*, or an eroded surface, persist after osteoclastic resorption until they are covered by newly formed bone. *(c)* The presence of osteoblasts (OB) and an osteoid (prebone [PB]) seems indicative of bone apposition. *(d)* Resting or quiescent bone surfaces are lined by bone-lining cells and a regular periosteum (ground sections; toluidine blue and basic fuchsin surface stain).

Remodeling of cortical bone. During the fourth month, the cortical bone entered its last phase of maturation, that is, haversian remodeling. Activation of bone metabolizing units led to the formation of resorption canals, which subsequently were filled with concentric lamellae (Figs 2-33a and 2-33b). The resulting secondary osteons were clearly distinguishable from primary osteons by the surrounding cement lines of the reversal type (Fig 2-33c). The remodeling process also started in the most mature part of the regenerate, close to the defect margins, and gradually progressed into the central portion of the defect space.

Modeling of the bony regenerate. At the end of the fourth month, growth and modeling of the bone within the membrane-confined space continued, particularly in the central portion. With the formation of a cortical bone layer, the periosteal and endosteal envelopes were also restored. They resumed their modeling activities by means of shape-deforming resorption and formation along the outer and inner cortical surfaces (Fig 2-34). As long as modeling was occurring, the bone surface was locally lined by osteoblasts and an osteoid seam or covered by osteoclasts or Howship lacunae as a sign of ongoing or past resorptive activity. In quiescent sites, the bone surface was smooth, and collagen was incorporated as Sharpey fibers in the mineralized bone matrix.

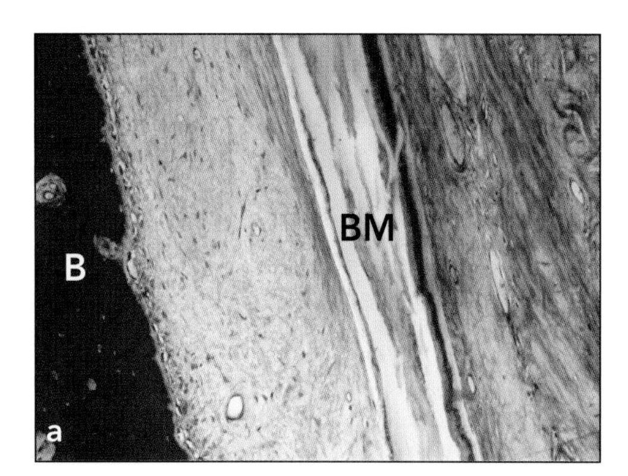

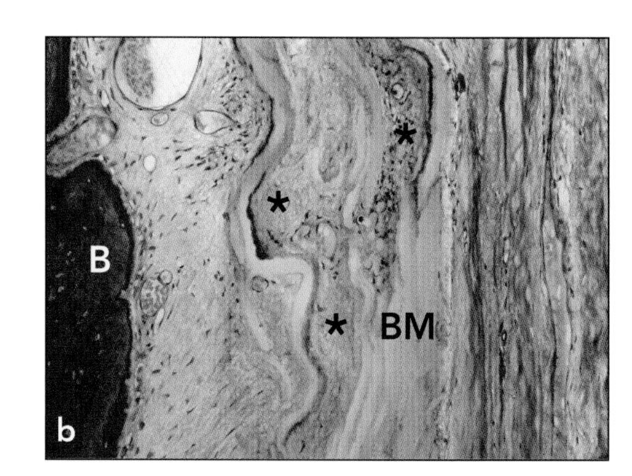

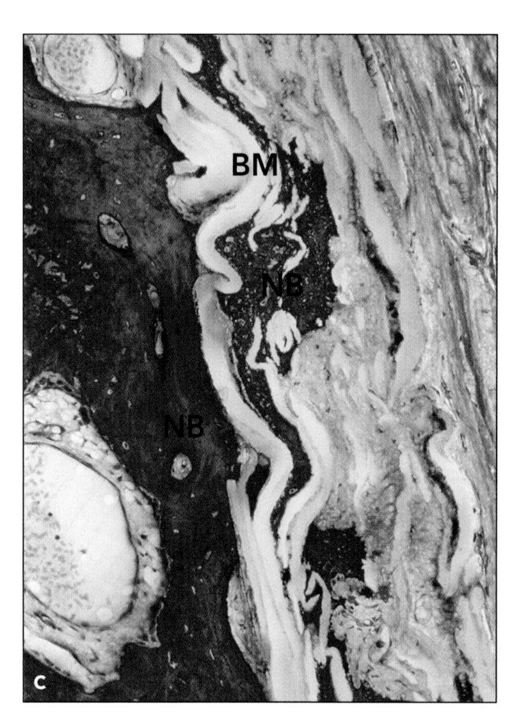

Fig 2-35 Soft and hard tissue compartments adjacent to an ePTFE barrier membrane (BM) (ground sections; toluidine blue and basic fuchsin surface stain). *(a)* The dense portion of the barrier membrane separates an outer, gingival compartment from an inner, soft connective tissue compartment that is mainly accessible from the bone (B) compartment. There are no signs of a foreign-body reaction. *(b)* The porous part of the barrier membrane *(asterisks)* allows ingrowth of blood vessels and cells into the membrane interstices. *(c)* Newly formed bone (NB) makes contact with the inner surface of the barrier membrane and grows into its interstitial pores.

In all modeling sites, the number of blood vessels increased. As a result, the cortex surface became more clearly defined and the intertrabecular spaces better interconnected. In this way, the maturation gradient was maintained, the central portion lagging somewhat behind with regard to overall height, bone density, and structural organization.

Soft tissue compartments. What remains to be discussed is the soft tissue integration of the membrane. The biocompatibility characteristics of the implanted material have an important effect on tissue integration (see chapter 3). The barrier membrane separates the soft tissue into an inner and an outer compartment (Fig 2-35a). During healing, both the chemical composition and the surface structure of the material influence connective tissue ingrowth or attachment to the membrane. Successful tissue integration is achieved with a material that does not provoke a foreign-body reaction that is too pronounced. If the material is porous and very biocompatible, the soft connective tissue may invade the membrane interstices (Fig 2-35b).

Moreover, even bone growth into the pores and interstices of the membrane may occur at sites where the membrane has come into close contact with bone (Fig 2-35c). Bone is directly deposited on the pore walls, fills the pores almost completely, and even penetrates through the membrane. This intramembranous ossification again demonstrates that the membrane consists of a perfectly bioinert material and may have osteoconductive properties.

A similar phenomenon is found in collagen-based barrier membranes, particularly if they are cross-linked. However, in the case of cross-linked collagen membranes, the modified collagen itself seems to trigger membrane ossification.[57,58]

Conclusion

Bone has the unique capability to rebuild its original structure and function in response to a defect or fracture. The pattern of bone healing closely resembles that of development and growth. Under stable mechanical conditions, bone is formed directly or primarily, provided that two essential conditions are present: an ample blood supply and a solid base for bone deposition. The solid base is provided by the surface of the fragment ends or by the bony margins of a defect.

Repair of bone defects closely resembles appositional growth. In the initial, rapid phase, a template of woven bone is constructed and gradually reinforced by lamellar bone. Depending on the local environment, this primary spongework is then transformed into compact cortical or trabecular bone. In the second phase, the regenerate undergoes profound remodeling and substitution by bone remodeling units (bone metabolizing units). In cortical bone, the remodeling units produce secondary osteons. In cancellous bone, the resulting bone structural units form packets.

While healing of bone defects has size limits in the range of a couple of millimeters, there are several means, alone or in combination, to promote bone regeneration:

- Osteoinduction by growth factors released from autologous bone particles or added as recombinant proteins in a carrier transplanted into the defect.
- Osteoconduction by autografts, allografts, xenografts, or alloplasts. Osteoconduction facilitates bridging of larger defects by offering a solid scaffold on which bone can be deposited. The substitution rate of the bone filler material varies greatly and depends on the bone graft or substitute material used.
- Transfer of stem cells or progenitor cells that differentiate into osteoblasts by using cancellous bone grafts or bone marrow aspirates.
- Distraction osteogenesis by canalizing bony callus formation into longitudinal compartments, confined by continuously stretched collagen fiber bundles. This technique yields impressive results.
- GBR, a well-established procedure based on the principle of protecting bone regeneration against overgrowth of tissues formed by rapidly proliferating nonosteogenic cells. It is successfully applied for alveolar ridge augmentations.

References

1. Bianco P. Structure and mineralization of bone. In: Bonucci E (ed). Calcification in Biological Systems. Boca Raton, FL: CRC Press, 1992:243–268.
2. Weiner S, Traub W, Wagner HD. Lamellar bone: Structure-function relations. J Struct Biol 1999;126: 241–255.
3. Frost HM. Micropetrosis. J Bone Joint Surg 1960; 42A:144–150.
4. Parfitt AM. The coupling of bone formation to bone resorption: A critical analysis of the concept and of its relevance to the pathogenesis of osteoporosis. Metab Bone Dis Relat Res 1982;4:1–6.
5. Marks SC Jr, Popoff SN. Bone cell biology: The regulation of development, structure, and function in the skeleton. Am J Anat 1988;183:1–44.
6. Candeliere GA, Liu F, Aubin JE. Individual osteoblasts in the developing calvaria express different gene repertoires. Bone 2001;28:351–361.
7. Qiu S, Rao DS, Palnitkar S, Parfitt AM. Relationships between osteocyte density and bone formation rate in human cancellous bone. Bone 2002;31:709–711.
8. Ferretti M, Muglia MA, Remaggi F, Cane V, Palumbo C. Histomorphometric study on the osteocyte lacuno-canalicular network in animals of different species. 2. Parallel-fibered and lamellar bones. Ital J Anat Embryol 1999;104:121–131.
9. Ham AW. Some histophysiological problems peculiar to calcified tissues. J Bone Joint Surg 1952; 34A:701–728.
10. Noble BS, Reeve J. Osteocyte function, osteocyte death and bone fracture resistance. Mol Cell Endocrinol 2000;159:7–13.
11. Jones SJ, Boyde A. Scanning electron microscopy of bone cells in cultures. In: Copp DH, Talmage RV (eds). Endocrinology of Calcium Metabolism. Amsterdam: Excerpta Medica, 1978:97–104.
12. Teitelbaum SL, Ross FP. Genetic regulation of osteoclast development and function. Nat Rev Genet 2003;4:638–649.
13. Minkin C. Bone acid phosphatase: Tartrate-resistant acid phosphatase as a marker of osteoclast function. Calcif Tissue Int 1982;34:285–290.
14. Nanci A. Content and distribution of noncollagenous matrix proteins in bone and cementum: Relationship to speed of formation and collagen packing density. J Struct Biol 1999;126:256–269.
15. Robey PG. Vertebrate mineralized matrix proteins: Structure and function. Connect Tissue Res 1996;35: 131–136.
16. Sodek J, McKee MD. Molecular and cellular biology of alveolar bone. Periodontol 2000 2000;24:99–126.
17. Butler WT. Noncollagenous proteins of bone and dentin: A brief overview. In: Goldberg M, Boskey A, Robinson C (eds). Chemistry and Biology of Mineralized Tissues. Rosemont, IL: American Academy of Orthopedic Surgeons, 2000:137–141.
18. Bosshardt DD. Are cementoblasts a subpopulation of osteoblasts or a unique phenotype? J Dent Res 2005;84:390–406.
19. Lamoureux F, Baud'huin M, Dulomb L, Heymann D, Rédini F. Proteoglycans: Key partners in bone cell biology. Bioessays 2007;29:758–771.
20. Hay ED. Collagen and other matrix glycoproteins in embryogenesis. In: Hay ED (ed). Cell Biology of Extracellular Matrix. New York: Plenum Press, 1991: 437–444.
21. Christoffersen J, Landis WJ. A contribution with review to the description of mineralization of bone and other calcified tissues in vivo. Anat Rec 1991;230: 435–450.
22. Aubin JE, Triffit J. Mesenchymal stem cells and the osteoblast lineage. In: Bilezikian LG, Raisz LG, Rodan GA (eds). Principles of Bone Biology. New York: Academic Press, 2002:59–81.
23. Yang X, Karsenty G. Transcription factors in bone: Developmental and pathological aspects. Trends Mol Med 2002;8:340–345.
24. Otto F, Thornell AP, Crompton T, et al. *Cbfa1*, a candidate gene for cleidocranial dysplasia syndrome, is essential for osteoblast differentiation and bone development. Cell 1997;89:765–771.
25. Bronckers AL, Engelse MA, Cavender A, Gaikwad J, D'Souza RN. Cell-specific patterns of *Cbfa1* mRNA and protein expression in postnatal murine dental tissues. Mech Dev 2001;101:255–258.
26. Suda T, Nakamura I, Jimi E, Takahashi N. Regulation of osteoclast function. J Bone Miner Res 1997;12: 869–879.
27. Mogi M, Otogoto J, Ota N, Togari A. Differential expression of RANKL and osteoprotegerin in gingival crevicular fluid of patients with periodontitis. J Dent Res 2004;83:166–169.
28. Aubin JE. Regulation of osteoblast formation and function. Rev Endocr Metab Disord 2001;2:81–94.
29. Harada S, Rodan GA. Control of osteoblast function and regulation of bone mass. Nature 2003;423: 349–355.
30. Hofbauer LC, Heufelder AE. Role of receptor activator of nuclear factor-κ B ligand and osteoprotegerin in bone cell biology. J Mol Med 2001;79: 243–253.
31. Goldring SR. Inflammatory mediators as essential elements in bone remodeling. Calcif Tissue Int 2003;73:97–100.
32. Clowes JA, Riggs BL, Khosla S. The role of the immune system in the pathophysiology of osteoporosis. Immunol Rev 2005;208:207–227.
33. Kearns AE, Khosla S, Kostenuik P. Receptor activator of nuclear factor B ligand and osteoprotegerin regulation of bone remodeling in health and disease. Endocr Rev 2008;29:155–192.
34. Enlow DH. Functions of the Haversian system. Am J Anat 1962;110:269–305.
35. Schenk R, Willenegger H. Morphological findings in primary fracture healing. In: Krompecher S, Kerner E (eds). Callus Formation: Symposium on the Biology of Fracture Healing. Symp Biol Hung 1967;7:75–86.

36. Jaworski ZF, Lok E. The rate of osteoclastic bone erosion in Haversian remodeling sites of adult dog's rib. Calcif Tissue Res 1972;10:103–112.
37. Schenk RK. Cytodynamics and histodynamics of primary bone repair. In: Lane JM (ed). Fracture Healing. Edinburgh: Churchill Livingstone, 1987:23–32.
38. Wolff J. Das Gesetz der Transformation der Knochen. Berlin: Hirschwalk, 1892.
39. Reddi AH. Cell biology and biochemistry of endochondral bone development. Coll Relat Res 1981;1: 209–226.
40. Johner R. Zur Knochenheilung in Abhängigkeit von der Defektgrösse. Helv Chir Acta 1972;39:409–411.
41. Schenk R, Willenegger H. Zur Histologie der primären Knochenheilung. Modifikationen und Grenzen der Spaltheilung in Abhängigkeit von der Defektgrösse. Unfallheilkunde 1977;80:155–160.
42. Harris WJ, White RE Jr, McCarthy JC, Walker PS, Weinberg EH. Bony ingrowth fixation of the acetabular component in canine hip joint arthroplasty. Clin Orthop 1983;176:7–11.
43. Berglundh T, Abrahamsson I, Lang NP, Lindhe J. De novo alveolar bone formation adjacent to endosseous implants. A model study in the dog. Clin Oral Implants Res 2003;14:251–262.
44. Abrahamsson I, Berglundh T, Linder E, Lang NP, Lindhe J. Early bone formation adjacent to rough and turned endosseous implant surfaces. An experimental study in the dog. Clin Oral Implants Res 2004;15:381–392.
45. Buser D, Broggini N, Wieland M, et al. Enhanced bone apposition to a chemically modified SLA titanium surface. J Dent Res 2004;83:529–533.
46. Urist MR. Bone: Formation by autoinduction. Science 1965;150:893–899.
47. Bang G, Urist MR. Bone induction in excavation chambers in matrix of decalcified dentin. Arch Surg 1967;94:781–789.
48. Urist MR, Strates BS. Bone morphogenetic protein. J Dent Res 1971;50:1392–1406.
49. Jung RE, Glauser R, Schärer P, Hämmerle CHF, Sailer HF, Weber FE. Effect of rhBMP-2 on guided bone regeneration in humans. A randomized, controlled clinical and histomorphometric study. Clin Oral Implants Res 2003;14:556–568.
50. Warnke PH, Springer IN, Wiltfang J, et al. Growth and transplantation of a custom vascularized bone graft in man. Lancet 2004;364:766–770.
51. Gautschi OP, Frey SP, Zellweger R. Bone morphogenetic proteins in clinical applications. ANZ J Surg 2007;77:626–631.
52. Finkemeier CG. Bone-grafting and bone graft substitutes. J Bone Joint Surg 2002;84:454–464.
53. Ziran BH, Smith WR, Morgan SJ. Use of calcium-based demineralized bone matrix/allograft for nonunions and posttraumatic reconstruction of the appendicular skeleton: Preliminary results and complications. J Trauma 2007;63:1324–1328.
54. Dai J, Rabie AB. VEGF: An essential mediator of both angiogenesis and endochondral ossification. J Dent Res 2007;86:937–950.
55. Schenk RK, Buser D, Hardwick WR, Dahlin C. Healing pattern of bone regeneration in membrane-protected defects: A histologic study in the canine mandible. Int J Oral Maxillofac Implants 1994;9:13–29.
56. Jackson L, Jones DR, Scotting P, Sottile V. Adult mesenchymal stem cells: Differentiation potential and therapeutic applications. J Postgrad Med 2007;53:121–127.
57. Connolly JM, Alferiev I, Clark-Gruel JN, et al. Triglycidylamine crosslinking of porcine aortic valve cusps or bovine pericardium results in improved biocompatibility, biomechanics, and calcification resistance: Chemical and biological mechanisms. Am J Pathol 2005;166:1–13.
58. Zubery Y, Goldlust A, Alves A, Nir E. Ossification of a novel cross-linked porcine collagen barrier in guided bone regeneration in dogs. J Periodontol 2007;78:112–121.

CHAPTER 3

Properties of Barrier Membranes

Michael M. Bornstein
Thomas von Arx
Dieter D. Bosshardt

The principle of physically sealing off an anatomical site for improved healing of a certain tissue type and directing tissue regeneration with some sort of mechanical barrier has been used in reconstructive surgery and for neural regeneration for spinal fusions since the mid-1950s.[1,2] In osseous reconstructive surgery, the placement of a barrier is used to prevent ingrowth of soft connective tissue into bone defects. In principle, the membrane is placed in direct contact with the surrounding bone surface, thereby placing the periosteum on the outer surface of the membrane. The mucoperiosteal flap is then repositioned and sutured, creating a secluded space into which only cells from the neighboring bone can migrate.[3]

The use of barrier membranes has become a standard of care in oral surgical procedures using guided bone regeneration (GBR) and guided tissue regeneration (GTR) for the treatment of periodontal bone defects and peri-implant defects as well as for bone augmentation procedures performed prior to or simultaneously with implant placement.[4,5] In the literature and in practice, the terms *GTR* and *GBR* are often confused and used synonymously or inappropriately. GTR describes the regeneration of the supporting periodontal apparatus, including cementum, periodontal ligament, and alveolar bone. GBR involves the promotion of bone formation only.

Basic Characteristics of Barrier Membranes

Clinicians today have access to a wide range of membrane materials for GBR and GTR procedures. To select the material best suited for a specific clinical application, it is necessary to understand the basic requirements for membrane materials used in these indications.[6] These basic characteristics include biocompatibility, cell occlusion, tissue integration, space making and space maintenance, clinical handling during surgery, and limited susceptibility to complications.[6,7]

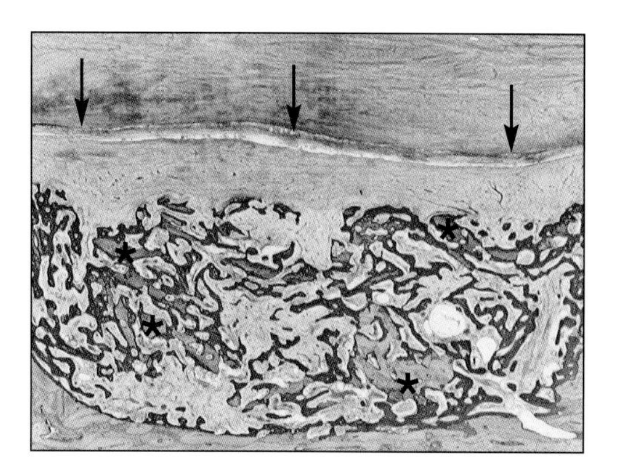

Fig 3-1 Bone defect created in the mandible of a minipig at 4 weeks. The defect was filled with autologous bone particles *(asterisks)* and covered with an expanded polytetrafluoroethylene (ePTFE) barrier membrane *(arrows)*. Note the separation of the underlying bone compartment from the soft connective tissue above the barrier membrane. Newly formed bone can be seen arising from the defect margins and extending between the autologous bone particles (undecalcified ground section; toluidine blue stain).

Biocompatibility

Biocompatibility is a fundamental requirement for acceptable function of any implantable medical device. The term defines the ability of a material to function in a specific application in the presence of an appropriate host response, and biocompatible materials must be free of any risks or significant safety concerns for the patient.[6] The biocompatibility of barrier membranes is characterized by many different parameters such as cytotoxicity, histocompatibility, genotoxicity, mutagenicity, and microbial effects. Therefore, it is impossible to characterize the biologic behavior of a certain material with a single method of testing.

On the contrary, the properties have to be investigated using a battery of in vitro and in vivo tests in a structured approach.[8] In principle, new and/or prototype materials should be subjected to a specific testing sequence, from the most simple to the most complex test method, ie, from in vitro to animal testing and from preclinical to clinical testing in humans.[9]

Clinicians who work with barrier membranes must be cognizant of the fact that inert materials (those that do not degrade in a physiologic environment) generally present a less complex safety situation than do degradable materials.[6] Degradable materials release breakdown products into the surrounding host tissue that can result in local and systemic adverse reactions.[10] The end products of such a degradation process must therefore be benign, and the intermediate breakdown products must be taken into account and controlled in the initial material design.

Cell occlusion

The primary aim of the membrane characteristic of cell occlusion is to exclude connective tissue cells from the region in which bone regeneration is intended to take place (Fig 3-1). This concept was extensively tested in the 1980s in periodontology, where exclusion of soft connective tissue and the dentogingival epithelium was intended to enable periodontal regeneration around the root surfaces of affected teeth (for review see Tatakis et al[11]).

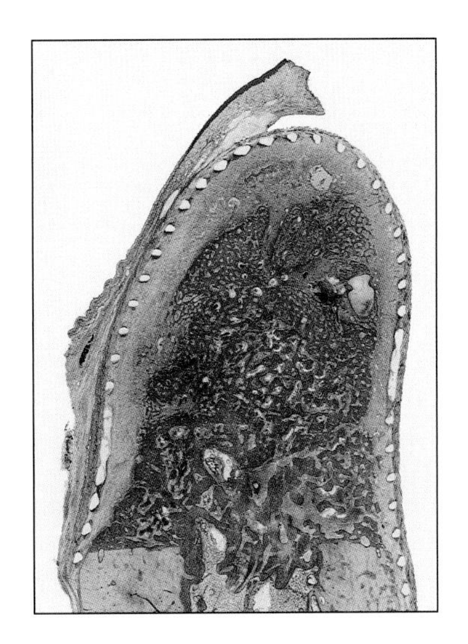

Fig 3-2 Buccolingual section 2 months after a bone defect was created in a dog mandible. The defect was filled with blood and covered with a prototype reinforced expanded polytetrafluoroethylene (ePTFE) membrane. Note the excellent preservation of the geometry of the mandible. Primary spongiosa fills most of the space confined by the membrane (undecalcified ground section; toluidine blue and basic fuchsin stain).

On the other hand, the theory of total cell occlusion has been challenged somewhat by the fact that nutrient transfer across the barrier membrane may be important for a successful regeneration process.[6,12] Other studies have found macroporous membranes to be more predictable for GTR procedures and to be more conducive to uncomplicated clinical management than occlusive barrier membranes.[13,14] Also, other local factors, such as an adequate vascular supply and source of osteogenic cells, both originating from the parent bone, may be of equal or even greater importance to the regeneration of bone than total cell occlusion provided by the barrier membrane.[15]

Tissue integration

The biocompatibility characteristics of a barrier membrane have an important effect on the tissue integration of the material. The surface topography, porosity, and chemical properties of a barrier membrane primarily determine whether ingrowth or surface bonding of tissue occurs during healing. A nonporous, nontextured biomaterial implanted in soft tissue results in the formation of a fibrous connective tissue capsule with no direct attachment to the material, resulting in decreased mechanical support of the wound during the healing period.[16] Membranes that have ideal tissue integration capacities provide increased mechanical stability of the augmented area in GBR and GTR procedures.[6,17]

Space making and space maintenance

The space-making ability of a membrane designed for GBR and GTR procedures can be defined as its capacity to resist collapse under in vivo conditions and therefore to create and maintain sufficient volume and geometry of space during the healing period[6] (Fig 3-2). An important factor determining the ability of a barrier membrane to resist collapse is the stiffness of the material used.

An important problem affecting bioresorbable barrier membranes is that degradable materials lose mechanical strength and, therefore, their space-making capability soon after insertion of the membrane.[18] Because of the somewhat unfavorable mechanical properties of bioresorbable membranes compared to reinforced nonresorbable barrier membranes, the use of supporting materials (eg, autologous block grafts, bone fillers) has been recommended to prevent barrier collapse.[19] Today, even titanium-reinforced polytetrafluoroethylene (PTFE) membranes are supported by grafting materials to achieve better results in GBR procedures.[20]

Clinical handling during surgery

During surgery, barrier membranes are often trimmed, cut, and shaped to fit and cover the augmented area. For a procedure to be completed in a timely manner, membranes must be easy to handle. Nonresorbable membranes, because of their stiffness and hydrophobic characteristics, have to be held in position by screws and pins.[21,22] Bioresorbable membranes, especially collagen membranes, are more supple, and because of their hydrophilicity, they even adhere to the surrounding bone and grafting material as soon as they are soaked with blood.[23]

Nonresorbable barrier membranes do not generally present a problem if removal is necessary because of premature exposure and site infection or in the case of stage-two surgery and implant placement. Nonresorbable membranes retain their structural integrity, which will enable the clinician to remove them completely. On the other hand, bioresorbable membranes can pose a problem when a premature membrane exposure with infection necessitates their removal: Because of fragmentation and the subsequent loss of material integrity, the removal of all remnants of the barrier membrane is sometimes quite problematic for the clinician.

Susceptibility to complications

Based on the nature of their material, barrier membranes exhibit different types of complications during the healing process. Nonresorbable membranes in particular have a significant risk of premature membrane exposure.[24] This may result in a wound infection and subsequently a poor outcome in terms of bone regeneration.[25] Bioresorbable membranes, especially if not cross-linked, are easier to manage and have a lower risk of premature membrane exposure. Inflammatory and foreign-body reactions are sometimes encountered during the resorption process of the barrier membrane when synthetic polymeric materials are used.[26]

Nonresorbable Membranes

Expanded polytetrafluoroethylene (ePTFE) was originally developed in 1969 and marketed in 1971 as Gore-Tex (Gore). Legend has it that W. L. Gore showed a piece of this material to a friend who was a cardiovascular surgeon. He demonstrated the ability of the material to retain water yet breathe, allowing smoke to pass through its porous framework.[27] This encounter triggered a cascade of events leading to the introduction of ePTFE in basic and animal research and in increasing clinical applications in cardiovascular, urogynecologic, fetal, reconstructive, oral, and general surgery.[28–32]

In chemistry, PTFE is a synthetic fluoropolymer that relies on an extremely strong bond between carbon and fluorine for its nondegradable, biologically inert properties. There is no known enzyme in the body capable of cleaving carbon-fluorine bonds.[33] The woven pattern of fibrils in the nonreinforced sheets, consisting of long chains of repeating units, allows the material to stretch in any dimension as well as to compress in thickness. Added rigidity of the material can be achieved by reinforcement with fluorinated ethylene propylene, resulting in ePTFE.

In dentistry, ePTFE membranes became a standard for GTR and GBR procedures in the 1980s and early 1990s.[11,21,22,31,32,34] Besides the ePTFE membrane, nonresorbable barriers are available as titanium-reinforced ePTFE.[35] In a classic article describing the GBR principle with nonresorbable barriers, Dahlin and coworkers[36] raised mucoperiosteal flaps and produced bilateral bone defects in the mandibular angles of 30 adult rats. On one side of the jaw, the defect was covered with an ePTFE membrane, whereas the defect on the other side served as a control. Histologic analysis after healing demonstrated that on the test (ePTFE) side, half of the animals showed complete bone healing after 3 weeks, and all animals showed complete healing after 6 weeks. Little or no signs of healing were evident on the control sides, even after an observation period of 22 weeks.

As these favorable results in animals are not necessarily transferable to the clinical situation because of the high potential for osteogenesis in rats, a similar study by the same group was performed using primates.[21] Through-and-through bone defects were produced bilaterally in edentulous areas of the mandible and in the maxilla in conjunction with apicoectomy of the lateral incisors. The defects on one side were covered buccally as well as lingually and palatally with ePTFE barrier membranes, whereas the defects on the other side served as controls (no membrane). Complete bone healing was seen at all test sites after a healing period of 3 months. At the control sites, bone healing was not complete, and various degrees of connective tissue ingrowth could be observed.

The bone healing events in the membrane-protected defects are described in chapter 2. The focus of this discussion is on the compartmentalization of the soft tissue space by the ePTFE membranes and their tissue integration. In a landmark experimental study in the canine mandible, Schenk and coworkers[37] reported descriptive histologic findings after GBR using ePTFE membranes. The soft tissues inside and outside of the barrier membrane were distinctly different (Fig 3-3a). The tissue outside the membrane consisted of soft connective tissue covered by a keratinizing epithe-

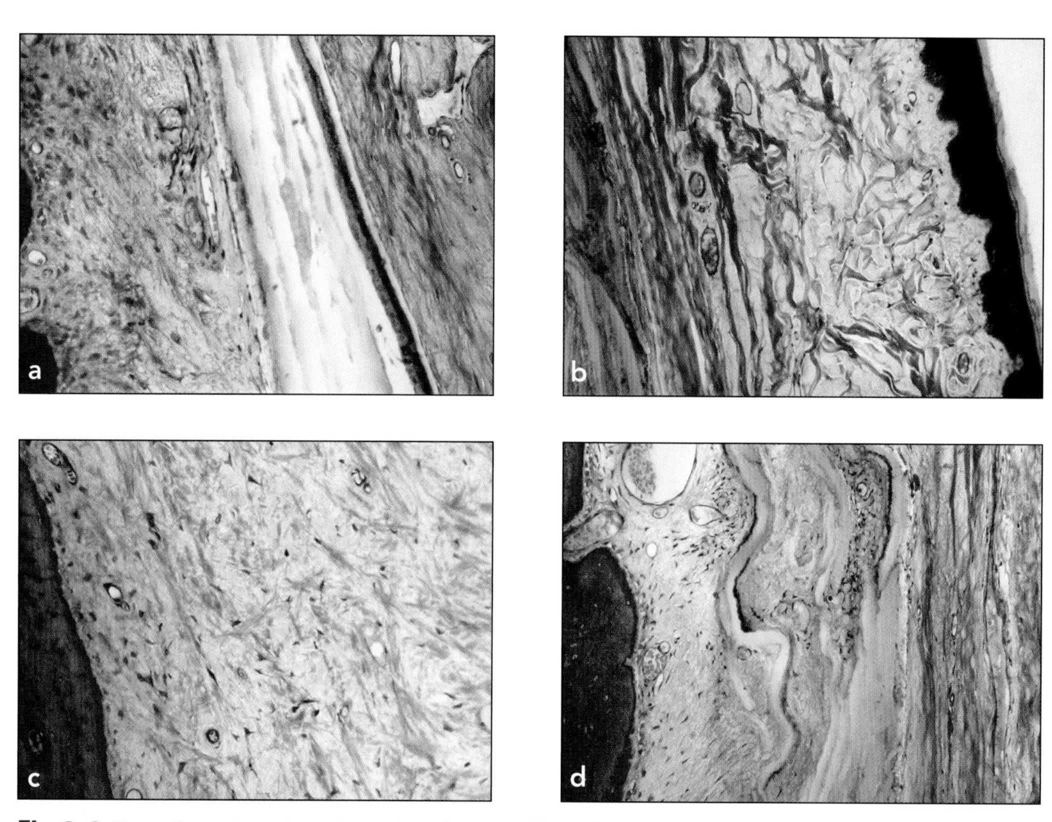

Fig 3-3 Buccolingual sections through a dog mandible showing a bone defect covered with an ePTFE membrane (undecalcified ground section; toluidine blue and basic fuchsin stain). *(a)* The dense central part of the membrane separates the outer soft connective tissue of the oral mucosa from an inner soft connective tissue of the bone compartment. Both fibrous tissues are in direct contact with the surfaces of the membrane. *(b)* The outer fibrous tissue compartment is characterized by a dense collagenous matrix, with collagen fibers increasing in diameter toward the membrane. *(c)* The inner compartment is in contact with the bone surface and consists of well-vascularized loose connective tissue. *(d)* The peripheral porous part of the membrane allows ingrowth of blood vessels and cells into the membrane interstices.

lium (Fig 3-3b). The density and diameter of the collagen fibers in the lamina propria increased toward the barrier membrane so that coarse bundles of collagen fibers were in contact with the surface of the ePTFE membrane.

In the inner compartment, loose connective tissue with delicate collagen fibers predominated (Fig 3-3c). This tissue, which was derived from bone marrow, was well vascularized, and the number of vessels increased toward the bone surface. Macrophages, lymphocytes, and granulocytes were extremely rare, even in contact with the inner surface of the membrane. These findings again provided proof of the excellent tissue compatibility of the ePTFE membrane.

The design of the ePTFE membranes used in the study by Schenk and coworkers[37] provided a certain porosity at the periphery, with communicating interstices reaching approximately 50 µm in diameter. This pore size allowed invasion by cells and small vessels, and it seems appropriate to define a third, intramembranous compartment because practically all porous parts were populated with living cells (Fig 3-3d). Most of these cells were fibroblasts, which were associated with thin collagen fibers and small capillaries.

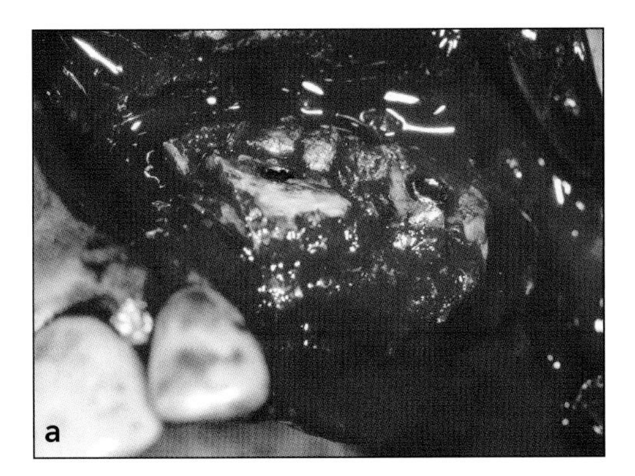

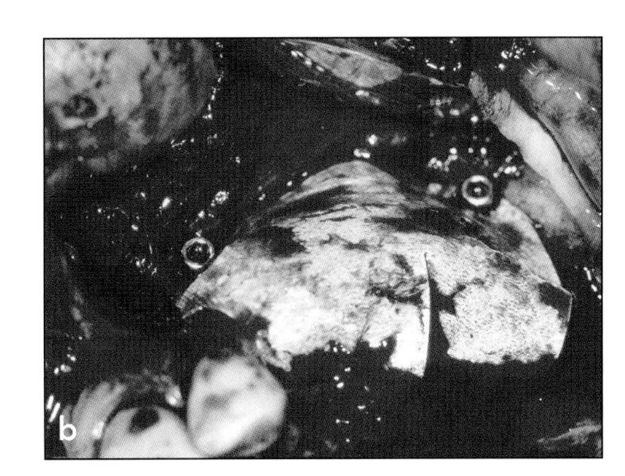

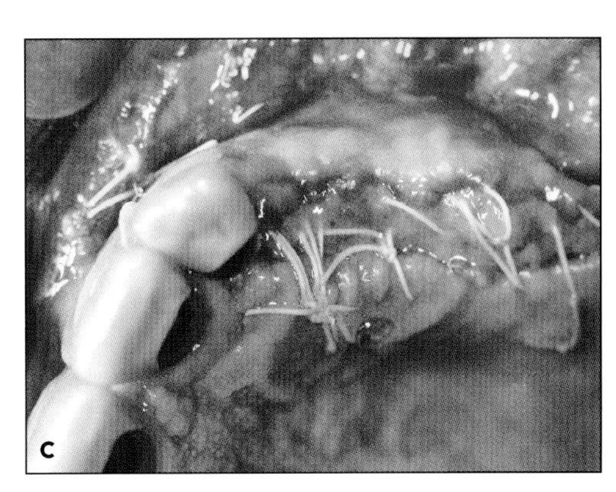

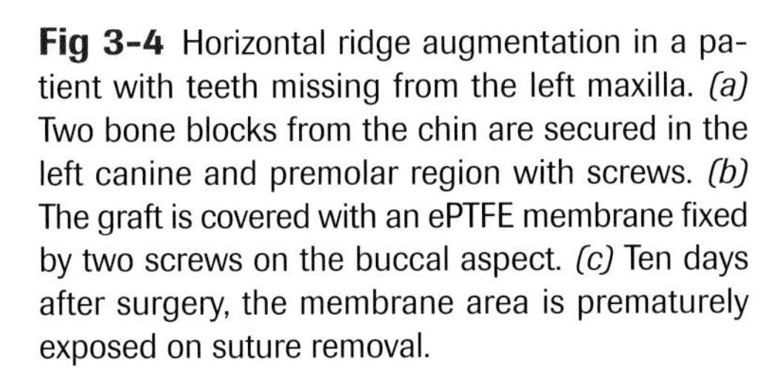

Fig 3-4 Horizontal ridge augmentation in a patient with teeth missing from the left maxilla. *(a)* Two bone blocks from the chin are secured in the left canine and premolar region with screws. *(b)* The graft is covered with an ePTFE membrane fixed by two screws on the buccal aspect. *(c)* Ten days after surgery, the membrane area is prematurely exposed on suture removal.

An experimental study in five beagle dogs compared the osteopromotive performance of titanium-reinforced ePTFE membranes to that of standard ePTFE barriers and no membrane (control) in large dehiscence and supracrestal bone deficits around dental implants placed in the mandibular alveolar process.[38] The histologic examination of the sections after a healing period of 6 months demonstrated large amounts of newly formed bone beneath both types of barrier membranes, with a superficial layer of connective tissue. Only the titanium-reinforced membranes exhibited bone formation superior to the top of an implant. The control sites without membrane placement revealed minimal supracrestal bone formation. The authors concluded that the reinforcement of ePTFE membranes with titanium provided superior preservation of the original form of the regenerate during the healing period.

Although clinical and experimental studies have shown excellent treatment results using nonresorbable membranes in GTR and GBR procedures,[11,21,22,31,32,34,39–41] the outcomes have been highly correlated with wound healing complications and, in particular, with dehiscences.[24,41,42] A number of studies have reported wound infection sequelae following the exposure of ePTFE membranes and subsequently a poor outcome in bone regeneration[25,43,44] (Fig 3-4). Simion and coworkers[41] have reported that bone gain around dental implants placed in fresh extraction sockets was significantly less when the membranes were exposed than when membranes were not exposed. Early exposure of barrier membranes to the oral environment and subsequent bacterial colonization can even necessitate premature retrieval of the membranes.[45,46] Another major disadvantage related to nonresorbable membranes is the need for a second surgery to remove the bioinert membrane.[47] This entails discomfort and increased costs for the patient, as well as the risk of losing some of the regenerated bone, because flap elevation results in a certain amount of crestal bone resorption.[48,49]

Bioresorbable Membranes

Because of the risk of early membrane exposure and the need for a second surgery to remove the nonresorbable membrane, clinicians and researchers alike have advocated the use of bioresorbable barrier membranes in GBR procedures. Advantages and characteristics of bioresorbable membranes described in the literature include elimination of the need for membrane removal surgery; a simplified surgical procedure with an implant system with a two-stage approach; a wider range of surgical techniques possible at abutment connection, which would coincide with membrane removal for bioinert membranes; greater cost-effectiveness; and decreased patient morbidity.[5]

Currently, two materials are mainly used to manufacture resorbable membranes: synthetic aliphatic polyesters and collagen derived from different animal sources.[50] Although both substances are considered biomaterials, each has distinctive features and biologic effects.[51,52] Important aspects of clinical significance are the longevity of barrier function and the tissue response (barrier biocompatibility), as related to membrane breakdown.

Polymeric membranes

Synthetic polyesters used as barrier membrane materials are polyglycolides (PGAs), polylactides (PLAs), or copolymers thereof. Other aliphatic polyesters used are polydioxanones[53] and trimethylene carbonates.[54] These synthetic materials can be prepared reproducibly under strictly controlled conditions and can be made available in almost unlimited quantities, which are clear advantages over naturally occurring materials such as collagen. Another advantage is the ability of PGA, PLA, and their copolymers to completely biodegrade to carbon dioxide and water via the Krebs cycle.[50]

Numerous factors are known to affect the degradation of biodegradable polymers in vitro and in vivo, such as their structure and chemical composition, molecular weight, shape, processing conditions, sterilizing process, physicochemical factors, and mechanism of hydrolysis.[55,56] The use of these polymers as bone plates, screws, and delivery vehicles for drugs and growth factors has been associated with inflammatory and foreign-body reactions in orthopedic and maxillofacial surgery and implant dentistry. In certain cases, even surgical debridement and removal of the material were required.[26,57–61]

The early tissue reactions to the insertion of PLA membranes were analyzed by Piattelli et al[62] in an experimental study in the rabbit tibia. After 1 week, the framework

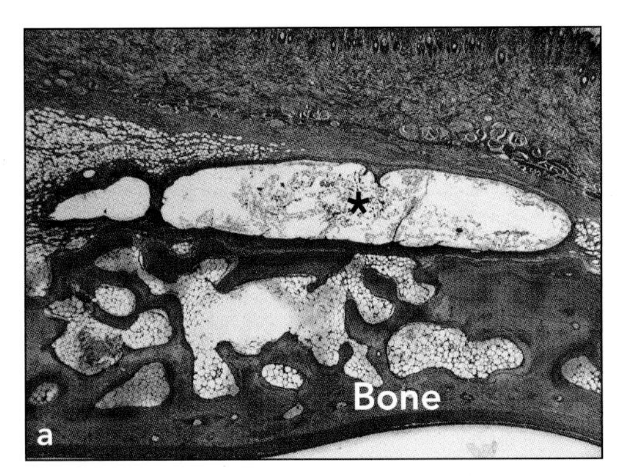

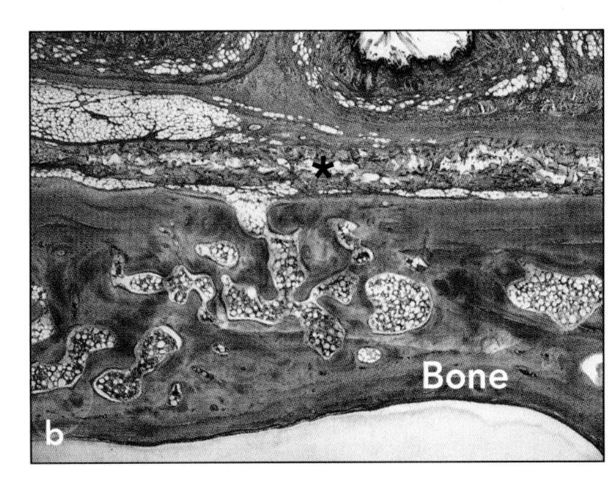

Fig 3-5 Durability of two synthetic barrier membranes 12 weeks after the creation of bone defects in the rabbit calvarium (undecalcified ground section; toluidine blue and basic fuchsin stain). *(a)* When a polylactide (Atrisorb, Tolmar) membrane was used, the shape and integrity of the membrane were preserved *(asterisk)*. *(b)* When a GLTC membrane (Osseoquest, Gore) was used, the membrane space was preserved, but the membrane material was partly replaced by an amorphous matrix *(asterisk)*.

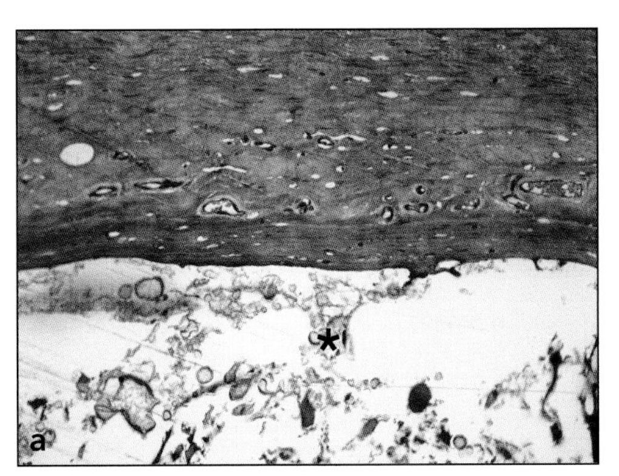

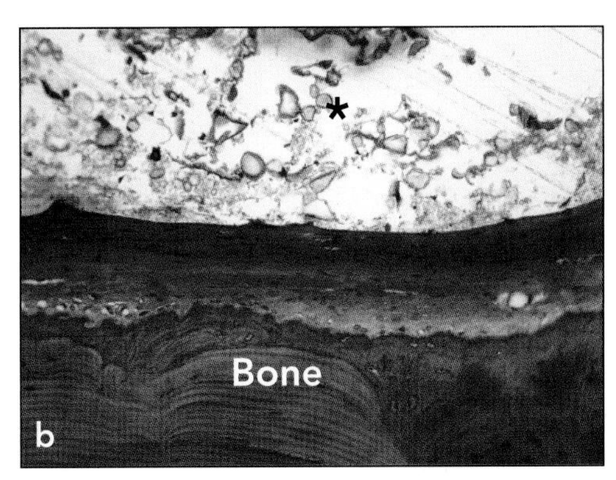

Fig 3-6 Polylactide membrane *(asterisk)* at 12 weeks (undecalcified ground section; toluidine blue and basic fuchsin stain). The membrane showed fibrous encapsulation, with minimal signs of inflammatory cell infiltration in the soft connective tissue outside the bone compartment *(a)* and interposed between the membrane and the bone *(b)*.

of the membrane was still recognizable, and there were no signs of fragmentation or resorption. However, the outer surface of the membrane appeared irregular, and macrophages and multinucleated giant cells were present. After 3 weeks, the membrane started to show signs of degradation, and a division into several fragments was present. Bone formation around the membrane exhibited two different characteristics: In some areas it was in direct contact with the membrane surface, while in other portions a small layer of multinucleated giant cells was interposed between the bone and the barrier membrane.

Extended barrier durability was also observed in another study by von Arx and coworkers[63] for both a PLA membrane and a glycolide-lactide–trimethylene carbonate (GLTC) membrane (Fig 3-5). The PLA membrane exhibited fibrous encapsulation on both sides of the membrane, with minimal signs of cell infiltration (Fig 3-6). At the GLTC membrane, an inflammatory cell infiltrate was present in the soft tissue encap-

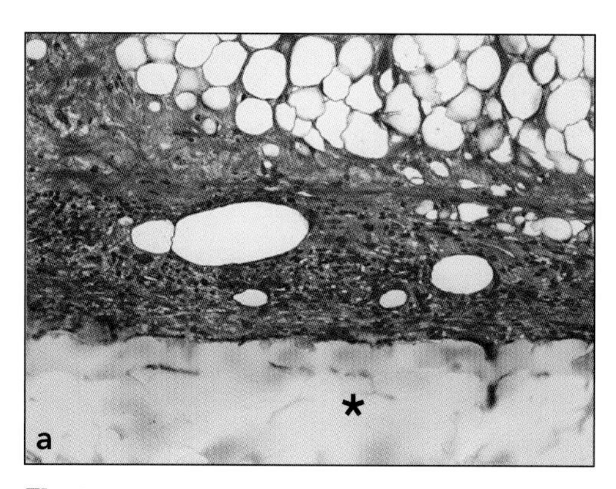

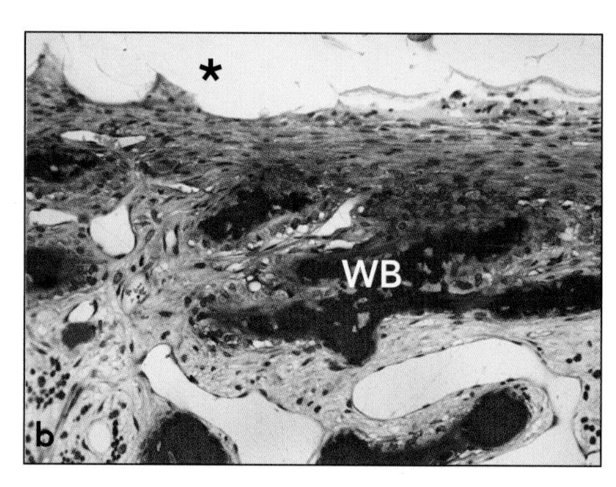

Fig 3-7 GLTC membrane *(asterisk)* at 2 weeks (undecalcified ground section; toluidine blue and basic fuchsin stain). The membrane showed fibrous encapsulation and a slight inflammatory cell infiltrate on both its sides, that is, in the soft connective tissues outside *(a)* and inside *(b)* the bone compartment. (WB) woven bone.

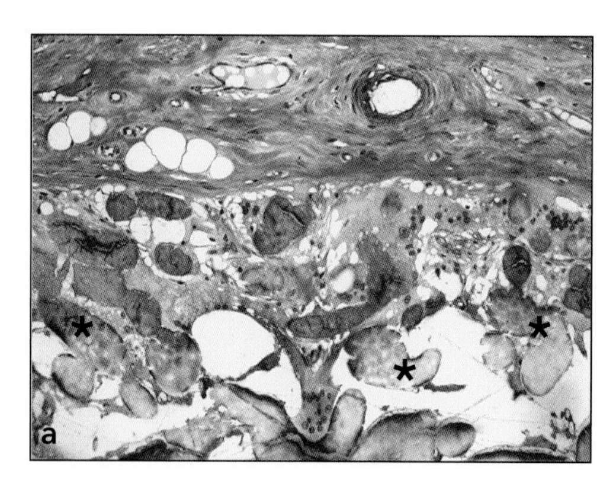

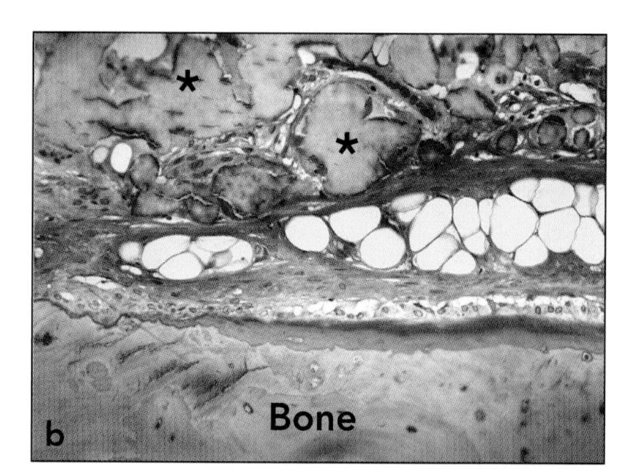

Fig 3-8 GLTC membrane at 12 weeks (undecalcified ground section; toluidine blue and basic fuchsin stain). The inflammatory cell infiltrate in the soft connective tissue adjacent to the membrane outside *(a)* and inside *(b)* the bone compartment was no longer apparent. The degradation of the membrane was quite advanced, and the membrane space was partly filled with an amorphous matrix *(asterisks)*.

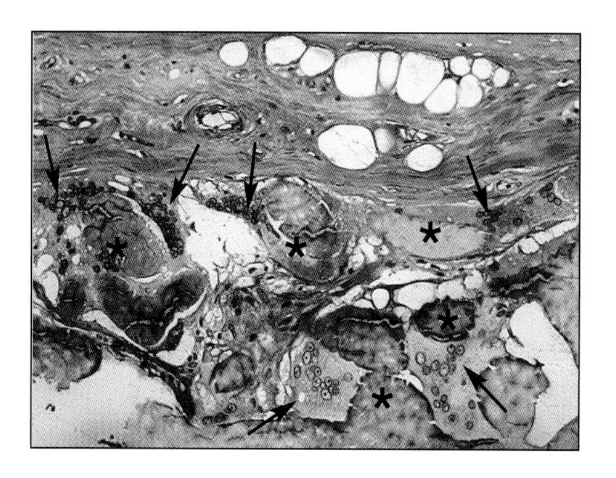

Fig 3-9 GLTC membrane at 12 weeks. Numerous large multinucleated giant cells *(arrows)* are interposed between an amorphous matrix *(asterisks)* that partly replaces the membrane material (undecalcified ground section; toluidine blue and basic fuchsin stain).

sulating the membrane at 2 weeks (Fig 3-7). At 12 weeks, when the degradation of the membrane was quite advanced, the inflammatory reaction in the soft tissue was no longer evident (Fig 3-8), but many multinucleated giant cells were found in the membrane space (Fig 3-9).

Studying premature exposure of barrier membranes to the oral cavity, Simion and coworkers[64] found that, once exposed, PLA/PGA membranes started to resorb almost instantly, and the resorption process was concluded after 3 to 4 weeks. The authors regarded this characteristic behavior as an advantage over nonresorbable barriers because it could lead to spontaneous healing and closure of the tissue. As a result, this would reduce the time of exposure of the affected membrane and wound area and could prevent bacterial invasion into the grafted site. On the other hand, a degradation process that is too fast could reduce the barrier function time and the space-making ability of the membrane. This could negatively affect the outcome of the whole GBR procedure.

Collagen membranes

Most of the commercially available collagen membranes have been developed from type I collagen, a predominant component of periodontal connective tissue, or from a combination of type I and type III collagen. The sources of the collagen in the barriers vary and include bovine tendon, bovine dermis, calf skin, or porcine dermis.[4] In the literature, several advantages of collagen materials have been mentioned, including hemostasis, chemotaxis for periodontal ligament fibroblasts[65] and gingival fibroblasts,[66] weak immunogenicity,[67] easy manipulation, a direct effect on bone formation,[68] and ability to augment tissue thickness.[69] Hence, collagen material appears to be an ideal choice for a bioresorbable GTR or GBR barrier.

On the other hand, while collagen membranes have been deemed more tissue-friendly, they have also been reported to have unfavorable mechanical properties[70] and to function inadequately as a barrier because of their fast biodegradation through the enzymatic activities of macrophages and polymorphonuclear leukocytes.[71–73] To prolong the barrier function of collagen membranes, several cross-linking technologies, such as ultraviolet radiation, glutaraldehyde, diphenylphosphoryl-azide, and hexamethylene diisocyanate, have been used.[74,75] The most widely used of these chemical cross-linking techniques, the glutaraldehyde technique, was reported to leave cytotoxic residue during the process.[76]

In an experimental study in the rabbit calvarium by von Arx et al,[63] three differently cross-linked prototype collagen membranes were compared to a non–cross-linked collagen and two synthetic polymer membranes in clinical use. Whereas fibrous encapsulation was observed for the two synthetic membranes tested, the GLTC membrane revealed a marginal inflammatory cell infiltrate at 2 weeks and multinucleated foreign-body giant cells in the fissures of the membrane at 12 weeks. In contrast, the non–cross-linked collagen membrane (Fig 3-10) and the three collagen prototype membranes (Fig 3-11) did not show signs of a foreign-body reaction. However, the soft tissue at the periphery of all types of collagen membranes was invaded by inflammatory cells.

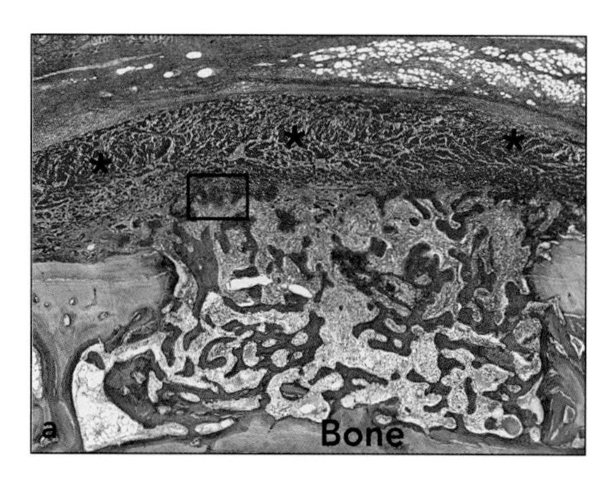

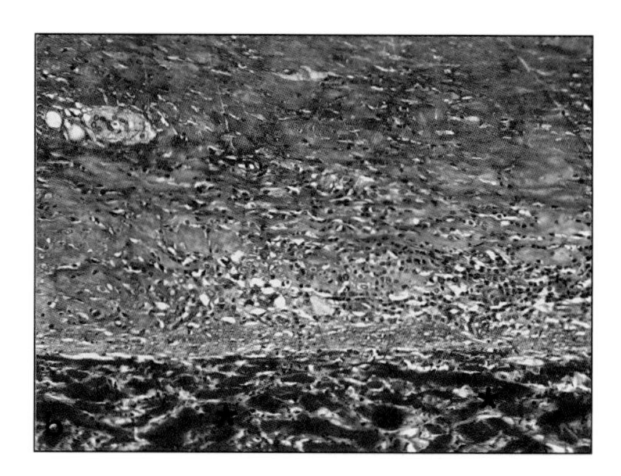

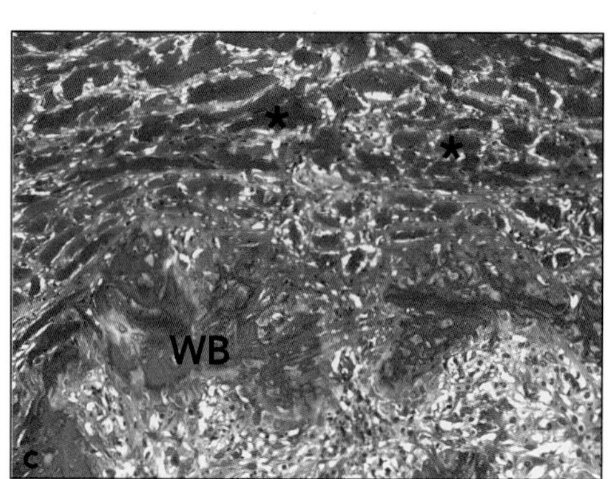

Fig 3-10 Degradation process of a non-cross-linked collagen membrane (Bio-Gide, Geistlich) *(asterisks)*, as shown in the rabbit calvarium 2 weeks after the creation of a bone defect (undecalcified ground section; toluidine blue and basic fuchsin stain). *(a)* The bony regenerate has partly filled the defect space and even surpassed the height of the original bone. *(b)* The outer part of the membrane is covered by a fibrous capsule that was infiltrated by some inflammatory cells. *(c)* Very close to the inner surface of the membrane *(increased magnification of inset in [a])*, woven bone (WB) formation occurs. The interstices of the membrane are populated by a mixed cell infiltrate.

This cell infiltration is interpreted as an event necessary for the cellular degradation of the collagen membranes. This view is supported by the fact that after 12 weeks, the cell infiltrate was no longer present. Cell invasion of the membrane at 2 weeks was clearly more advanced in the non–cross-linked membrane (compare Figs 3-10 and 3-11). The non–cross-linked collagen membrane and two prototype collagen membranes demonstrated histologic signs of biodegradation at 6 weeks and had disappeared after 12 weeks (Fig 3-12). In contrast, components of one of the chemically modified prototype membranes were still visible in the 12-week specimens[63] (Fig 3-13).

In a recent experimental study, five commercially available and three experimental collagen membranes were evaluated in rats.[77] The authors stated that cross-linking of bovine- and porcine-derived collagen types I and III was associated with prolonged biodegradation, decreased tissue integration, and decreased vascularization. In a follow-up investigation from the same group, the angiogenesis patterns of native and cross-linked collagen membranes were evaluated in rats.[78] The membranes that were analyzed exhibited a transmembranous formation of blood vessels in the first 2 to 8 weeks following implantation.

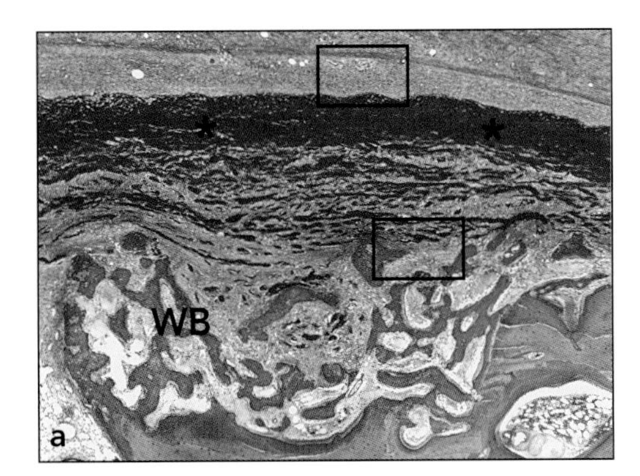

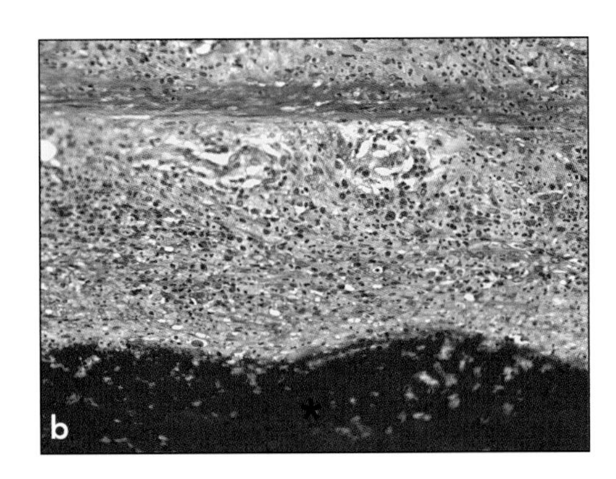

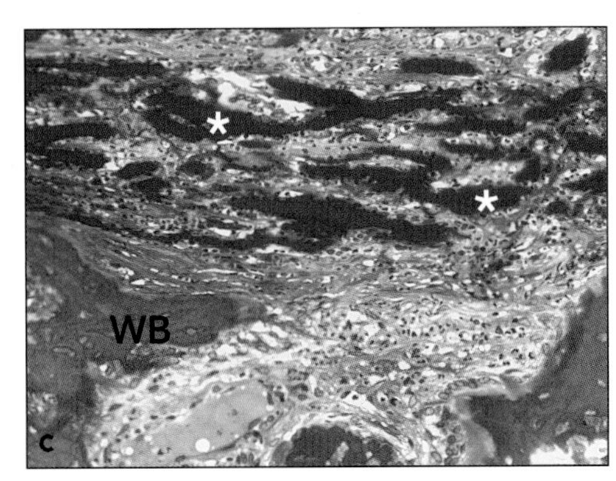

Fig 3-11 Prolonged durability of a prototype cross-linked collagen membrane *(asterisks)* as seen in the rabbit calvarium 2 weeks after the creation of a bone defect (undecalcified ground section; toluidine blue and basic fuchsin stain). *(a)* Most of the membrane layer is compact and lacks cell infiltration. Newly formed woven bone (WB) can be seen in the bone defect area underneath the membrane. *(b)* The soft connective tissue above the membrane (*increased magnification of top inset in [a]*) shows a cell infiltrate. *(c)* Woven bone (WB) formation can be seen very close to the inner surface of the membrane (*increased magnification of bottom inset in [a]*). The more porous inner portion of the barrier membrane shows a mixed cell infiltrate.

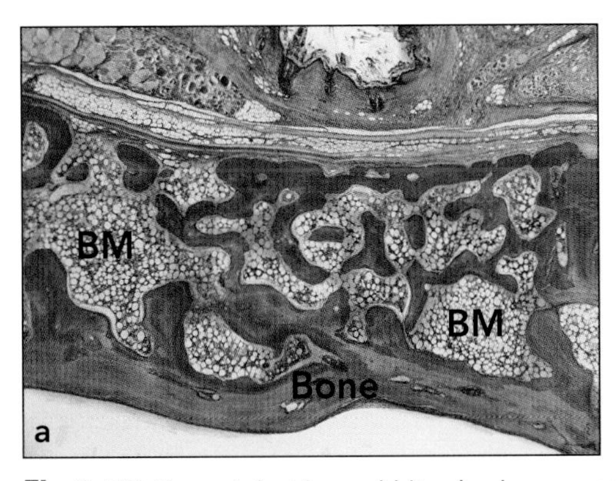

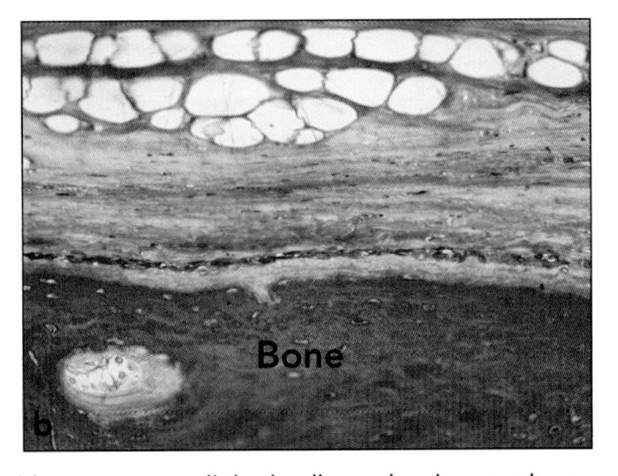

Fig 3-12 Bone defect in a rabbit calvarium covered with a non-cross-linked collagen barrier membrane at 12 weeks (undecalcified ground section; toluidine blue and basic fuchsin stain). *(a)* The bone filling the defect area consists of thick trabeculae with interposed bone marrow (BM). *(b)* A collagen-rich soft connective tissue covers the outer bone surface. Differentiation between membrane and host collagen is virtually impossible.

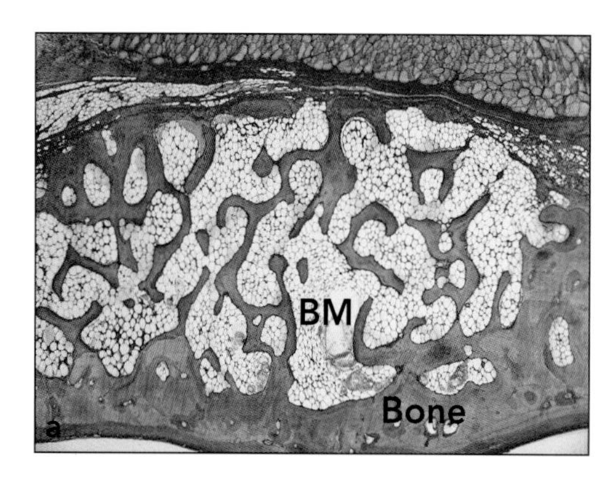

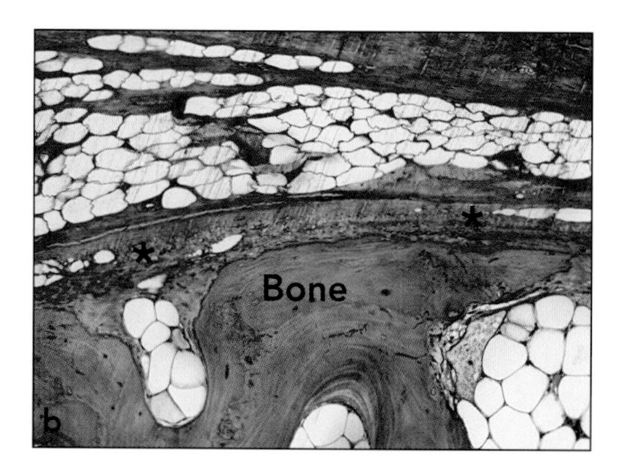

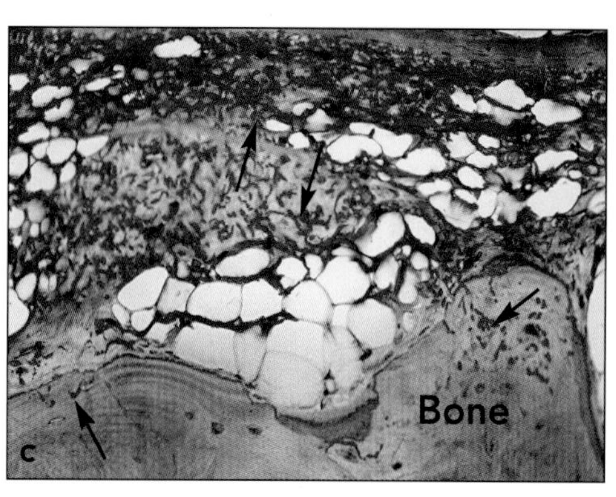

Fig 3-13 Bone defect in a rabbit calvarium covered with a cross-linked collagen barrier membrane at 12 weeks (undecalcified ground section; toluidine blue and basic fuchsin stain). *(a)* The bone filling the defect area consists of thick trabeculae with interposed bone marrow (BM). *(b)* A collagen-rich soft connective tissue covers the outer bone surface *(asterisks)*. Some remnants of the barrier membrane are barely visible within the host tissue. *(c)* At higher magnification, some remnants of the barrier membrane *(arrows)* can occasionally be seen in the soft connective tissue and even in the mineralized bone matrix.

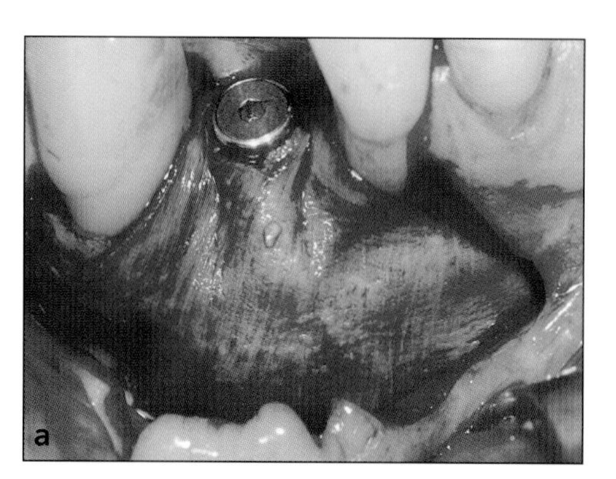

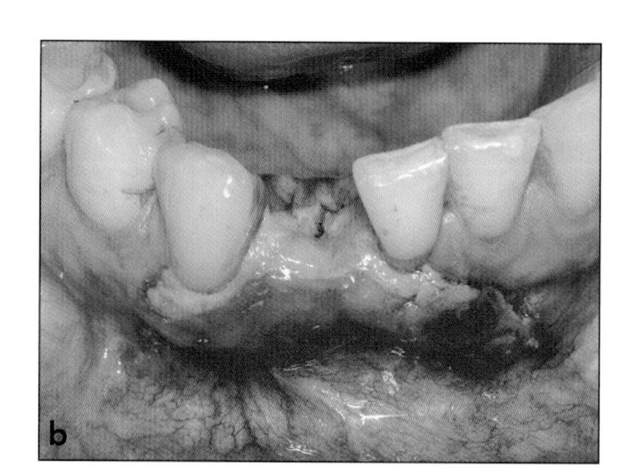

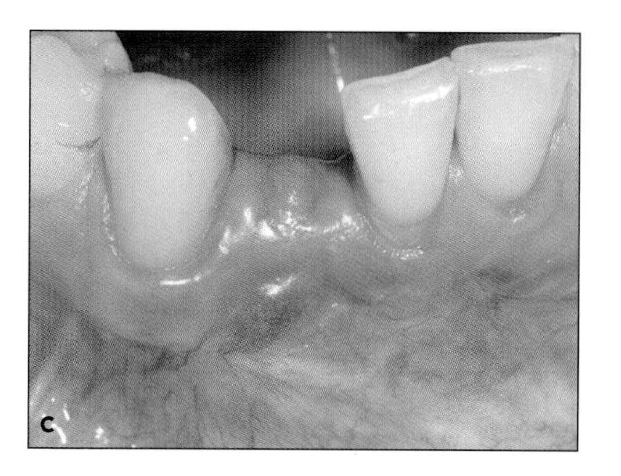

Fig 3-14 Missing lateral incisor replaced by a single dental implant in a 34-year-old woman. *(a)* During surgery, the buccal aspect of the implant is covered with bone chips, particulate bovine bone mineral, and a bioresorbable collagen membrane. *(b)* Ten days after surgery there is a premature membrane exposure at the site of implantation. The management of this complication consists of local disinfection with a chlorhexidine gel (0.2%) and weekly control visits. *(c)* Two months after surgery the site has healed with secondary wound closure and without an infection.

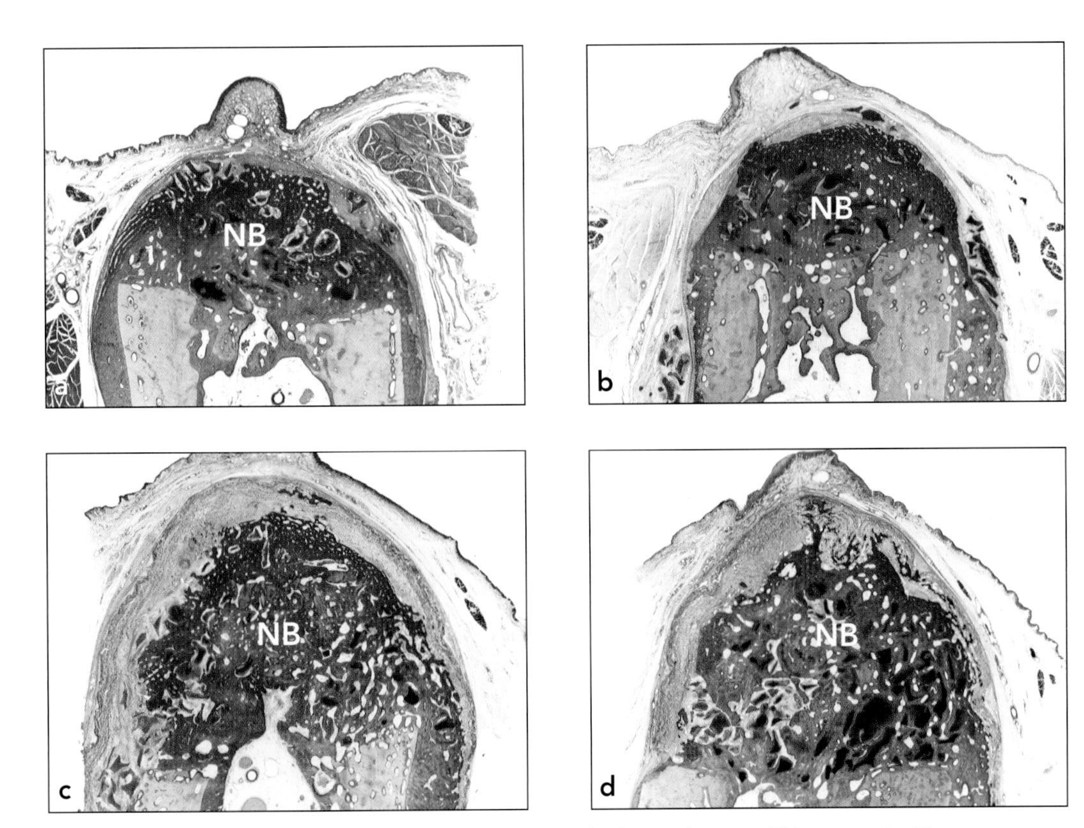

Fig 3-15 Buccolingual sections through bone defects in the canine mandible covered with a non–cross-linked *(a and b)* and a prototype cross-linked *(c and d)* membrane after healing times of 8 *(a and c)* and 16 *(b and d)* weeks. All defect sites show new bone (NB) formation and well-preserved surface contours (undecalcified ground section; toluidine blue and basic fuchsin stain).

Clinically, the rapid degradation of non–cross-linked collagen membranes following exposure to the oral cavity has been reported to be an advantage in horizontal ridge augmentation procedures[23] (Fig 3-14). In that study, 3 of 42 patients developed a small membrane exposure shortly after ridge augmentation. All sites showed normal healing, with spontaneous reepithelialization within 2 to 4 weeks, and it was possible to place an implant in all sites at the reentry surgery.

In an experimental study testing a prototype cross-linked collagen membrane (types I and III collagen) for bone regeneration in saddle-type bone defects in dog mandibles, three standardized defects were created on each side of the mandible.[79] The defects were filled with bone chips and deproteinized bovine bone mineral and covered with one of three different modalities: no membrane (control), collagen membrane, or prototype cross-linked collagen membrane. Each side of the mandible was allocated to one of two healing periods: 8 or 16 weeks (Fig 3-15).

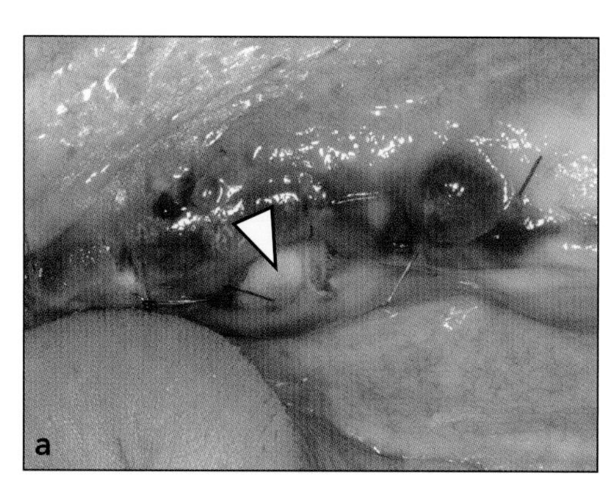

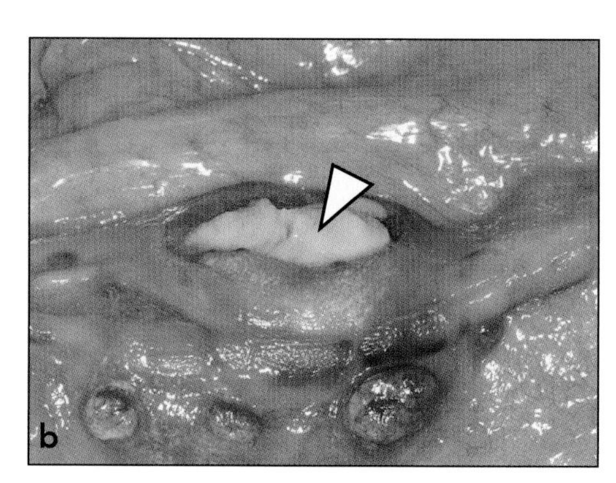

Fig 3-16 Premature exposures with signs of inflammation in the right *(a)* and left *(b)* mandible 1 week after placement of a prototype cross-linked collagen membrane over bone defects created in the canine mandible. The cross-linked collagen membranes *(arrowheads)* are clearly visible in the exposed areas. (Reprinted from Bornstein et al[79] with permission.)

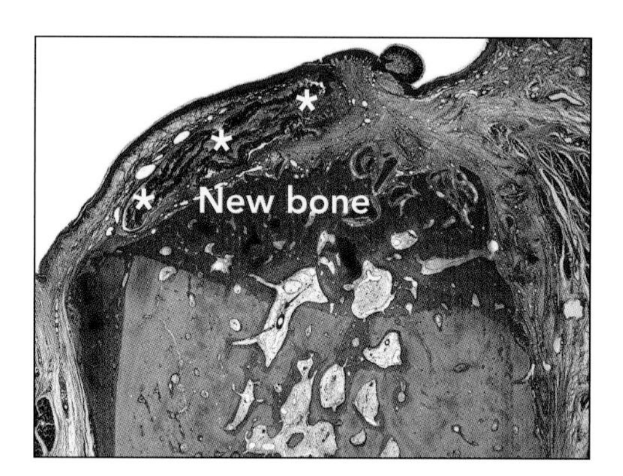

Fig 3-17 Buccolingual section of one saddle-type bone defect created in the canine mandible and covered with a prototype cross-linked collagen membrane. The membrane was exposed (see Fig 3-16) to the oral cavity prior to the end of the healing period of 8 weeks. The histology shows discontinuous membrane coverage of the bony regenerate. A large piece of membrane *(asterisks)* is visible between the bone surface and the epithelial lining of the oral mucosa (undecalcified ground section; toluidine blue and basic fuchsin stain).

In the 8-week healing group, two dehiscences occurred with the cross-linked collagen membrane (Fig 3-16). These two premature membrane exposures resulted in severely compromised amounts of bone regenerate, and the values of the regenerate were even lower than the values for most of the control and non–cross-linked collagen membranes (Fig 3-17). In addition, a cell infiltrate was found in association with the membrane matrix (Fig 3-18). The authors speculated that the cross-linking technology gave the tested membrane the capacity to withstand bacterial collagenolytic degradation when prematurely exposed, thus resulting in severe inflammation and resorption of the grafted area.[79]

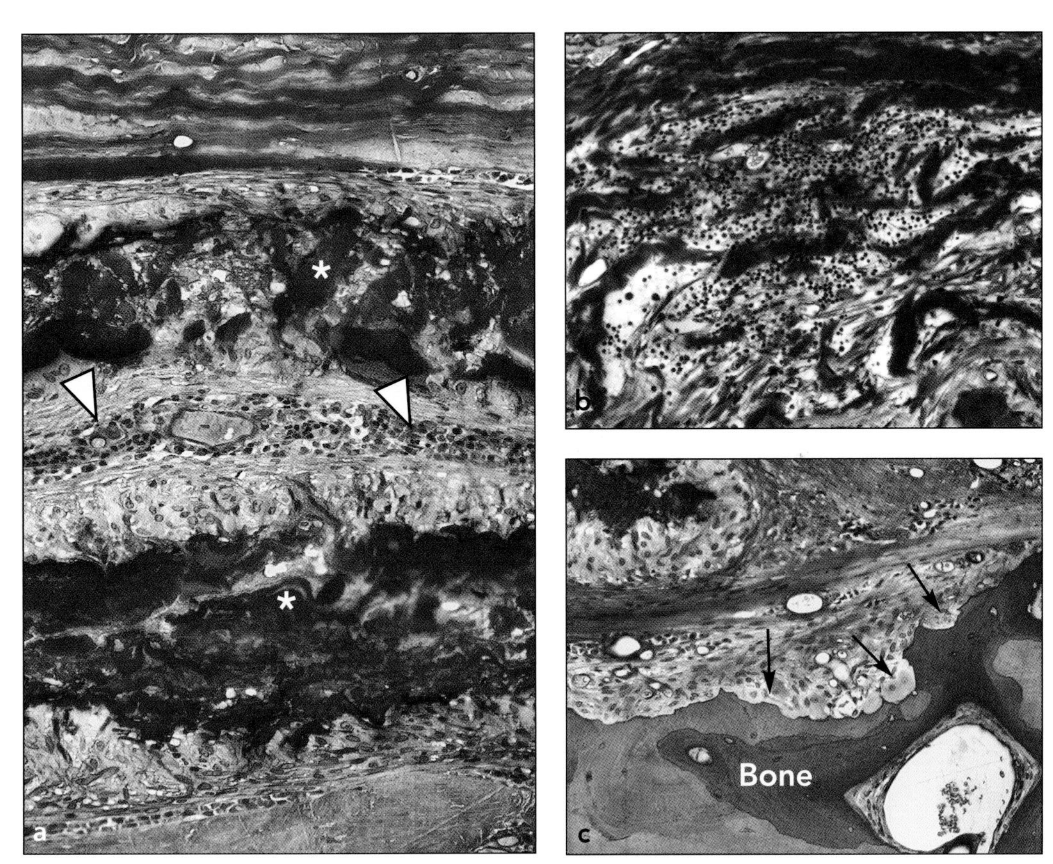

Fig 3-18 Details of the exposed cross-linked collagen membrane shown in Fig 3-17 (undecalcified ground section; toluidine blue and basic fuchsin stain). *(a)* The presence of two separate membrane layers *(asterisks)* suggests displacement and folding of the collagen membrane. The tissue surrounding the membrane layers consists of a mixed cell population, blood vessels, and few collagen fibers and is distinctly different from the surrounding soft connective tissues above and underneath the barrier membrane space. A thin strand of inflammatory cells *(arrowheads)* occupies the central space between the two membrane layers. *(b and c)* Loose portions of the collagen membrane are occasionally infiltrated with inflammatory cells *(b)* and bone resorption *(arrows)* occasionally occurs adjacent to the infiltrated membrane *(c)*. Both infiltration of the membrane and bone resorption may be related to a bacterial contamination of the previously exposed collagen membrane.

In contrast to these results, a case series study with an enzymatically cross-linked bovine type I collagen membrane reported secondary healing taking place in all prematurely exposed sites within 4 weeks, whereas exposed ePTFE membranes showed no healing tendency.[80] The barrier in this study remained intact over a period of 6 months, still promoting good bone regeneration in the cases of premature membrane exposure.

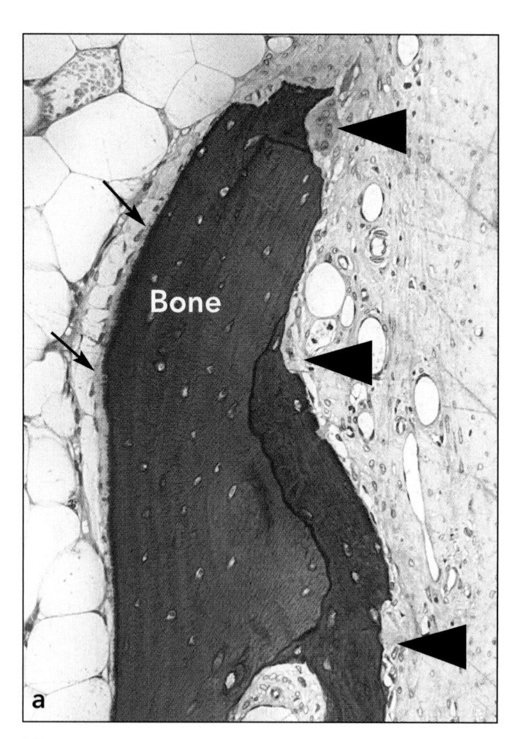

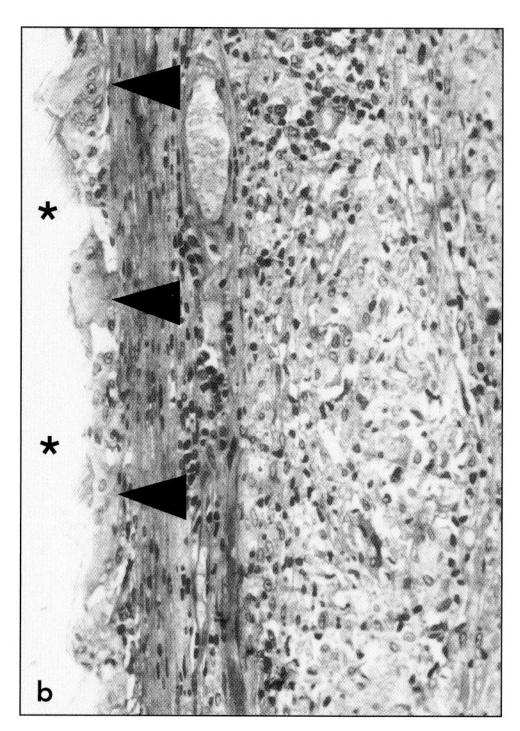

Fig 3-19 Hard and soft tissue responses adjacent to a disintegrating prototype trilayer membrane, consisting of two collagen layers and an internal polylactide layer, 3 months after lateral ridge augmentation in the canine mandible. *(a)* The surface of a newly formed bone plate facing the tissue under the membrane is subject to osteoclastic resorption *(arrowheads)*, whereas the opposite side of this plate is lined by an osteoid seam and osteoblasts indicating lamellar bone apposition *(arrows)* (undecalcified ground section; toluidine blue stain). *(b)* Multinucleated (foreign-body) giant cells *(arrowheads)* are present at the interface between the barrier membrane *(asterisks)* and the soft connective tissue, which is infiltrated by inflammatory cells (microtome section; toluidine blue stain).

Combination membranes

In an experimental study in dogs, a bioresorbable prototype trilayer membrane consisting of two collagen layers and an internal PLA layer was evaluated by von Arx et al[81] for lateral ridge augmentation in conjunction with two different bone grafting materials. For most trilayer membrane sites, histologic specimens demonstrated moderate infiltration of lymphocytes and plasma cells adjacent to empty spaces corresponding to PLA fragments. In addition, these reactions appeared to provoke subsequent resorption of newly formed bone (Fig 3-19). No such findings were observed in the control ePTFE sites. Although it would appear tempting to combine the advantages of collagen and synthetic polyesters in one bioresorbable membrane, the authors concluded that the tested prototype membrane could not be recommended for clinical applications.

Membrane support

Both collagen materials and synthetic polyesters, because of their somewhat unfavorable mechanical properties compared to (reinforced) nonresorbable barrier membranes, need supporting materials (autologous bone grafts or bone substitute materials) to prevent barrier collapse. When grafting materials are used in combination with bioresorbable membranes, the results of GBR procedures are generally favorable and are even comparable to the results achieved with nonresorbable ePTFE barriers.[82–85] Grafting material alone seems to be less effective than the combination of a supporting material and a barrier. Lundgren and coworkers[82] reported results that were clearly in favor of the coverage of the bone graft particles with a bioresorbable barrier, with respect to both the height and the volume of the augmented bone.

Future Directions

Future developments and research in the field of barrier membranes for GBR procedures will most likely follow two pathways.[5] One is a mechanical approach aimed at facilitating the surgical intervention for the surgeon and reducing the morbidity for the patient. The other is a biologic approach, focused on cellular and even molecular mechanisms of the wound healing process—that is, on the natural regeneration and repair of bone in the human body. The goal of this approach will be to apply new findings of these central biologic mechanisms to clinical practice and the way GBR procedures are performed today.

In the mechanical approach, a liquid bioresorbable barrier membrane consisting of polyethylene glycol (PEG) hydrogels has recently been described as a potential material for forming resorbable membranes for GBR procedures in situ.[86] PEG hydrogels are known for their biocompatibility and are already used in other medical fields such as neurosurgery and vascular surgery.[87,88] Nevertheless, future research is needed to assess the clinical indications for this new technique. Possibly, a PEG hydrogel matrix could be combined with growth and differentiation factors to bring grafting material and barrier membrane together in a single device.

A primarily biologic approach is the search for new barrier materials to achieve better GTR and GBR results. One new material being investigated is acellular dermal matrix, a material obtained from human skin, which has been used as a membrane for GBR in edentulous ridges and in association with immediate implants.[89,90] Future controlled clinical studies are necessary to evaluate its potential for fulfilling the requirements of a barrier membrane for GTR and GBR procedures.

Conclusion

Non–cross-linked collagen membranes are currently the membrane of choice for most GBR procedures. The philosophy of the Department of Oral Surgery and Stomatology at the University of Bern, Switzerland, is to use bioresorbable collagen membranes for all horizontal GBR and all sinus floor elevation surgeries. Nonresorbable ePTFE membranes are used only for selected vertical augmentation procedures. This philosophy is based on the following clear advantages of collagen membranes:

- They have favorable clinical handling characteristics during surgery, including their hydrophilic quality.
- In comparison with nonresorbable ePTFE membranes, they have a low risk of postoperative complications that impair bone regeneration, such as a premature membrane exposure.
- They eliminate the need for a second surgery to remove the membrane.

When this philosophy is applied in daily clinical practice, the following disadvantages of bioresorbable collagen membranes have to be taken into account:

- Because of their somewhat unfavorable mechanical properties, supporting materials (eg, autologous block or particulate grafts, bone fillers) are needed to prevent barrier collapse.
- A grafting material with a prolonged resorption time is needed to overcome the short barrier function of collagen membranes (see chapter 4).

References

1. Bassett CA, Campbell JB, Girado JM, Rossi JP, Seymour RJ. Application of monomolecular filter tubes in bridging gaps in peripheral nerves and for prevention of neuroma formation; A preliminary report. J Neurosurg 1956;13:635–637.
2. Hurley LA, Stinchfield FE, Bassett AL, Lyon WH. The role of soft tissues in osteogenesis. An experimental study of canine spine fusions. J Bone Joint Surg Am 1959;41A:1243–1254.
3. Dahlin C. Scientific background of guided bone regeneration. In: Buser D, Dahlin C, Schenk RK (eds). Guided Bone Regeneration in Implant Dentistry. Chicago: Quintessence, 1994:31–48.
4. Bunyaratavej P, Wang HL. Collagen membranes: A review. J Periodontol 2001;72:215–229.
5. Hämmerle CHF, Jung R. Bone augmentation by means of barrier membranes. Periodontology 2000 2003;33:36–53.
6. Hardwick R, Scantlebury TV, Sanchez R, Whitley N, Ambruster J. Membrane design criteria for guided bone regeneration of the alveolar ridge. In: Buser D, Dahlin C, Schenk RK (eds). Guided Bone Regeneration in Implant Dentistry. Chicago: Quintessence, 1994:101–136.
7. McAllister BS, Haghighat K. Bone augmentation techniques. J Periodontol 2007;78:377–396.
8. Hauman CHJ, Love RM. Biocompatibility of dental materials used in contemporary endodontic therapy: A review. 1. Intracanal drugs and substances. Int Endod J 2003;36:75–85.
9. Autian J. The use of rabbit implants and tissue culture tests for the evaluation of dental materials. Int Dent J 1970;20:481–490.
10. Ignatius AA, Claes LE. In vitro biocompatibility of bioresorbable polymers: Poly(L, DL-lactide) and poly(L-lactide-co-glycolide). Biomaterials 1996;17:831–839.
11. Tatakis DM, Promsudthi A, Wikesjö OM. Devices for periodontal regeneration. Periodontol 2000 1999;19:59–73.

12. Boyne PJ. Restoration of osseous defects in maxillofacial casualities. J Am Dent Assoc 1969;78:767–776.
13. Zellin G, Linde A. Effects of different osteopromotive membrane porosities on experimental bone neogenesis in rats. Biomaterials 1996;17:695–702.
14. Wikesjö UME, Lim WH, Thomson RC, Hardwick WR. Periodontal repair in dogs: Gingival tissue occlusion, a critical requirement for GTR? J Clin Periodontol 2003;30:655–664.
15. Majzoub Z, Berengo M, Giardino R, Aldini NN, Cordioli G. Role of intramarrow penetration in osseous repair: A pilot study in the rabbit calvaria. J Periodontol 1999;70:1501–1510.
16. Claffey N, Motsinger S, Ambruster J, Egelberg J. Placement of a porous membrane underneath the mucoperiosteal flap and its effect on periodontal wound healing in dogs. J Clin Periodontol 1989; 16:12–16.
17. Haney JM, Nilvéus RE, McMillan PJ, Wikesjö UM. Periodontal repair in dogs: Expanded polytetrafluoroethylene barrier membranes support wound stabilization and enhance bone regeneration. J Periodontol 1993;64:883–890.
18. Lundgren D, Sennerby L, Falk H, Friberg B, Nyman S. The use of a new bioresorbable barrier for guided bone regeneration in connection with implant installation. Case reports. Clin Oral Implants Res 1994;5:177–184.
19. von Arx T, Kurt B. Implant placement and simultaneous ridge augmentation using autogenous bone and a microtitanium mesh: A prospective clinical study with 20 implants. Clin Oral Implants Res 1999;10:24–33.
20. Lorenzoni M, Pertl C, Polansky R, Jakse N, Wegscheider W. Evaluation of implants placed with barrier membranes. A retrospective follow-up study up to five years. Clin Oral Implants Res 2002;13: 274–280.
21. Dahlin C, Gottlow J, Linde A, Nyman S. Healing of maxillary and mandibular bone defects using a membrane technique. An experimental study in monkeys. Scand J Plast Reconstr Surg Hand Surg 1990;24:13–19.
22. Buser D, Dula K, Belser U, Hirt HP, Berthold H. Localized ridge augmentation using guided bone regeneration. 1. Surgical procedures in the maxilla. Int J Periodontics Restorative Dent 1993;13:29–45.
23. von Arx T, Buser D. Horizontal ridge augmentation using autogenous block grafts and the guided bone regeneration technique with collagen membranes: A clinical study with 42 patients. Clin Oral Implants Res 2006;17:359–366.
24. Machtei EE. The effect of membrane exposure on the outcome of regenerative procedures in humans: A meta-analysis. J Periodontol 2001;72:512–516.
25. Nowzari H, Slots J. Microbiologic and clinical study of polytetrafluoroethylene membranes for guided bone regeneration around implants. Int J Oral Maxillofac Implants 1995;10:67–73.
26. Dupoirieux L, Pourquier D, Picot MC, Neves M. Comparative study of three different membranes for guided bone regeneration of rat cranial defects. Int J Oral Maxillofac Surg 2001;30:58–62.
27. Hanel KC, McCabe C, Abbott WM, Fallon J, Megerman J. Current PTFE grafts: A biomechanical, scanning electron, and light microscopic evaluation. Ann Surg 1982;195:456–463.
28. Schoenrock LD, Chernoff WG. Subcutaneous implantation of Gore-Tex for facial reconstruction. Otolaryngol Clin North Am 1995;28:325–340.
29. Singh S, Baker JL Jr. Use of expanded polytetrafluoroethylene in aesthetic surgery of the face. Clin Plast Surg 2000;27:579–593.
30. Bordenave L, Fernandez P, Rémy-Zolghardi M, Villars S, Daculsi R, Midy D. In vitro endothelialized ePTFE prostheses: Clinical update 20 years after the first realization. Clin Hemorheol Microcirc 2005; 33:227–234.
31. Becker W, Lynch SE, Lekholm U, et al. A comparison of ePTFE membranes alone or in combination with platelet-derived growth factors and insulin-like growth factor-I or demineralized freeze-dried bone in promoting bone formation around immediate extraction socket implants. J Periodontol 1992;63: 929–940.
32. Becker W, Dahlin C, Lekholm U, et al. Five-year evaluation of implants placed at extraction and with dehiscences and fenestration defects augmented with ePTFE membranes: Results from a prospective multicenter study. Clin Implant Dent Relat Res 1999;1: 27–32.
33. Ham J, Miller PJ. Expanded polytetrafluoroethylene implants in rhinoplasty: Literature review, operative techniques, and outcome. Facial Plast Surg 2003;19: 331–339.
34. Buser D, Dula K, Belser U, Hirt HP, Berthold H. Localized ridge augmentation using guided bone regeneration. 2. Surgical procedures in the mandible. Int J Periodontics Restorative Dent 1995;15:10–29.
35. Jovanovic SA, Nevins M. Bone formation utilizing titanium-reinforced barrier membranes. Int J Periodontics Restorative Dent 1995;15:57–70.
36. Dahlin C, Linde A, Gottlow J, Nyman S. Healing of bone defects by guided tissue regeneration. Plast Reconstr Surg 1988;81:672–676.
37. Schenk RK, Buser D, Hardwick WR, Dahlin C. Healing pattern of bone regeneration in membrane-protected defects: A histologic study in the canine mandible. Int J Oral Maxillofac Implants 1994;9: 13–29.
38. Jovanovic SA, Schenk RK, Orsini M, Kenney EB. Supracrestal bone formation around dental implants: An experimental dog study. Int J Oral Maxillofac Implants 1995;10:23–31.
39. Buser D, Ruskin J, Higginbottom F, Hardwick R, Dahlin C, Schenk RK. Osseointegration of titanium implants in bone regenerated in membrane-protected defects: A histologic study in the canine mandible. Int J Oral Maxillofac Implants 1995;10: 666–681.
40. Buser D, Dula K, Hirt HP, Schenk RK. Lateral ridge augmentation using autografts and barrier membranes: A clinical study with 40 partially edentulous patients. J Oral Maxillofac Surg 1996;54:420–432.

41. Simion M, Baldoni M, Rossi P, Zaffe D. A comparative study of the effectiveness of ePTFE membranes with and without early exposure during the healing period. Int J Periodontics Restorative Dent 1994; 14:167–180.
42. Zitzmann NU, Näf R, Schärer P. Resorbable versus nonresorbable membranes in combination with Bio-Oss for guided bone regeneration. Int J Oral Maxillofac Implants 1997;12:844–852.
43. Gher ME, Quintero G, Assad D, Monaco E, Richardson AC. Bone grafting and guided bone regeneration for immediate dental implants in humans. J Periodontol 1994;65:881–891.
44. Augthun M, Yildirim M, Spiekermann H, Biesterfeld S. Healing of bone defects in combination with immediate implants using the membrane technique. Int J Oral Maxillofac Implants 1995;10:421–428.
45. Selvig KA, Kersten BG, Chamberlain ADH, Wikesjö UME, Nilvéus RE. Regenerative surgery of intrabony periodontal defects using ePTFE barrier membranes: Scanning electron microscopic evaluation of retrieved membranes versus clinical healing. J Periodontol 1992;63:974–978.
46. Tempro PJ, Nalbandian J. Colonization of retrieved polytetrafluoroethylene membranes: Morphological and microbiological observations. J Periodontol 1993;64:162–168.
47. Nevins M, Mellonig JT. Enhancement of the damaged edentulous ridge to receive dental implants: A combination of allograft and the Gore-Tex membrane. Int J Periodontics Restorative Dent 1992;12: 96–111.
48. Philstrom BL, McHugh RB, Oliphant TH, Ortiz-Campos C. Comparison of surgical and nonsurgical treatment of periodontal disease. J Clin Periodontol 1983;10:524–541.
49. Rasmusson L, Sennerby L, Lundgren D, Nyman S. Morphological and dimensional changes after barrier removal in bone formed beyond the skeletal borders at titanium implants. A kinetic study in the rabbit tibia. Clin Oral Implants Res 1997;8:103–116.
50. Hutmacher DW, Hürzeler MB, Schliephake H. A review of material properties of biodegradable and bioresorbable polymers and devices for GTR and GBR applications. Int J Oral Maxillofac Implants 1996;11:667–678.
51. Zellin G, Gritli-Linde A, Linde A. Healing of mandibular defects with different biodegradable and non-biodegradable membranes: An experimental study in rats. Biomaterials 1995;16:601–609.
52. Aaboe M, Schou S, Hjørting-Hansen E, Helbo M, Vikaer D. Osseointegration of subperiosteal implants using bovine bone substitute and various membranes. Clin Oral Implants Res 2000;11:51–58.
53. Ray AJ, Doddi N, Regula D, Williams JA, Melveger A. Polydioxanone (PDS), a novel monofilament synthetic absorbable suture. Surg Gynecol Obstet 1981;153:497–507.
54. Hürzeler MB, Quinones CR, Hutmacher D, Schüpbach P. Guided bone regeneration around dental implants in the atrophic alveolar ridge using a bioresorbable barrier. An experimental study in the monkey. Clin Oral Implants Res 1997;8:323–331.
55. Vert M, Li S, Garreau H. New insights on the degradation of bioresorbable polymeric devices based on lactic and glycolic acids. Clin Mater 1992;10:3–8.
56. Vert M, Mauduit J, Li S. Biodegradation of PLA/GA polymers: Increasing complexity. Biomaterials 1994; 15;1209–1212.
57. Böstman OM. Osteolytic changes accompanying degradation of absorbable fracture fixation implants. J Bone Joint Surg Br 1991;73:679–682.
58. Bergsma EJ, Rozema FR, Bos RR, de Bruijn WC. Foreign body reactions to resorbable poly(L-lactide) bone plates and screws used for the fixation of unstable zygomatic fractures. J Oral Maxillofac Surg 1993;51:666–670.
59. Gotfredsen K, Nimb L, Hjørting-Hansen E. Immediate implant placement using a biodegradable barrier, polyhydroxybutyrate-hydroxyvalerate reinforced with polyglactin 910. Clin Oral Implants Res 1994;5:83–91.
60. Schliephake H, Dard M, Planck H, Hierlemann H, Jakob A. Guided bone regeneration around endosseous implants using a resorbable membrane vs. a PTFE membrane. Clin Oral Implants Res 2000;11: 230–241.
61. Schmitz JP, Lemke RR, Zardeneta G, Hollinger JO, Milam SB. Isolation of particulate degradation debris 1 year after implantation of a Guidor membrane for guided bone regeneration: Case report. J Oral Maxillofac Surg 2000;58:888–893.
62. Piattelli A, Scarano A, Coraggio F, Matarasso S. Early tissue reactions to polylactic acid resorbable membranes: A histological and histochemical study in rabbit. Biomaterials 1998;19:889–896.
63. von Arx T, Broggini N, Jensen SS, Bornstein MM, Schenk RK, Buser D. Membrane durability and tissue response of different bioresorbable barrier membranes: A histologic study in the rabbit calvarium. Int J Oral Maxillofac Implants 2005;20:843–853.
64. Simion M, Maglione M, Iamoni F, Scarano A, Piattelli A, Salvato A. Bacterial penetration through Resolut resorbable membrane in vitro. An histological and scanning electron microscopic study. Clin Oral Implants Res 1997;8:23–31.
65. Postlethwaite AE, Sayer JM, Kang AH. Chemotactic attraction of human fibroblasts to type I, II, and III collagens and collagen-derived peptides. Proc Natl Acad Sci U S A 1978;75:871–875.
66. Locci P, Calvitti M, Belcastro S, et al. Phenotype expression of gingival fibroblasts cultured on membranes used in guided tissue regeneration. J Periodontol 1997;68:857–863.
67. Schlegel AK, Möhler H, Busch F, Mehl A. Preclinical and clinical studies of a collagen membrane (Bio-Gide). Biomaterials 1997;18:535–538.
68. Rothamel D, Schwarz F, Sculean A, Herten M, Scherbaum W, Becker J. Biocompatibility of various collagen membranes in cultures of human PDL fibroblasts and human osteoblast-like cells. Clin Oral Implants Res 2004;15:443–449.
69. Pitaru S, Tal H, Soldinger M, Noff M. Collagen membranes prevent apical migration of epithelium and support new connective tissue attachment during periodontal wound healing in dogs. J Periodontal Res 1989;24:247–253.

70. Hürzeler MB, Kohal RJ, Naghshbandi J, et al. Evaluation of a new bioresorbable barrier to facilitate guided bone regeneration around exposed implant threads. An experimental study in the monkey. Int J Oral Maxillofac Surg 1998;27:315–320.
71. Miller N, Penaud J, Foliguet B, Membre H, Ambrosini P, Plombus M. Resorption rates of 2 commercially available bioresorbable membranes. A histomorphometric study in a rabbit model. J Clin Periodontol 1996;23:1051–1059.
72. Zhao S, Pinholt EM, Madsen JE, Donath K. Histological evaluation of different biodegradable and non-biodegradable membranes implanted subcutaneously in rats. J Craniomaxillofac Surg 2000;28: 116–122.
73. Owens KW, Yukna RA. Collagen membrane resorption in dogs: A comparative study. Implant Dent 2001;10:49–56.
74. Minabe M, Kodama T, Hori T, Watanabe Y. Effects of atelocollagen on the wound healing reaction following palatal gingivectomy in rats. J Periodontal Res 1989;24:178–185.
75. Quteish D, Dolby AE. The use of irradiated-crosslinked human collagen membrane in guided tissue regeneration. J Clin Periodontol 1992;24: 476–484.
76. Speer DP, Chvapil M, Ekelson CD, Ulreich J. Biological effects of residual glutaraldehyde in glutaraldehyde-tanned collagen biomaterials. J Biomed Mater Res 1980;14:753–764.
77. Rothamel D, Schwarz F, Sager M, Herten M, Sculean A, Becker J. Biodegradation of differently cross-linked collagen membranes: An experimental study in the rat. Clin Oral Implants Res 2005;16:369–378.
78. Schwarz F, Rothamel D, Herten M, Sager M, Becker J. Angiogenesis pattern of native and cross-linked collagen membranes: An immunohistochemical study in the rat. Clin Oral Implants Res 2006;17: 403–409.
79. Bornstein MM, Bosshardt D, Buser D. Effect of two different bioresorbable collagen membranes on guided bone regeneration. A comparative histomorphometric study in the dog mandible. J Periodontol 2007;78:1943–1953.
80. Friedman A, Strietzel FP, Maretzki B, Pitaru S, Bernimoulin JP. Histological assessment of augmented jaw bone utilizing a new collagen barrier membrane compared to a standard barrier membrane to protect a granular bone substitute material. A randomized clinical trial. Clin Oral Implants Res 2002;13: 587–594.
81. von Arx T, Cochran DL, Schenk RK, Buser D. Evaluation of a prototype trilayer membrane (PTLM) for lateral ridge augmentation: An experimental study in the canine mandible. Int J Oral Maxillofac Surg 2002;31:190–199.
82. Lundgren AK, Sennerby L, Lundgren D, Taylor A, Gottlow J, Nyman S. Bone augmentation at titanium implants using autologous bone grafts and a bioresorbable barrier. An experimental study in the rabbit tibia. Clin Oral Implants Res 1997;8:82–89.
83. Lundgren AK, Lundgren D, Sennerby L, Taylor A, Gottlow J, Nyman S. Augmentation of skull bone using a bioresorbable barrier supported by autologous bone grafts. An intra-individual study in the rabbit. Clin Oral Implants Res 1997;8:90–95.
84. Simion M, Misitano U, Gionso L, Salvato A. Treatment of dehiscences and fenestrations around dental implants using resorbable and nonresorbable membranes associated with bone autografts: A comparative clinical study. Int J Oral Maxillofac Implants 1997;12:159–167.
85. Donos N, Kostopoulos L, Karring T. Alveolar ridge augmentation using a resorbable copolymer membrane and autogenous bone grafts. An experimental study in the rat. Clin Oral Implants Res 2002;13: 203–213.
86. Jung RE, Zwahlen R, Weber FE, Molenberg A, van Lenthe GH, Hämmerle CHF. Evaluation of an in situ formed synthetic hydrogel as a biodegradable membrane for guided bone regeneration. Clin Oral Implants Res 2006;17:426–433.
87. Boogaarts JD, Grotenhuis JA, Bartels RH, Beems T. Use of a novel absorbable hydrogel for augmentation of dural repair: Results of a preliminary clinical study. Neurosurgery 2005;57(1 suppl):146–151.
88. Wallace DG, Cruise GM, Rhee WM, et al. A tissue sealant based on reactive multifunctional polyethylene glycol. J Biomed Mater Res 2001;58:545–555.
89. Fowler EB, Breault LG. Ridge augmentation with a folded acellular dermal matrix allograft: A case report. J Contemp Dent Pract 2001;15:31–40.
90. Novaes AB Jr, Papalexiou V, Luczyszyn SM, Muglia VA, Souza SL, Taba M Jr. Immediate implant in extraction socket with acellular dermal matrix graft and bioactive glass: A case report. Implant Dent 2002;11:343–348.

CHAPTER 4

Bone Grafts and Bone Substitute Materials

Simon Storgård Jensen
Dieter D. Bosshardt
Daniel Buser

Bone filler materials may serve several purposes in guided bone regeneration (GBR) procedures:

- Support the membrane to avoid membrane collapse
- Act as a scaffold for bone ingrowth from the recipient site
- Stimulate bone ingrowth from the recipient site
- Supply a mechanical shield against pressure from the overlying soft tissues
- Protect the augmented volume from resorption

Moreover, the clinical indications for using bone filler materials range from grafting minor peri-implant defects to the regeneration of large continuity defects.

Considering this wide range of purposes, it is to be expected that one single material cannot fulfill all requirements. Therefore, it will often be necessary to combine two or more materials to obtain a successful and predictable treatment outcome. The characteristics of the most commonly used bone grafts and bone substitute materials will be discussed in this chapter.

Bone filler materials can be derived either from the person being treated (autogenous bone grafts or autografts) or from an external source (bone substitute materials). Figure 4-1 provides a classification of available bone grafting materials. Both autografts and bone substitute materials can be used as block grafts or as particulate grafts.

Irrespective of the origin or production method, the bone grafting material should meet certain demands and demonstrate some defined material characteristics to be suitable for bone augmentation procedures. A bone substitute material must be safe and biocompatible to avoid the risk of disease transmission or immunologic reactions. This is not an issue with autografts unless they are improperly handled during surgery.

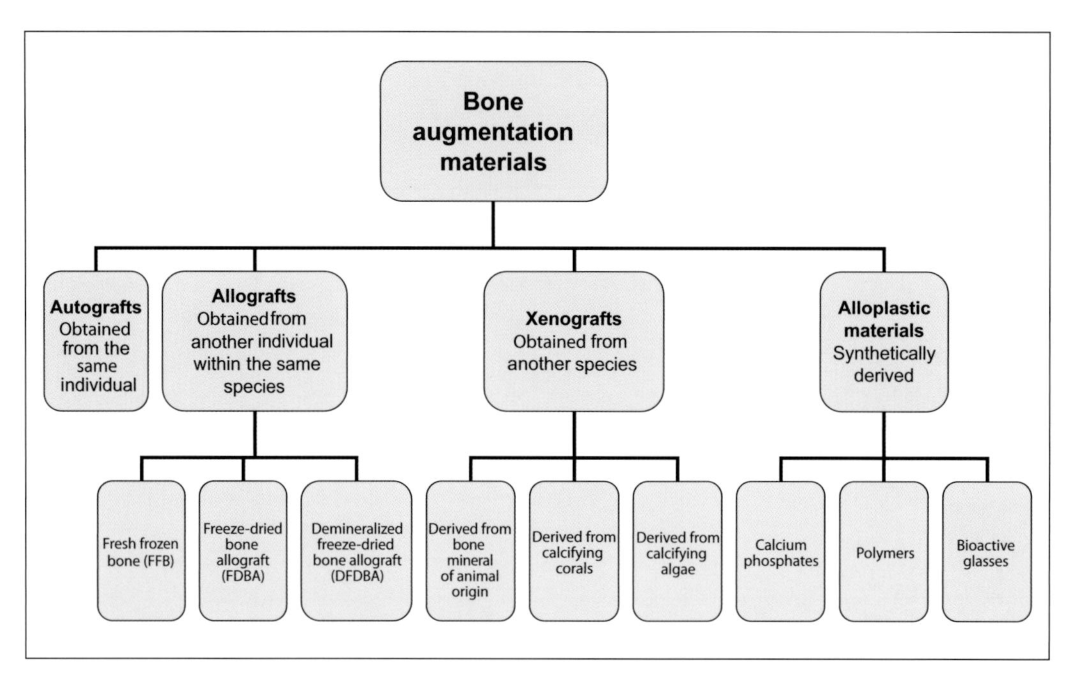

Fig 4-1 Classification of bone augmentation materials.

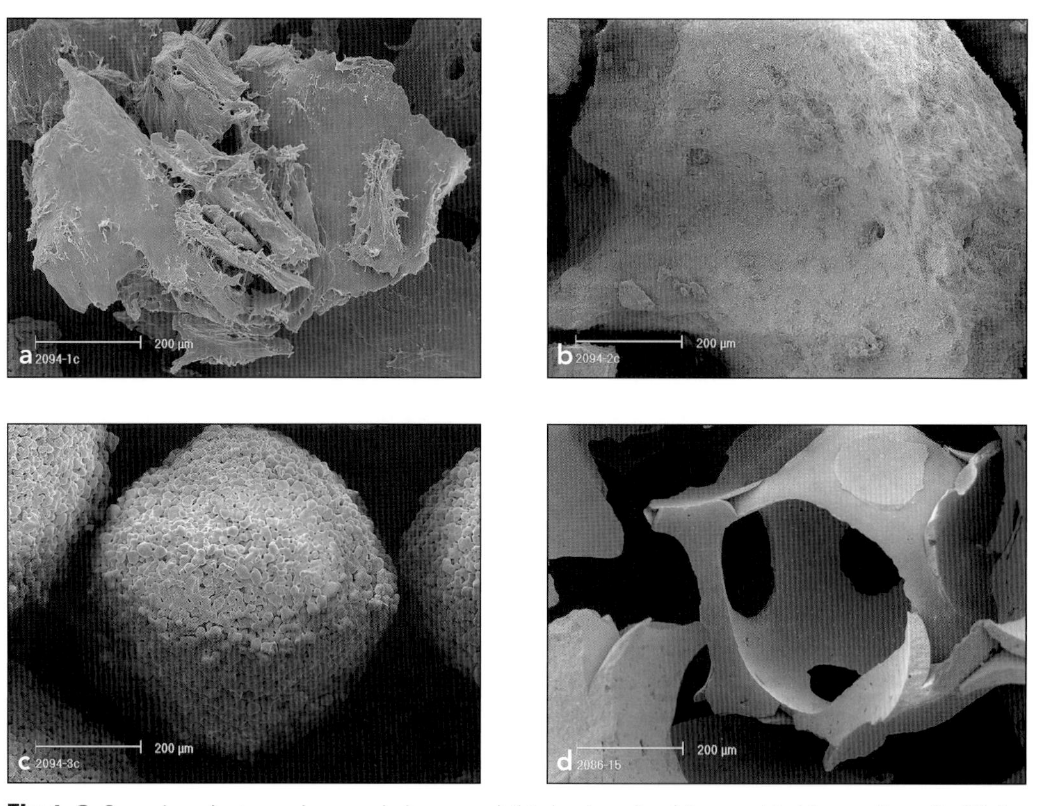

Fig 4-2 Scanning electron microscopic images of *(a)* demineralized freeze-dried bone allograft, *(b)* deproteinized bovine bone mineral, *(c)* nonporous synthetic calcium phosphate, and *(d)* porous synthetic calcium phosphate. (Courtesy of R. Christ, Institut Straumann, Basel, Switzerland.)

The geometry should favor the ingrowth of blood vessels, which is crucial for the formation of bone inside the material. This means that the material needs not only to be porous but also to have macropores that are interconnected.[1] There have been conflicting reports regarding the optimal macropore size, but it is believed to lie within the range of 100 to 500 µm.[2] The macroporosity is presumably most important in revascularization of bone filler materials used in the form of blocks. When particulate grafts are used, the vascular ingrowth is more likely to take place between the graft particles. It is therefore important not to compress the bone filler material too tightly into the grafted area, thus allowing unhindered revascularization of the augmented volume.

The surface characteristics of bone substitute materials are determined by their chemical composition, microporosity, surface roughness, crystallinity, and crystal size. These surface characteristics are of great importance for initial protein adsorption, attachment of osteoblasts and osteoclasts, and deposition of osteoid and therefore for the direct apposition of newly formed bone on the material surface (osteoconduction)[3–8] (Fig 4-2).

Finally, the handling properties of the grafting material should facilitate clinical application. Additional desired material characteristics depend on the clinical indication: If the bone filler material is applied in areas in which implants are to be placed later, such as extraction sockets, the material should preferably be resorbed along with the formation of new bone or during remodeling, thus allowing the implants to be placed in vital bone alone. In other situations, a low substitution rate or even a nonresorbable material may be more favorable. This can be the case in esthetic sites where the bone filler material is used to reestablish the contour of the alveolar process and functions as a resorption barrier to maintain the support of the soft tissues, thereby contributing to a successful long-term esthetic outcome.[9,10]

All these material characteristics should be carefully evaluated before a new bone substitute material is introduced in the clinic. In the laboratory, in vitro studies using osteoblastic cell lines can reveal how the main target cells react to the material with regard to cell proliferation, differentiation, and extracellular matrix production. It can also be determined whether osteoclasts are able to develop resorption pits on the material surface or if physicochemical dissolution may take place. Experimental documentation should include data from standardized comparative studies with other well-documented bone augmentation materials.

Buser and coworkers developed an experimental model in the mandibles of minipigs that has proven valuable for comparing biomaterials.[7,11–13] The minipig is used because of its close similarity to humans in terms of bone structure and bone metabolism.[14,15] Three to four standardized bone defects can be prepared on each side of the mandible. The defects are not critical-sized defects[16] and would thus be expected with time to heal by themselves, without the introduction of any grafting material. The model is suitable for studying the bone healing dynamics of new bone fillers and especially for direct comparison with other bone fillers. Comparisons can be made from deposition of the first osteoid to complete healing of the defects with mature lamellar bone (Figs 4-3 and 4-4).

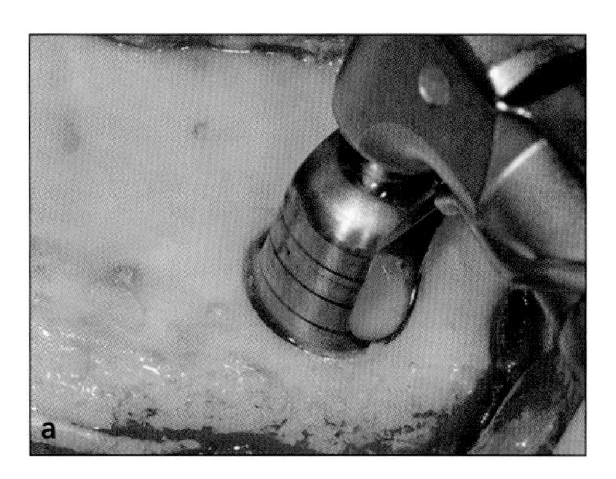
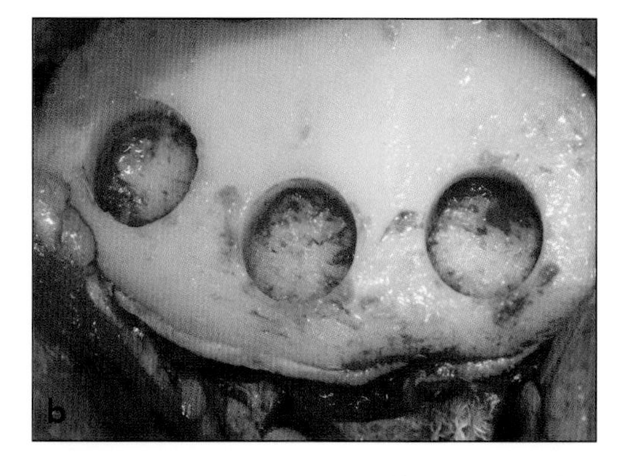
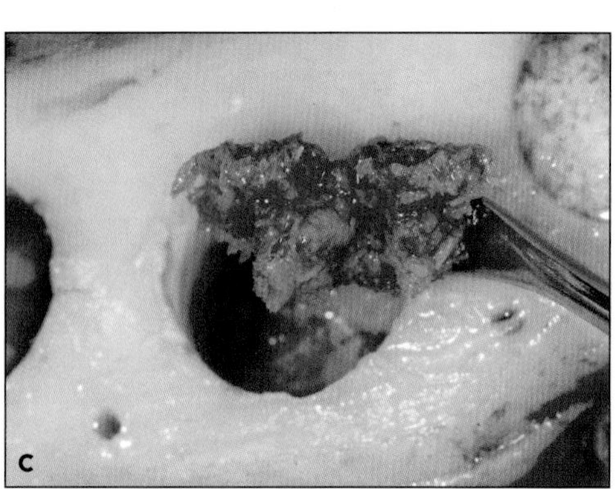
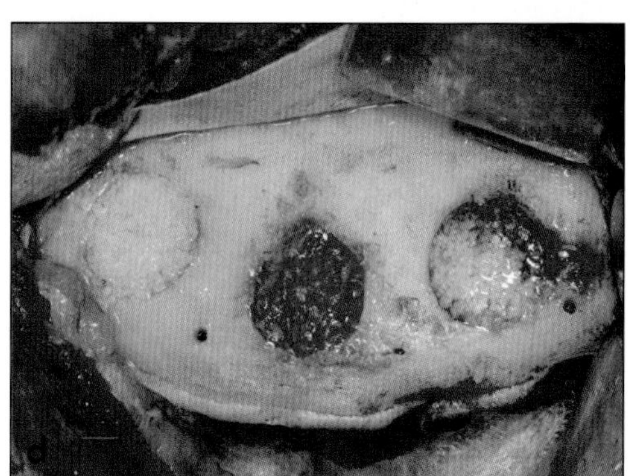
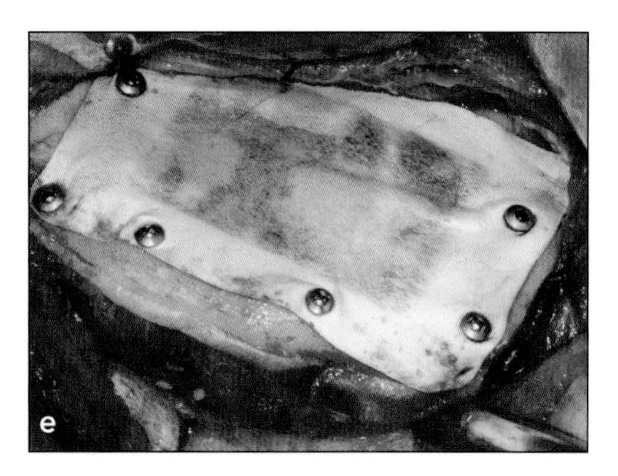

Fig 4-3 Non-critical-sized defect model in the mandible of minipigs. This has proven to be a valuable experimental to study bone formation in association with biomaterials. *(a)* A bone defect is prepared in the mandibular angle of a minipig; a trephine (9 mm in diameter) is used with copious saline irrigation. *(b)* Three standardized monocortical defects are shown before grafting. *(c)* A defect is grafted with particulated autogenous bone. *(d)* The center defect has been grafted with particulated autogenous bone, and the other two defects have been grafted with alloplastic calcium phosphate bone substitute materials. *(e)* The grafted defects are covered with an expanded polytetrafluoroethylene (ePTFE) membrane to exclude ingrowth of fibrous tissue and stabilized with fixation screws to delineate the border of the defects in the later histologic sections.

The bone fillers that perform best in these comparative screening studies should be examined further in experimental studies with clinically more relevant bone defect models. Materials for GBR procedures are often tested in lateral ridge augmentations in dogs (see chapter 3). Clinical data should include prospective documentation of the outcome, preferably with data for 1 year or more, and histologic short- and long-term observations.

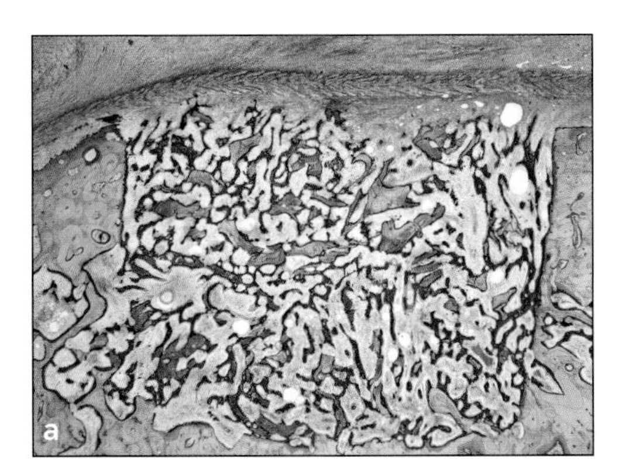
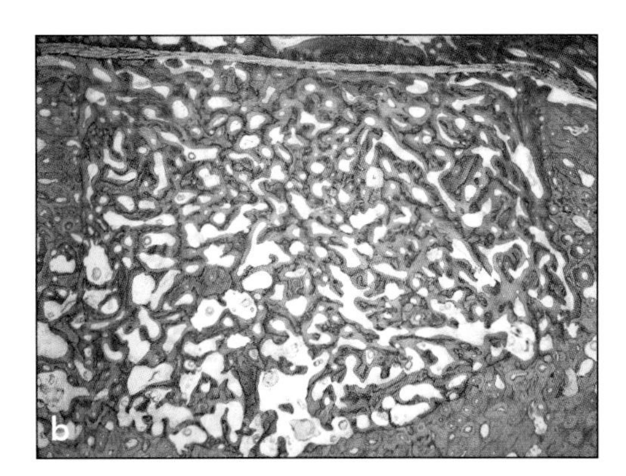

Fig 4-4 Histologic overview sections of bone defects created in the mandible of minipigs. The defects were grafted with autogenous particulate bone and covered with an ePTFE barrier membrane (undecalcified ground sections; toluidine blue stain). *(a)* After 2 weeks of healing, woven bone has formed throughout the defect area up to the level of the membrane. *(b)* After 6 months, osseous healing, as demonstrated by the presence of lamellar bone, extends to the membrane. Parallel-fibered bone and remnants of woven bone are still present.

All available documentation from in vitro and in vivo studies should be carefully evaluated before a new material is introduced. In the field of implant dentistry, however, new bone substitute materials are often launched on the market without sufficient documentation.

Autogenous Bone Grafts

Autografts may be harvested from intraoral or extraoral donor sites (Table 4-1). Autogenous bone is composed of approximately 30% organic and 70% inorganic compounds. Of the organic compounds, 90% to 95% is collagen (type I), and the rest is noncollagenous proteins such as osteocalcin, calcitonin, osteopontin, and sialoproteins. The inorganic component is composed of calcium phosphate, predominantly in the form of crystalline hydroxyapatite (HA).

With transplantation of autogenous bone, bone-stimulating growth factors and viable osteogenic cells are brought to the recipient site.[17] The amount of cells and the concentration of growth factors demonstrate great interindividual and intraindividual variation and depend largely on patient age, the presence of systemic diseases, and location of the donor site.

The growth factors comprise bone morphogenetic proteins (BMPs), transforming growth factor β, insulin-like growth factors I and II, platelet-derived growth factor, and fibroblast growth factors A and B. They are mainly present in the bone matrix and are released during resorption of the autografts. The higher the absolute surface area of the autograft, the faster the growth factors are set free. This means that blocks of cancellous bone more readily release growth factors than blocks of compact bone and that particulated autografts demonstrate faster release of bone-stimulating growth factors than do blocks.[18]

Table 4-1 Donor sites for autografts

Region	Geometry	Volume	Resorption
Intraoral			
Chin	Corticocancellous*	++	++
Mandibular body/ramus	Cortical	++	+
Nasal spine	Corticocancellous*	+	+++
Maxillary tuberosity	Corticocancellous†	+	+++
Zygomatic body	Corticocancellous†	+	+++
Extraoral			
Iliac crest, anterior/posterior	Corticocancellous†	+++	++
Tibial condyle	Cancellous	++	+++
Calvaria	Cortical	++	+
Fibula (vascularized)	Corticocancellous†	+++	+

Volume: + = Sufficient bone for augmenting a one-tooth gap; ++ = sufficient bone for up to two sinus augmentations; +++ = sufficient bone for major inlay and onlay augmentations and reconstruction of continuity defects.
Resorption: + = minimal; ++ = moderate; +++ = pronounced.
*More cortical than cancellous bone.
†More cancellous than cortical bone.

The cells harbored in bone tissue are osteocytes, osteoblasts, osteoclasts, and predominantly bone-lining cells. The cells of primary interest in GBR procedures are the osteogenic cells (osteoblasts, preosteoblasts, and pluripotent stem cells). These cells are most numerous in trabecular bone, whereas compact bone demonstrates the least amount of osteogenic cells. The osteogenic potential in young healthy individuals is greater than that in elderly patients mainly because of a decreased proliferative capacity of osteoprogenitor cells in older individuals rather than compromised function of the osteoblasts present.[19] There is no evidence that transplanted osteocytes resting in their lacunae play any role in bone formation, but the presence of living osteocytes in bone biopsies after GBR procedures confirms that cells can survive the transplantation procedure.

The geometry of cortical and cancellous autografts varies greatly and mainly with patient age and location of the donor site (see Table 4-1). Autografts can be harvested at different locations and can be used in different forms (see chapter 5). The expected biologic behavior of the different types of autografts is discussed in the following sections.

Autogenous block grafts

Autogenous block grafts are the only grafts that offer mechanical stability against pressure from the overlying soft tissue, assuming that they are immobilized with fixation screws. The rate of revascularization depends on the geometry of the block graft and, therefore, primarily on the donor site.[20] The use of a cell-occlusive membrane to cover the block graft may decelerate revascularization,[21] but if the cortical plate at the recipient site is penetrated with a small bur, the ingrowth of new blood vessels can be facilitated.[22] Compact blocks, eg, from the mandibular body, demonstrate slower revascularization than corticocancellous blocks from the iliac crest.[17] The same is true

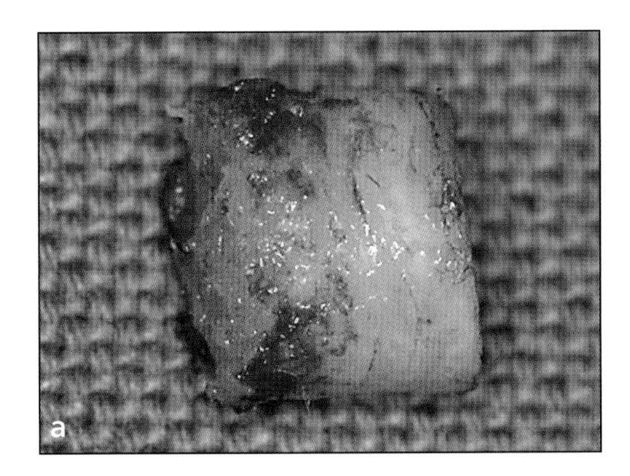

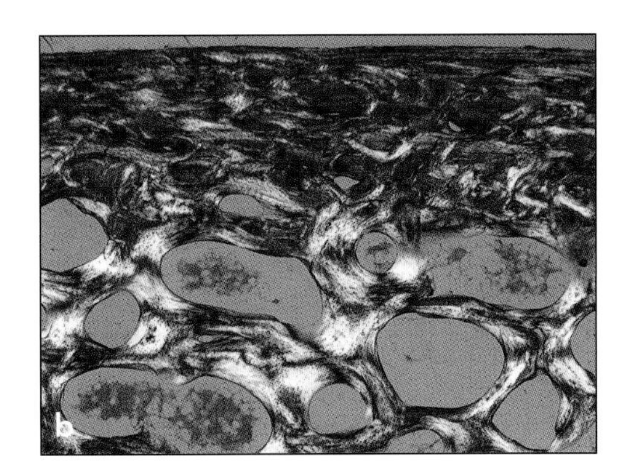

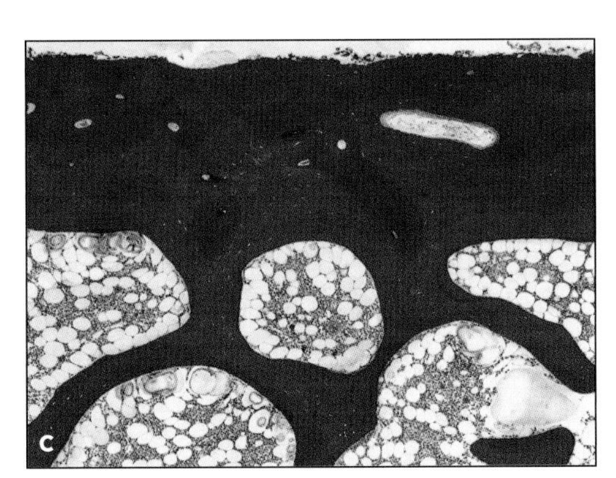

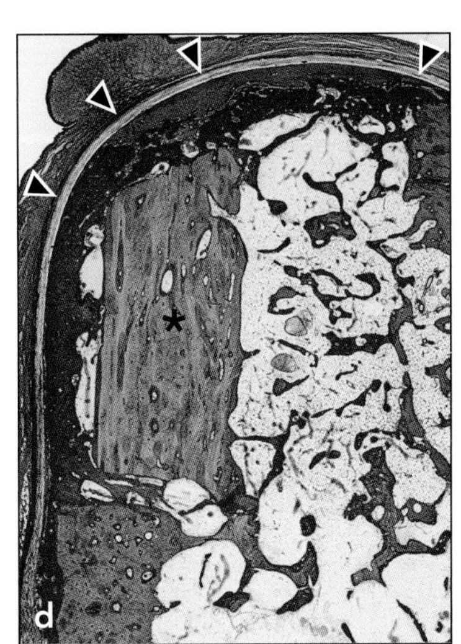

Fig 4-5 Autogenous block grafts. *(a)* Human corticocancellous block graft harvested with a trephine from the chin. *(b)* Histologic section of a human corticocancellous block graft harvested from the calvaria before transplantation (undecalcified ground section viewed under polarized light). *(c)* Histologic section of a human corticocancellous block graft harvested from the iliac crest before transplantation. Note the cortical bone layer and the fine network of trabeculae. The bone marrow is rich in hematopoietic cells (undecalcified ground section; basic fuchsin and toluidine blue stain). *(d)* Histologic section of an extended, chronic bone defect in the canine mandibular alveolar ridge grafted with an autogenous corticocancellous block graft *(asterisk)* and an ePTFE barrier membrane *(arrowheads)*. Note the excellent healing result with a well-preserved ridge profile after a healing period of 6 months (undecalcified ground section; basic fuchsin and toluidine blue stain).

regarding the rate of resorption. Corticocancellous blocks may demonstrate resorption of up to 60% of the initial volume within 6 months.[23,24] Cortical blocks from cranial donor sites also undergo resorption but to a lesser extent.[25]

Over the years, the block grafts will be substituted by newly formed bone in what is termed *creeping substitution*. In this remodeling-like process, the bone-stimulating growth factors harbored in the graft matrix are exposed, causing additional remodeling (Fig 4-5).

Autogenous particulate grafts

Autogenous particulate grafts demonstrate greater osteoinduction and osteoconduction than do block grafts because a much larger area of exposed graft surface presents growth factors.[18] Whereas the osteogenic potential of an autograft increases if it is particulated, the total amount of osteogenic cells decreases through the mechanical manipulation of the graft.[26] This means that the number of cells is higher in a block from the iliac crest than it is in the particulate material after the same block is particulated in a bone mill (Fig 4-6). However, if the blocks are particulated, the possibility of fixating the graft disappears, and the mechanical stability of the graft is thereby decreased. In addition, the resorption rate increases considerably.[27]

A vast body of scientific evidence from experimental and clinical studies documents the suitability of particulate autografts for bone augmentation procedures where a highly osteogenic graft is needed. Numerous experimental studies have documented that particulate autografts are considerably more osteogenic than any bone substitute material on the market today[7,11,13] (Fig 4-7).

Autogenous bone from bone scrapers

Autogenous bone from bone scrapers has been advocated over the past few years for minor bone regeneration procedures, such as extraction sockets and localized sinus floor elevation procedures, or coverage of dehiscence-type defects, either alone or in combination with bone substitute materials.[28–30] With this technique, small particles of cortical bone are harvested by scraping the bone surface—a simple intraoral approach with which up to 5 cm^3 of bone can be obtained.[28] Viable osteocytes have been shown to survive the grafting procedure in their lacunae, but because of the cortical nature of the graft, very few osteoblasts and osteoblast precursors can be expected to be present. The resistance toward resorption is presumably low because of the small "particle" size (1.0 to 1.3 $\times$ 0.2 $\times$ 0.1 mm).[30] Data on the content of growth factors are not yet available (Fig 4-8).

Autogenous bone from bone collectors

Autogenous bone obtained with bone collectors is a harvesting method by which bone dust is collected through a filter that is connected to the suction device used during preparation of the implant bed. The philosophy is intriguing because the acquisition of the autogenous bone graft causes no additional discomfort for the patient. There are several different bone collectors on the market with different collection efficiencies,[31] but the amount of bone that can be collected can only be expected to cover small peri-implant defects.

The graft material frequently is contaminated with bacteria from the oral cavity. This contamination can be reduced, but not eliminated, by having the patient rinse preoperatively with chlorhexidine; by using a stringent suction protocol with two suction

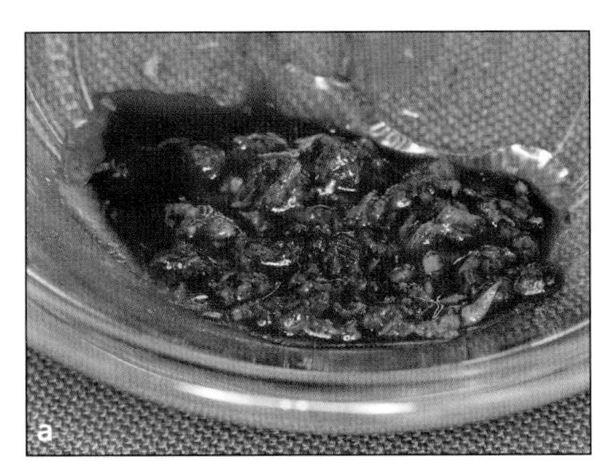

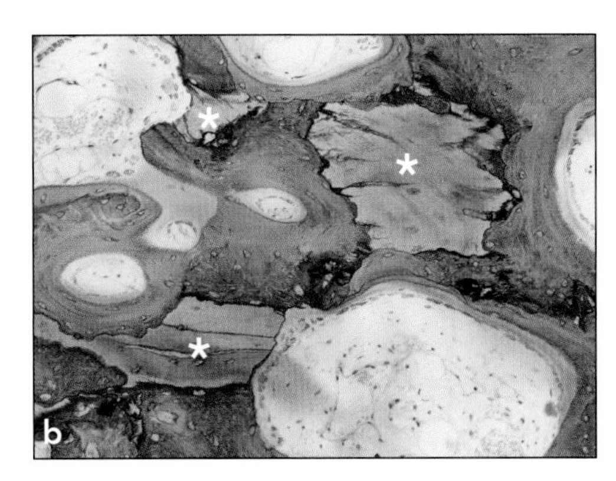

Fig 4-6 Particulate bone autograft. *(a)* Human particulate bone graft obtained by grinding a corticocancellous block in a bone mill. *(b)* Histologic section showing bone formation around autogenous bone graft particles *(asterisks)* (toluidine blue surface stain).

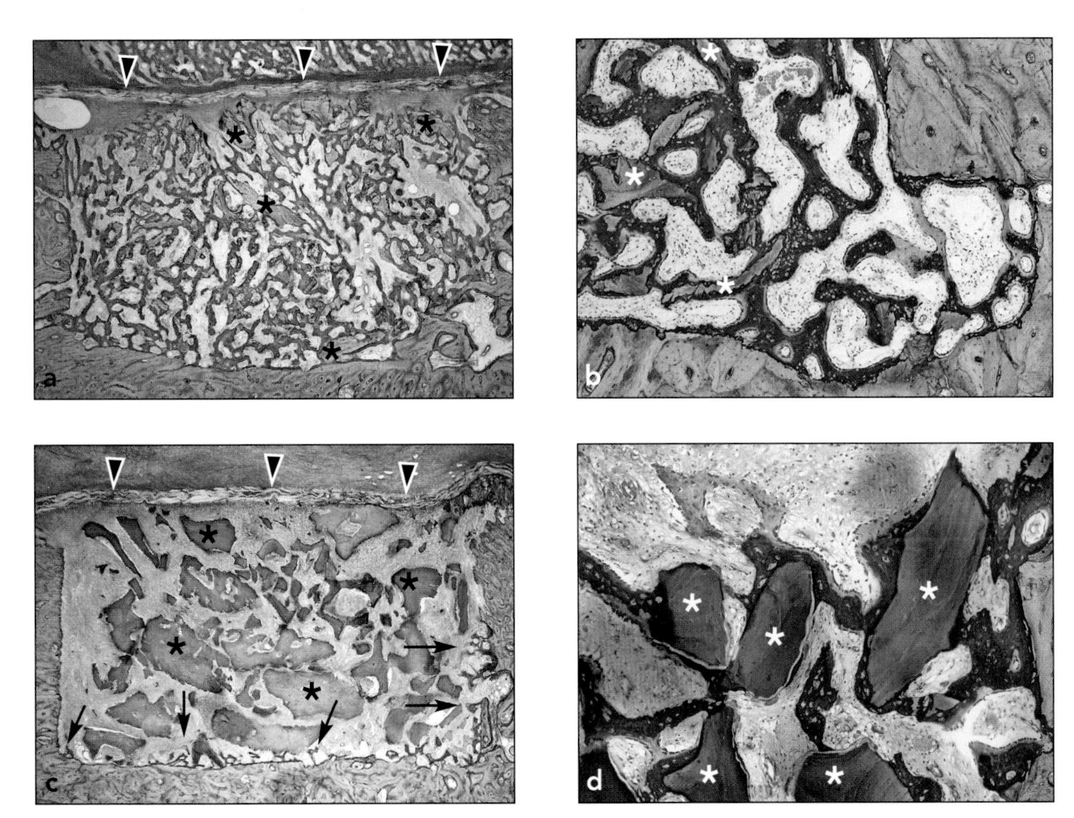

Fig 4-7 Micrographs comparing the osteoconductive property of autogenous particulate bone graft *(a and b, asterisks)* and deproteinized bovine bone mineral *(c and d, asterisks)*, a bone substitute material. The bone fillers were placed in bone defects created in the mandible of minipigs and covered with an ePTFE barrier membrane *(arrowheads)*. The healing time was 2 weeks (undecalcified ground sections; toluidine blue stain). *(a and b)* Note the dense network of newly formed bone trabeculae around and between the autograft particles. *(c and d)* In contrast, there is little new bone formation at the margins of the bone defect *(arrows)* where the xenogeneic bone substitute material was used.

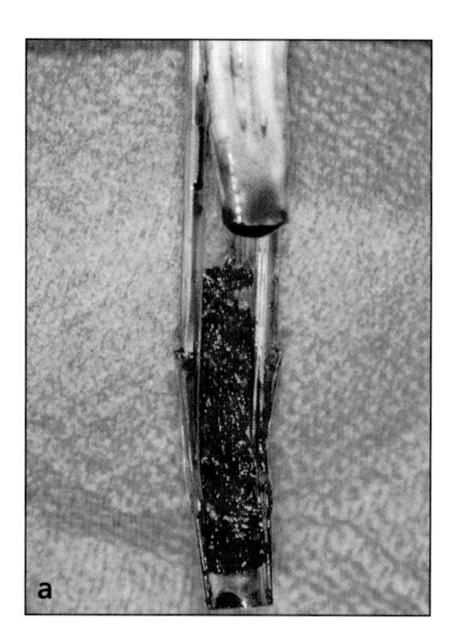

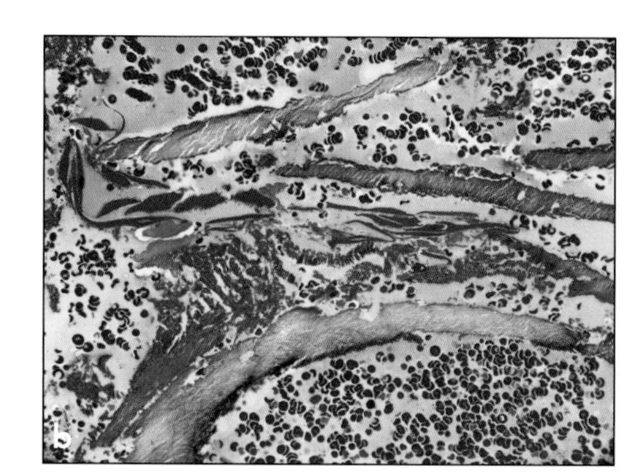

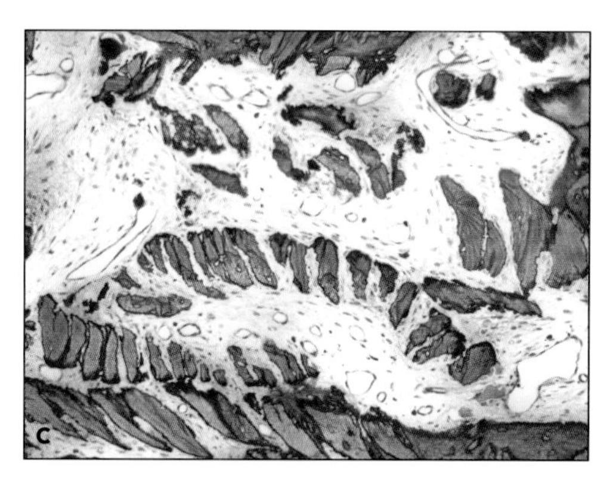

Fig 4-8 Autogenous cortical bone chips. *(a)* Cortical autogenous bone chips harvested with a bone scraper. *(b)* Histologic section of autogenous bone chips immediately after harvesting with a bone scraper (ex vivo). Note the presence of blood plasma and many blood cells among the bone chips (thin section of decalcified tissue; toluidine blue stain). *(c)* Histologic section of autograft particles harvested with a bone scraper. Note tissue integration of the bone chips and no obvious signs of resorption (undecalcified ground sections; toluidine blue stain).

devices so that the one with the collector is used exclusively during bone drilling; and by rinsing the collected bone with chlorhexidine.[32,33] However, it is not known how rinsing with chlorhexidine affects the osteogenic potential of the graft.

Viable osteocytes and osteoblast-like cells that express alkaline phosphatase and osteocalcin have been identified in grafts from bone collectors. These cells are, however, present in clearly lower numbers than in other autografts and have only limited growth potential.[26,34] The resorption resistance and mechanical stability of grafts from bone collectors have not been investigated but should be expected to be almost nonexistent because of the dustlike particle size (Fig 4-9).

An overview of possible indications for the different forms of autografts is given in Table 4-2.

Autografts are still considered the gold standard in osseous reconstructive surgery.[35] However, significant drawbacks related to the use of autografts have intensified the search for alternatives. First, there is the unpredictable resorption of up to 60% of corticocancellous block grafts.[24] If uniform resorption could be expected, it would be simple to perform a standardized overcompensation of the augmented volume. Second, there is donor site morbidity. This is most pronounced in relation to extraoral donor sites[36] but may also be significant in intraoral grafting procedures (see chapter 5). Finally, it can be a problem that autogenous bone is not available in unlimited quantities.

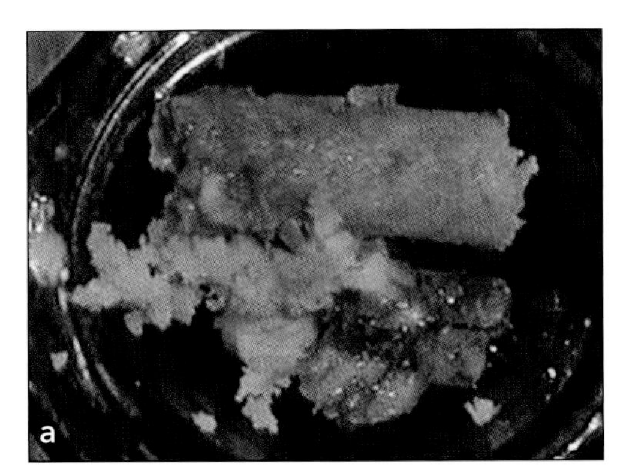

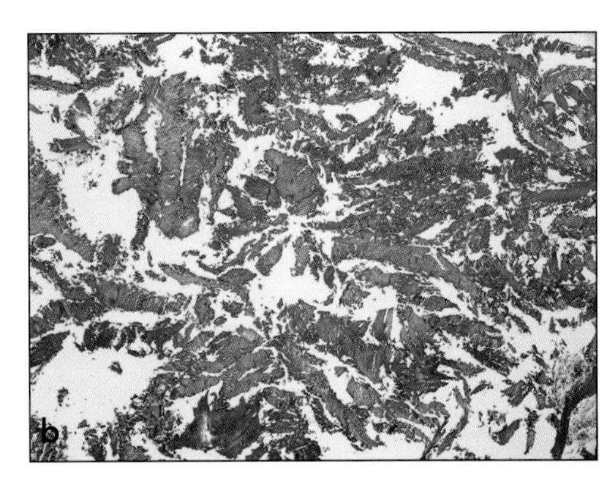

Fig 4-9 Autogenous bone dust. *(a)* Bone dust collected during preparation of implant bed with a bone trap. (Courtesy of Prof Dr S. Hillerup, University of Copenhagen, Denmark.) *(b)* Histologic section of bone dust immediately after harvesting with a bone trap (ex vivo). Note the lack of both blood plasma and cells among the bone dust particles (thin section of decalcified tissue; toluidine blue stain).

Table 4-2 Characteristics of autografts and their indications

Graft type	Osteogenic cells	Growth factors	Mechanical stability	Resorption	Indications
Cortical block	++	++++	+++++	+	Lateral and vertical ridge augmentation in a staged approach
Corticocancellous block	++++	+++	++++	++	Lateral and vertical ridge augmentation in a staged approach
Cortical particles	+	+++	+++	+++	Minor lateral augmentations, peri-implant defects, fenestrations, and dehiscence-type defects simultaneous with implant placements Sinus augmentation procedures Packing around blocks Mixing with bone substitute materials
Cancellous particles	+++	++	++	++++	Minor lateral augmentations, peri-implant defects, fenestrations, and dehiscence-type defects simultaneous with implant placements Sinus augmentation procedures Packing around blocks Mixing with bone substitute materials
Bone from bone scraper	+	++	++	++++	Minor lateral augmentations, peri-implant defects, fenestrations, and dehiscence-type defects simultaneous with implant placements Minor sinus augmentation procedures Mixing with bone substitute materials
Bone from bone collector	+	+	+	+++++	Mixing with bone substitute materials

Osteogenic cells and Growth factors: + = few; ++ = moderate number; +++ = many; ++++ = abundant.
Mechanical stability and Resorption: + = minimal; ++ = limited; +++ = moderate; ++++ = substantial; +++++ = pronounced.

With the main goal of reducing or even eliminating the shortcomings of autografts, the search for appropriate bone substitute materials has been ongoing for the past 40 years.

Allografts

Allografts consist of bone obtained from a donor and used in another individual within the same species. Transplantation of bone from one individual to another has been performed in orthopedic surgery for more than 120 years.[37]

Allografts are usually stored in bone banks, and may be used as fresh frozen bone (FFB), freeze-dried bone allograft (FDBA), or demineralized freeze-dried bone allograft (DFDBA). FFB is rarely used in GBR procedures because of a high risk of immunologic rejection and disease transmission, whereas the freeze drying of FDBA and DFDBA is reported to reduce the immunogenicity of the material, potentially improving the clinical outcome. Allografts are available as blocks or in particulate forms from both cortical or cancellous origins.[38,39]

FDBA and DFDBA have been shown to be biocompatible and to contain osteoinductive molecules such as BMPs.[40] Demineralization of allografts is intended to expose the BMPs additionally to increase their immediate osteoinductive potential. However, during the demineralization process, FDBA loses some of its mechanical stability, and DFDBA should therefore be used in combination with a space-maintaining material if used in bone defects that are not self-contained. Different batches of DFDBA have been shown to contain very different concentrations of BMPs,[41,42] and the osteoinductivity may, therefore, be expected to vary correspondingly.

Histologic evidence from an experimental comparative study in the mandibles of minipigs showed that allografts decelerated new bone formation in comparison to autografts (positive control) and coagulum (negative control).[11] DFDBA showed osteoconductive properties, but an effect of possible osteoinductive potential could not be demonstrated[11] (Figs 4-10 and 4-11). Therefore, FFB, FDBA, and DFDBA indisputably contain osteoinductive molecules. However, it is still debatable whether the concentrations of these BMPs are sufficient to elicit a clinically relevant osteoinductive potential and whether they are present in an active form.

Allografts are widely used in the United States, whereas local regulations in Europe restrict the collection of human bone, which has limited their widespread popularity among clinicians. Compared to the limitations of autografts, donor site morbidity is not an issue, and allografts are available in abundant quantities. However, resorption is reported to take place, as is seen with autografts.[38]

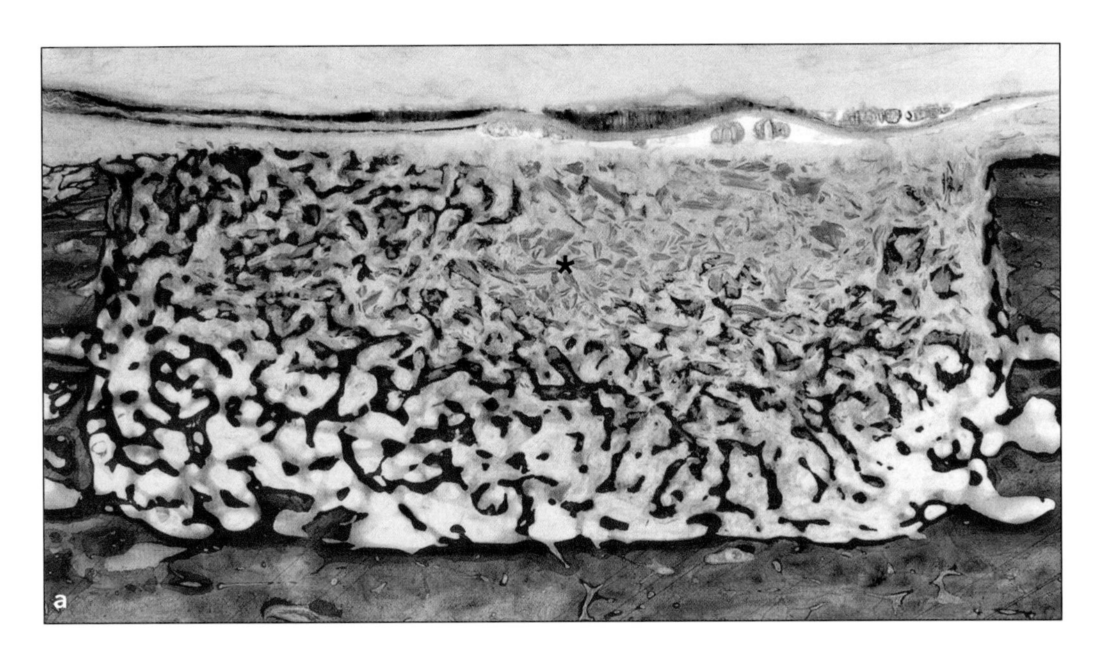

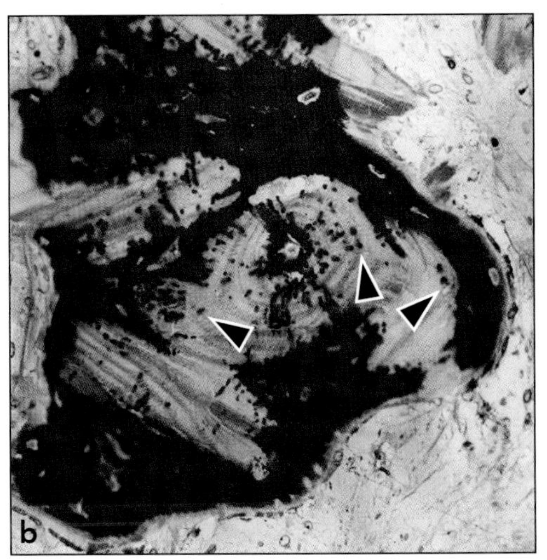

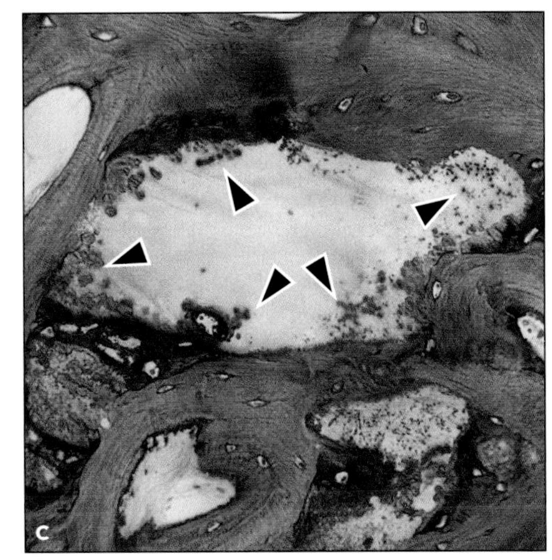

Fig 4-10 DFDBA particulate used as a bone filler in bone defects covered with a barrier membrane in the mandible of minipigs. *(a)* The overview micrograph taken at 4 weeks after filling with DFDBA shows that bone formation started from the defect walls. The central defect area underneath the barrier membrane *(asterisk)* contains only DFDBA particles embedded in granulation tissue. *(b and c)* At 4 *(b)* and 12 *(c)* weeks, histologic signs of recalcification of the DFDBA particles are apparent *(arrowheads)*. The recalcification process seems to have progressed from the bone-graft interface toward the center of the DFDBA particles (undecalcified ground sections; *[a and b]* basic fuchsin and toluidine blue stain; *[c]* toluidine blue stain alone).

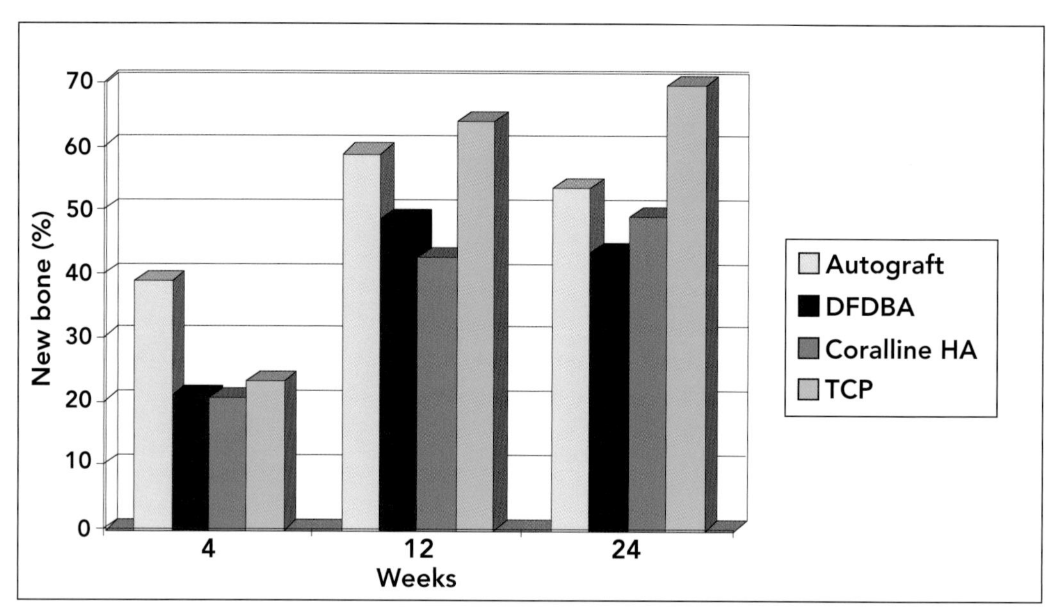

Fig 4-11 Percentage of new bone in standardized bone defects in the mandibles of minipigs grafted with particulated autograft, demineralized freeze-dried bone allograft (DFDBA), xenogeneic coral-derived hydroxyapatite (coralline HA), or alloplastic β-tricalcium phosphate (TCP). (Data from Buser et al.[11])

Xenografts

Xenografts, or xenogeneic bone substitutes, consist of bone mineral derived from animals or bonelike minerals derived from calcifying corals or algae from which the organic component has been removed to eliminate the risk of immunogenic reactions or transmission of diseases.

Coral- and algae-derived bonelike minerals

Coral-derived bone substitutes gained popularity in orthopedic and craniofacial surgery in the late 1980s. Different species of calcifying corals were found to have a calcium carbonate skeleton with a geometry similar to that of human cancellous bone, with interconnected macropores of 200 to 600 μm (Fig 4-12). The coralline calcium carbonate is transformed into HA by a hydrothermal exchange reaction with phosphorus. Although the coralline HA is almost identical to the mineral component of bone, experimental studies have demonstrated that the osteoconductive potential is less than that of other bone substitute materials[11,43] (Fig 4-13). Today, coralline HA is seldom used for onlay grafts in GBR procedures because of a high rate of late complications.[44]

When used as a particulate, the granules tend to migrate, and the ones that are kept at the augmented site predominantly become encapsulated by fibrous tissue. The blocks, on the other hand, most often show bone formation throughout the augmented volume but are prone to develop late dehiscences[45] (Fig 4-14).

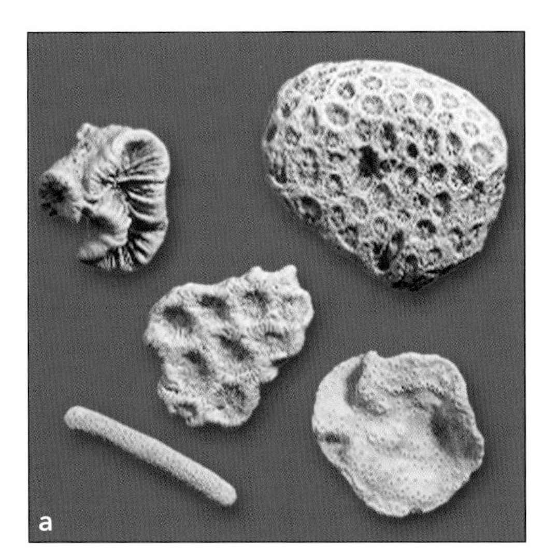

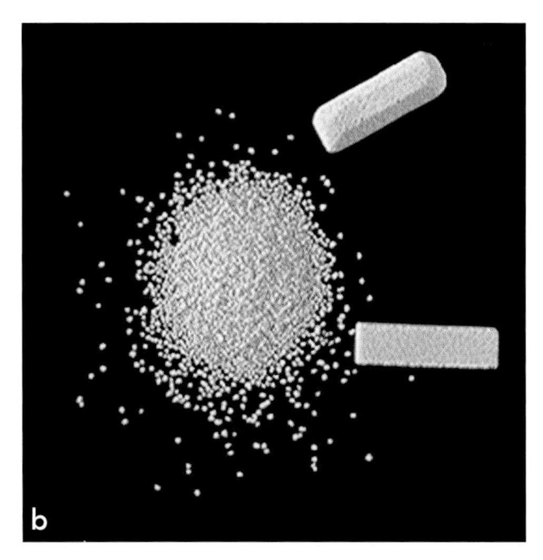

Fig 4-12 Xenogeneic coral-derived bone substitutes. *(a)* Calcifying corals (genus *Porites*) in their natural shapes. *(b)* Xenogeneic HA blocks and particles derived from calcifying corals. (Courtesy of Dr N. Worsaae, Copenhagen University Hospital, Denmark.)

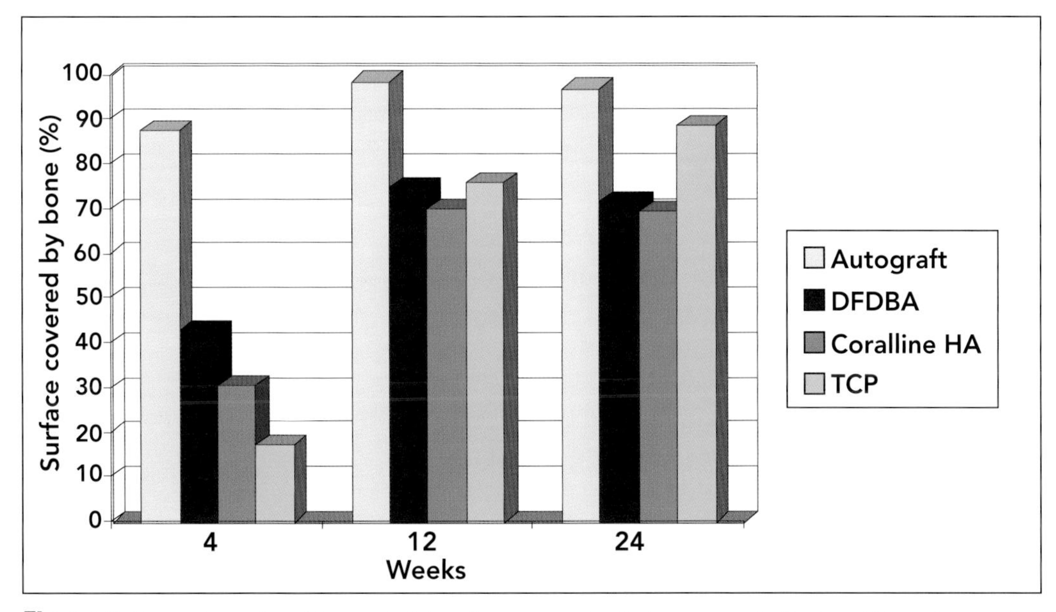

Fig 4-13 Percentage of grafting material surface covered with bone as an indicator of the osteoconductive potential of particulated autograft, demineralized freeze-dried bone allograft (DFDBA), xenogeneic coral-derived hydroxyapatite (coralline HA), or alloplastic β-tricalcium phosphate (TCP) in standardized bone defects in the mandibles of minipigs. (Data from Buser et al.[11])

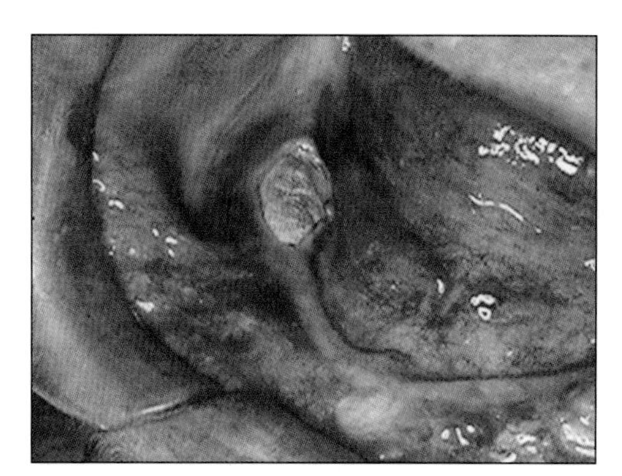

Fig 4-14 Mucosal dehiscence of a coral-derived xenogeneic block 4 years after augmentation of an edentulous mandible. (Courtesy of Dr N. Worsaae, Copenhagen University Hospital, Denmark.)

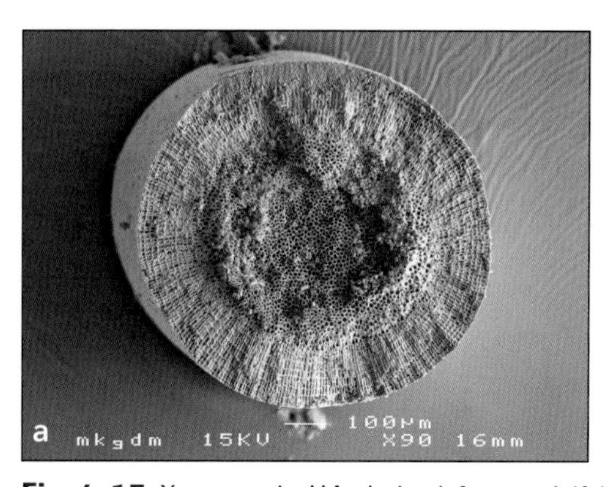

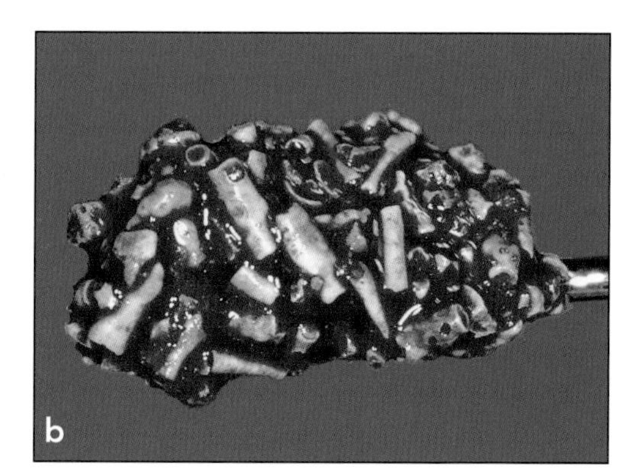

Fig 4-15 Xenogeneic HA derived from calcifying algae. *(a)* Scanning electron microscopic image. *(b)* Algae-derived xenograft mixed with blood just before clinical application.

There is also a group of marine algae that consists of a calcified exoskeleton made of calcium carbonate. The natural material is converted into fluorhydroxyapatite through an exchange reaction with ammonium phosphate at around 700°C. The morphologic structure is built up of pores arranged in parallel with a mean diameter of 10 µm and connected through microperforations (Fig 4-15). The pore configuration is thus not ideal for vascular ingrowth, but cellular invasion of the pores and bone deposition directly on the material surface have been documented.[46,47] Neovascularization is instead expected to take place between the bone substitute particles. In contrast to coralline HAs, phycogenic fluorapatite undergoes slow resorption by enzymatic and cellular degradation but at a lower rate than autografts.[46]

Animal-derived bone minerals

Xenografts derived from natural bone sources have been extensively investigated in multiple experimental and clinical studies. In particular, cancellous bovine bone has been used as a source for these bone substitute materials because of its close simi-

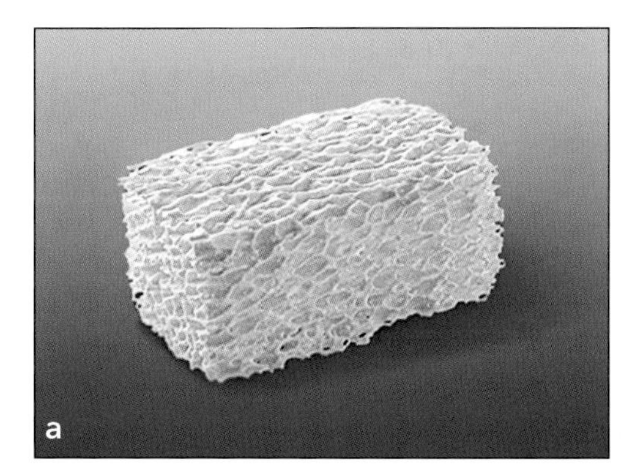

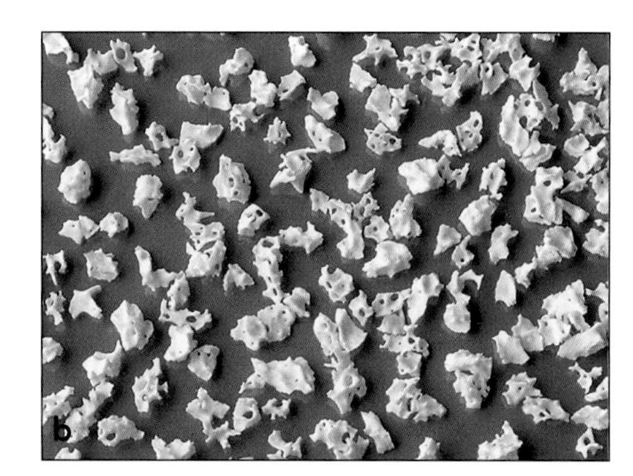

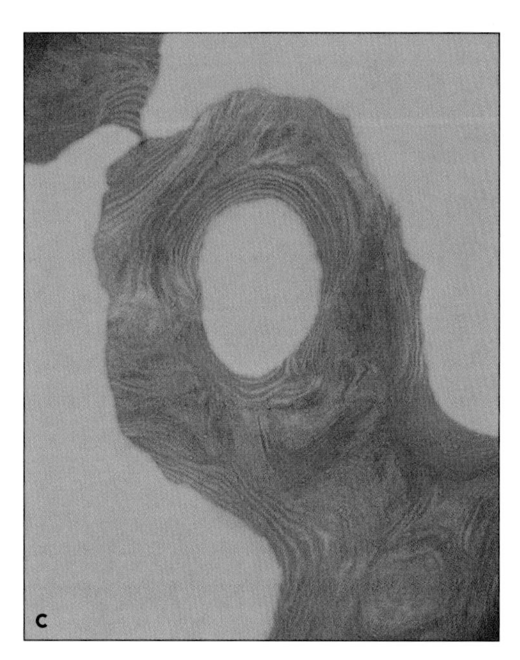

Fig 4-16 Deproteinized bovine bone mineral (DBBM), a xenogeneic bone substitute. *(a)* Cancellous block of DBBM. *(b)* DBBM in particulate form. *(c)* Histologic section of particulate DBBM before implantation. The lamellar bone pattern is visualized with polarized light microscopy.

larity to cancellous human bone (Fig 4-16). The organic component is removed by heat treatment, by a chemical extraction method, or by a combination of the two to eliminate the risk of immunologic reactions and disease transmission. Since the first reports of bovine spongiform encephalopathy, there has been a particular focus on the ability of these extraction methods to completely eliminate all protein from the bovine bone source.[48,49] However, despite the hypothetical risk of organic remnants in bovine bone substitutes, there have been no reports of disease transmission from these materials. In contrast, a few cases of transmission of human immunodeficiency virus and hepatitis related to allogeneic materials have been reported.[50]

Deproteinized bovine bone minerals (DBBMs) are in general known to be biocompatible and osteoconductive, although the production methods have a strong impact on their biologic behavior. Two bovine bone substitutes derived from bovine cancellous bone, one deproteinized by high temperatures and the other mainly by chemi-

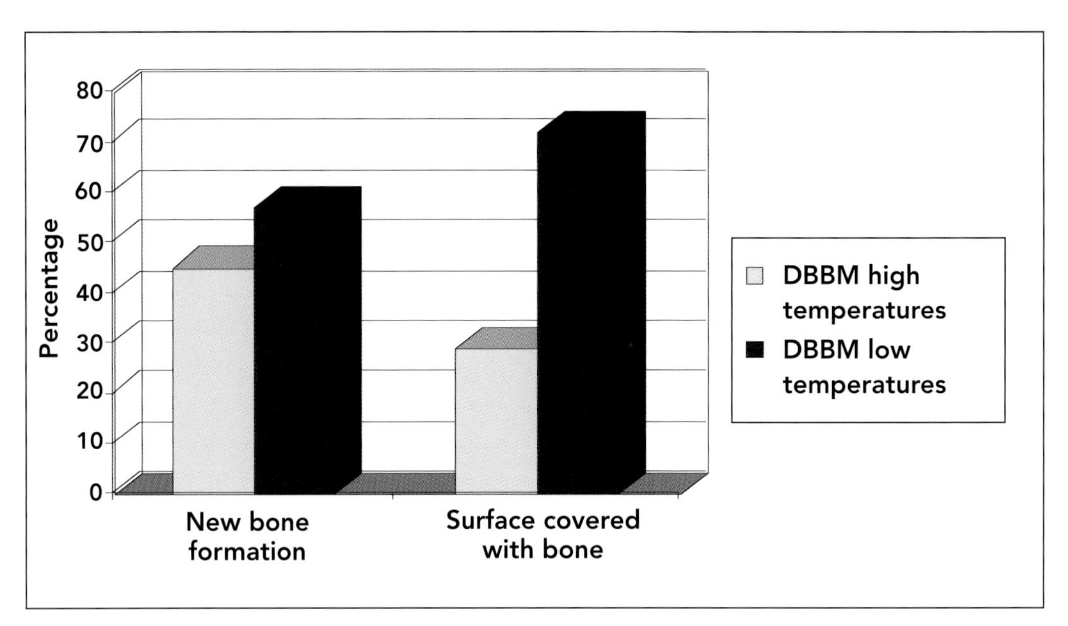

Fig 4-17 Percentage of new bone formation and percentage of grafting material covered with bone for two deproteinized bovine bone minerals (DBBMs) deproteinized in different ways. The difference in amount of new bone is not statistically significant, whereas the material deproteinized using low temperatures shows significantly higher ($P < .01$) osteoconductive capacity than does the one treated with high temperatures. (Data from Jensen et al.[43])

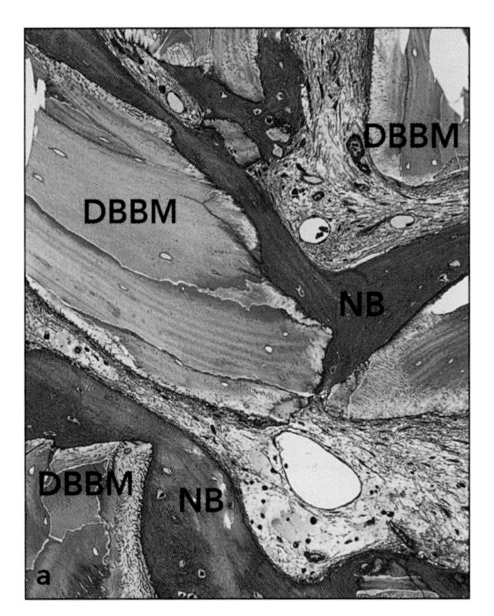

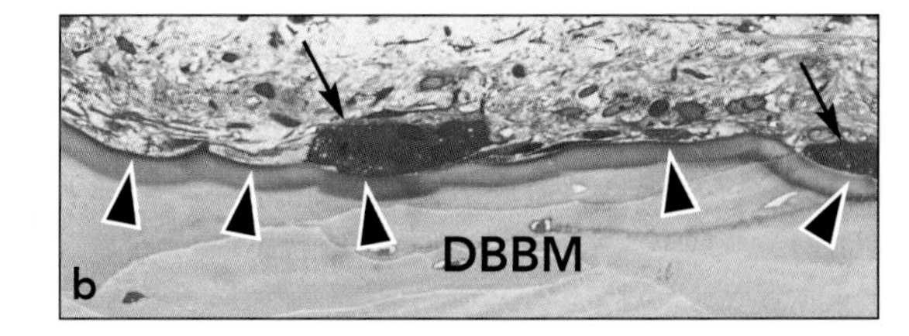

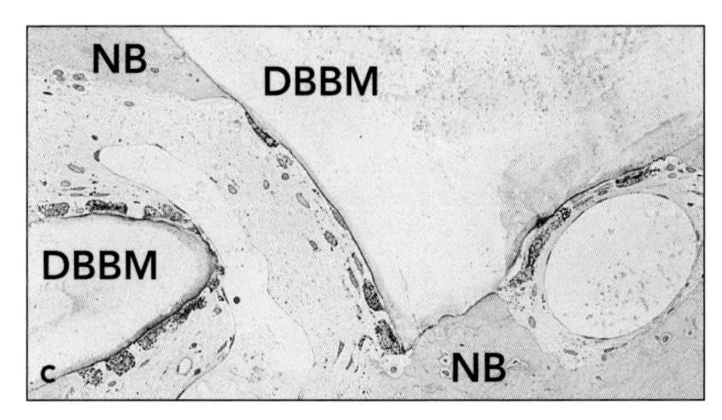

Fig 4-18 Histologic sections of human biopsy specimens grafted with deproteinized bovine bone mineral (DBBM) (thin sections of decalcified tissue). *(a)* The DBBM particles show good tissue integration. Newly formed bone (NB) covers part of the bone substitute surface and bridges neighboring DBBM particles (basic fuchsin and toluidine blue stain). *(b)* Osteoclast-like, multinucleated giant cells *(arrows)* are frequently seen lining the DBBM surface, which occasionally shows shallow resorption depressions *(arrowheads)* (toluidine blue stain alone). *(c)* Staining for tartrate-resistant acid phosphatase (TRAP) (red staining) identifies osteoclast-like, multinucleated giant cells on the surface of the DBBM particles (stained for TRAP and counterstained with toluidine blue).

cal extraction methods, display very different osteoconductive and resorptive properties in vivo and in vitro[43,47,51] (Fig 4-17). This difference most likely reflects production-related changes in surface characteristics. Temperatures exceeding 1,000°C cause a sintering of the natural HAs, by which the apatite crystals grow and the intercrystalline spaces to a large extent disappear.[4] This reduces the microroughness and porosity of the bone substitute and increases the crystallinity.

Controversy remains as to whether DBBM is truly resorbable.[52] It has been shown in vitro that osteoclast progenitor cells are able to proliferate on DBBM surfaces and later, as osteoclast-like cells, produce resorption pits. Compared with native bovine bone, however, DBBM has fewer and smaller osteoclasts, and its resorption pits are less pronounced.[51] Experimental in vivo studies have also demonstrated multinucleated cells on DBBM surfaces that stain positive for tartrate-resistant acid phosphatase (TRAP)[7,8,53] (Fig 4-18). This suggests that these cells have osteoclast-like properties. However, the same studies histomorphometrically fail to demonstrate any reduction in DBBM volume over observation periods of up to 1 year.[8] Human biopsies after sinus augmentation confirm that particles of bovine-derived bone substitutes can still be found up to 10 years postoperatively.[52] Thus in daily practice, xenografts must be considered close to nonresorbable.

Alloplastic Bone Substitutes

The advantage of alloplastic bone substitutes is that, because of their completely synthetic nature, they bear no risk of disease transmission. The other main reason why alloplasts have gained increasing scientific and clinical attention over the past 40 years is the theoretic possibility of designing every single material characteristic individually for a specific clinical indication. Today, the chemical composition of the materials can be controlled down to the molecular level; the size and interconnectivity of the macropores can be optimized for vascular ingrowth; the phase distribution between crystalline and amorphous material can be varied; and the morphology of the blocks and granules can be tailored.

However, not all characteristics of the ideal alloplastic bone substitute have been identified. It is, for example, believed that the initial adsorption of proteins and other macromolecules from the serum is of crucial importance for the attachment of osteogenic cells and their precursors. This applies also to other bone substitute materials (Fig 4-19). However, knowledge of the surface characteristics responsible for this material-tissue interaction is limited.[54] In addition, technical limitations have, so far, made it impossible to reproduce desired material characteristics. It has thus until now not been possible to prepare a macroporous material with a surface roughness that simulates natural bone mineral. This is in contrast to advances in the titanium implant surface technology.[55–57]

The materials on the market today can be categorized into three groups: calcium phosphates, bioactive glasses, and polymers (see Fig 4-1). Of these, calcium phosphates, and especially HA and β–tricalcium phosphate (TCP), have been most intensively studied because of their composition, which closely resembles the inorganic phase of bone.[58] A

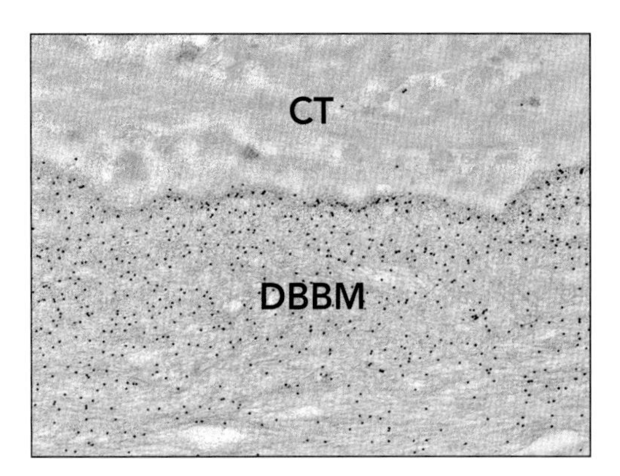

Fig 4-19 Ultrathin section of a human biopsy retrieved from a bony site augmented with deproteinized bovine bone mineral (DBBM) and embedded in acrylic resin. High resolution postembedding immunocytochemistry performed with an antibody against a typical bone-related noncollagenous protein. Visualization with protein A-gold shows gold particle labeling preferentially at the periphery of a DBBM particle. This finding indicates protein adsorption from the wound environment to DBBM after its implantation into a bony site. (CT) soft connective tissue.

wide array of materials has emerged on the market, and many of them have disappeared just as quickly. Many of the "dropouts" may have failed because of the false assumption that having a chemical composition close to that of natural bone mineral is sufficient to make a material suitable as a bone substitute. Increased understanding of the importance of the different material characteristics, such as microporosity, crystallinity, crystal size, and surface roughness, has helped clarify why materials with identical chemical compositions and macromorphologies have performed so biologically differently in vivo.

In general, however, HA is considered to be osteoconductive and nonresorbable, whereas TCP also demonstrates osteoconductive properties but resorbs rapidly. In protected bone defects, TCP-based bone substitute materials show faster bone healing than HA-based materials[7,11,13] (Figs 4-11, 4-20, and 4-21). The explanation for this is that calcium and phosphate ions are released from the TCP material during the degradation process and are used as "raw material" for new bone formation. In addition, the resorption of TCP makes space for the healing bone through the process of creeping substitution. However, in more demanding defect morphologies, such as lateral ridge augmentations, the resorption rate of TCP is too high to allow the formation of new bone. The space-making capacity of the TCP material simply fades away before the newly formed bone has stabilized the augmented volume.[59]

Therefore, combinations of HA and TCP—biphasic calcium phosphates—have been investigated to benefit from both the stable space-maintaining properties of HA and the osteogenic, resorbable properties of TCP.[60] In experimental animal studies, it has thus been possible to modulate the substitution rate and bioactivity of these materials by changing the HA-TCP ratio.[7,8] Future perspectives involve applying these findings to develop a selection of two to three biphasic calcium phosphates to fit individual clinical indications.

Although calcium phosphates in general are considered to be osteoconductive (Fig 4-22), the optimal surface characteristics still need to be identified to attain the osteoconductivity of the natural cancellous bone surface (Fig 4-23). They are, however, a valuable alternative for clinicians and patients who hesitate to have implanted material of human or animal origin.

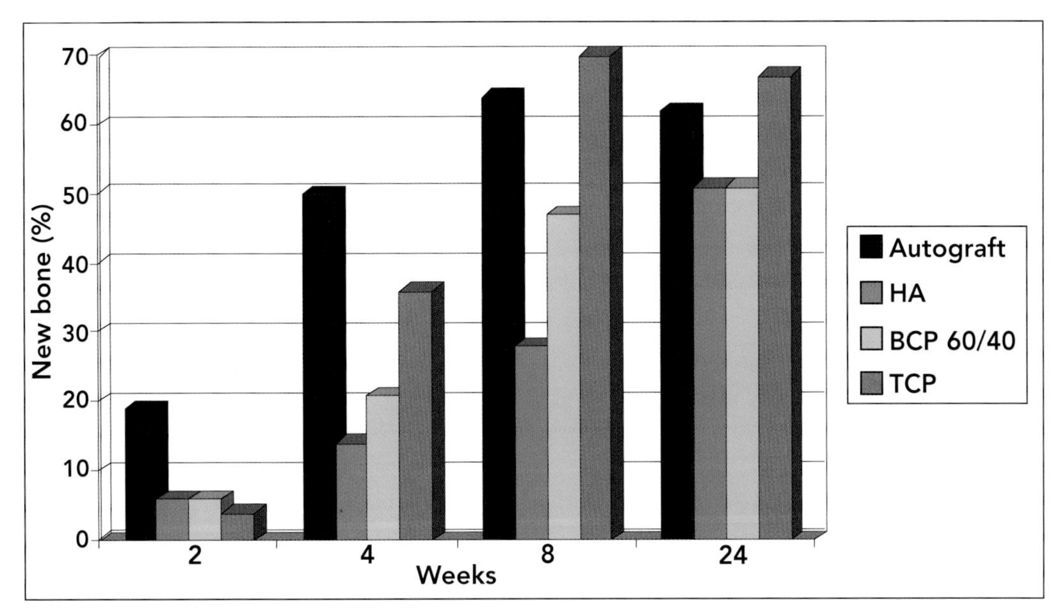

Fig 4-20 Percentage of new bone formation in standardized bone defects in the mandibles of minipigs grafted with particulated autograft, hydroxyapatite (HA), biphasic calcium phosphate (BCP), or β-tricalcium phosphate (TCP). The three bone substitute materials have identical material characteristics except for the chemical composition. In the early healing phases, more new bone formation was observed in defects grafted with TCP than with BCP, which resulted in more new bone formation than HA. (Data from Jensen et al.[7])

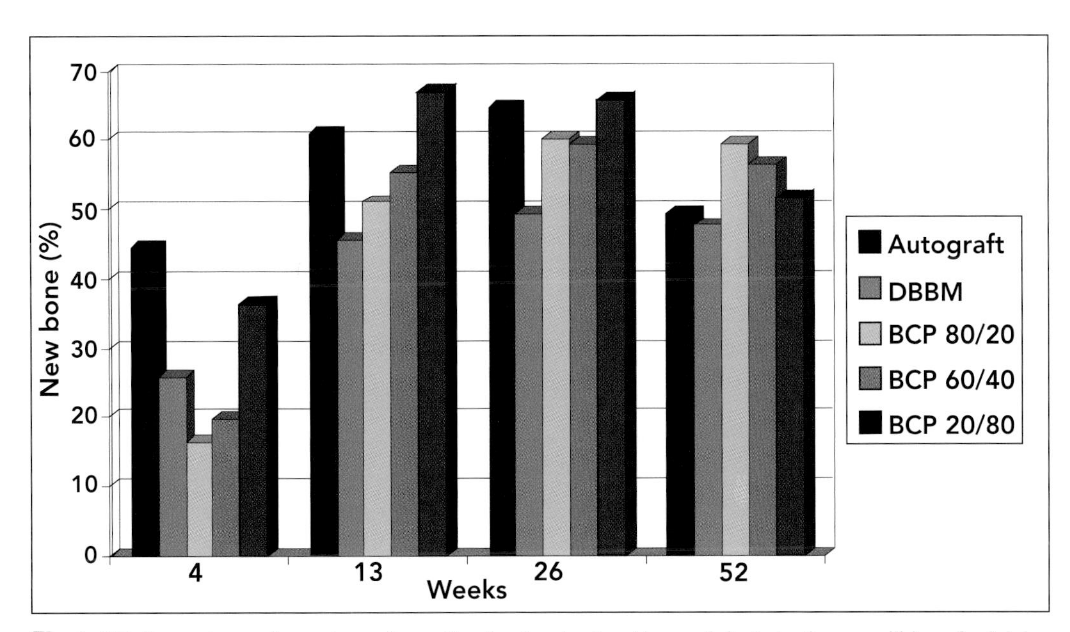

Fig 4-21 Percentage of new bone formation in standardized bone defects in the mandibles of minipigs grafted with particulated autograft, deproteinized bovine bone mineral (DBBM), or biphasic calcium phosphate (BCP) with three different ratios of hydroxyapatite and β-tricalcium phosphate (TCP). In the early healing phases, more new bone formation is seen in defects grafted with BCPs with high TCP content. (Data from Jensen et al.[8])

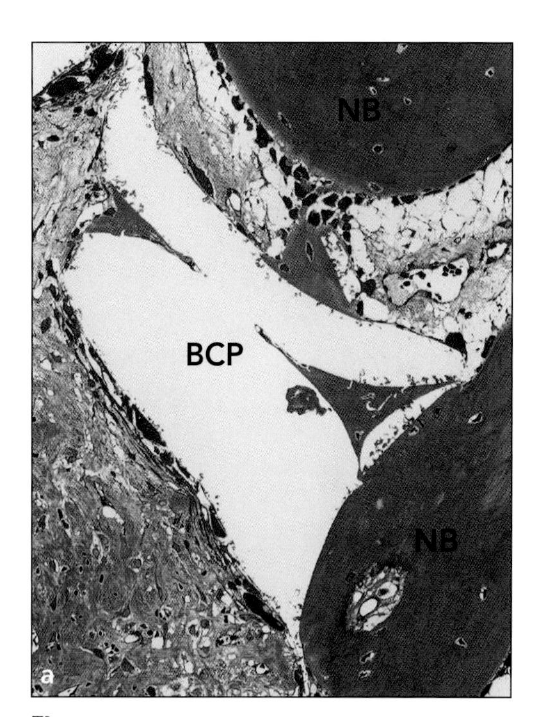

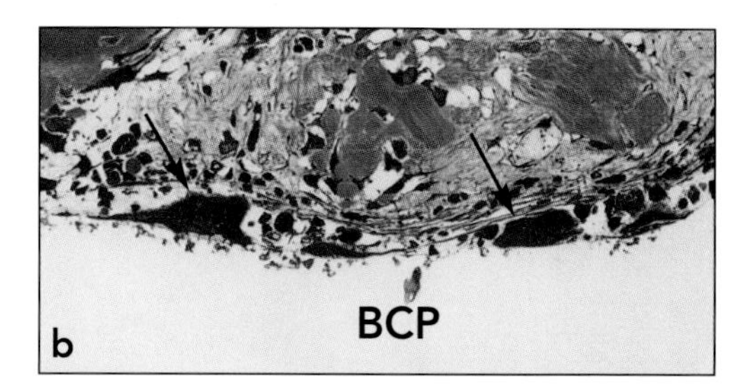

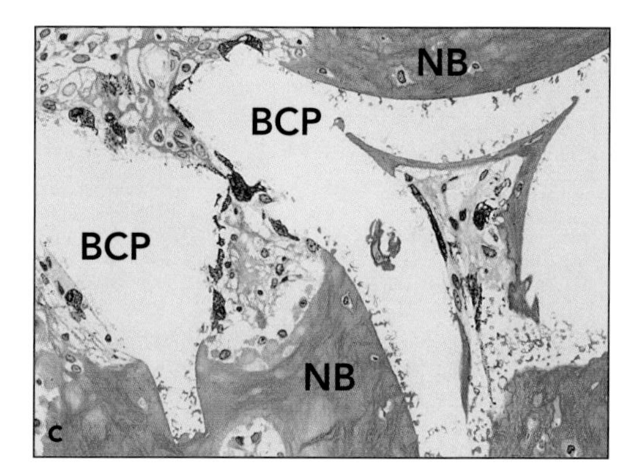

Fig 4-22 Histologic sections of human biopsy specimens harvested from sites grafted with a biphasic calcium phosphate (BCP) consisting of HA and TCP (thin sections of decalcified tissues; *[a and b]* basic fuchsin and toluidine blue stain; *[c]* stained for TRAP and counterstained with toluidine blue). *(a)* The alloplastic bone substitute particles show good tissue integration. Newly formed bone (NB) covers part of the particle surface and bridges neighboring BCP particles. *(b)* Numerous osteoclast-like, multinucleated giant cells cover the BCP particles *(arrows)*. *(c)* Staining for TRAP (red staining) identifies numerous osteoclast-like, multinucleated giant cells on the surface of the BCP particles.

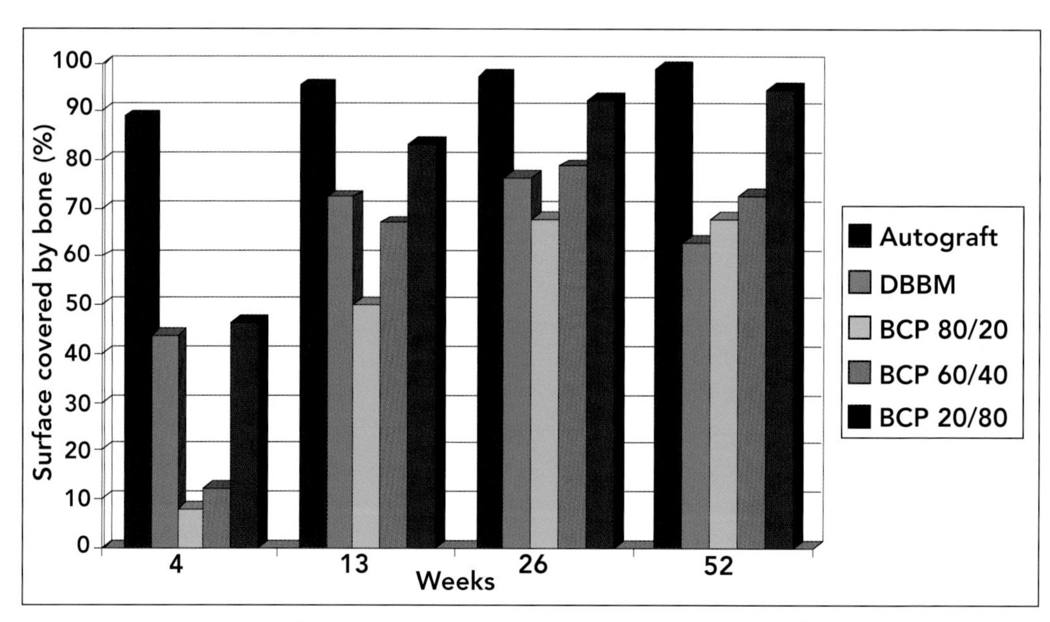

Fig 4-23 Percentage of grafting material surface covered with bone in standardized bone defects in the mandibles of minipigs. (DBBM) deproteinized bovine bone mineral; (BCP) biphasic calcium phosphate with three different ratios of hydroxyapatite and β-tricalcium phosphate. (Data from Jensen et al.[8])

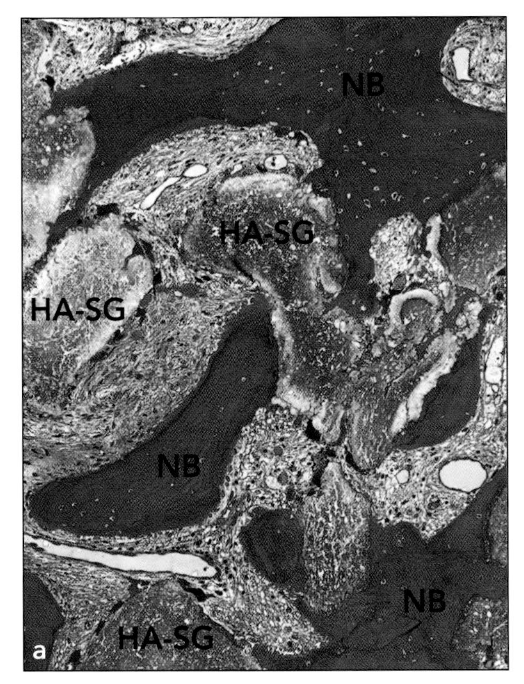

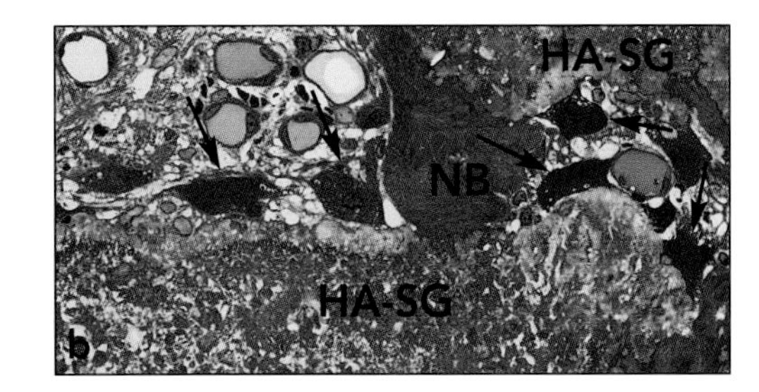

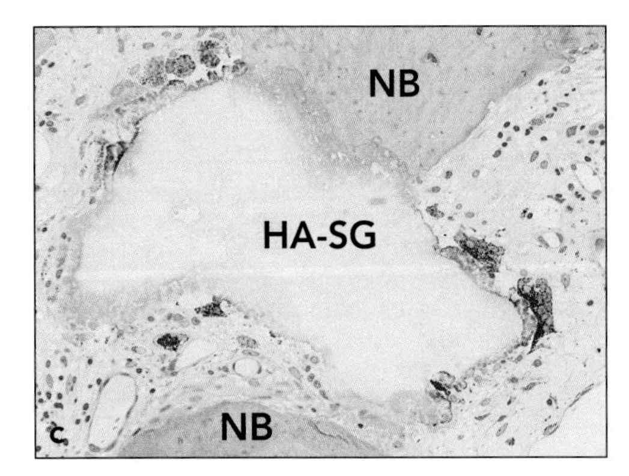

Fig 4-24 Micrographs from sections of human biopy specimens harvested from sites grafted with a composite material consisting of nonsintered, nanocrystalline hydroxyapatite (HA) embedded in a matrix of silica gel (SG) (thin sections of decalcified tissues; *[a and b]* basic fuchsin and toluidine blue stain; *[c]* stained for TRAP and counterstained with toluidine blue). *(a)* The alloplastic bone substitute particles show good tissue integration. Newly formed bone (NB) covers part of the particle surface and bridges neighboring HA-SG particles. *(b)* Numerous osteoclast-like, multinucleated giant cells cover the HA-SG particles *(arrows)*. *(c)* Staining for TRAP (red staining) identifies numerous osteoclast-like, multinucleated giant cells on the surface of the HA-SG particles.

Bioglasses are silica-based materials that were first introduced in the early 1970s. These glasses exhibit bone bonding as a result of the surface-reactive silica, calcium, and phosphate groups that are characteristic of these materials. Silica is believed to play a critical role in bioactivity. Bioactive glasses are very biocompatible materials. There are some experimental data supporting their use in GBR procedures such as ridge preservation and sinus augmentation. However, there are inherent limitations in the bioglass products that are currently available. Because of their granular and nonporous nature, they cannot reliably serve as space-maintaining devices, although the first macroporous glass ceramic recently has been presented.[61]

Composites of silica- and HA-based alloplastic bone substitutes are also available on the dental market. One such material consists of nonsintered, nanocrystalline HA embedded in a matrix of silica gel. Like DBBM, it is predisposed to take up proteins because of its high porosity with interconnecting pores.[62] Abundant new bone formation is observed in association with this bone substitute material. Biopsies from both humans and animals have shown multinucleated giant cells, which stain positive for TRAP, on the surface of the material (Fig 4-24), which becomes partly replaced by bone over time. This suggests that these osteoclast-like cells participate in its degradation, although other degradation processes such as dissolution must also be taken into consideration.

Conclusion

Bone grafts and bone substitute materials play important roles in GBR procedures, with the indications ranging from minor implant fenestration defects to bridging major continuity defects in the facial skeleton.

Autografts are the only grafting materials with well-documented osteoinductive potential. The immediate availability of the bone-stimulating molecules harbored in autografts is increased by particulating the graft and thereby enhancing the surface area. However, resistance toward graft resorption is reduced when the size of the autogenous particles decreases. Unpredictable resorption, donor site morbidity, and limited quantities available are the main drawbacks related to the use of autografts in bone augmentation procedures.

As a result of the drawbacks of autografts, much effort has been invested in the search for suitable alternatives. Like autografts, allografts contain osteoinductive molecules. However, it is debatable whether the concentration and activity of these molecules is of clinical significance. In addition, allografts have the same drawbacks as autografts except that they are available in abundant quantities.

Xenografts are, today, mainly used in the form of DBBM. The production process preserves the original cancellous geometry and natural surface characteristics, but the organic material is removed to exclude the risk of disease transmission. DBBM is well-documented as an osteoconductive material that should be considered close to non-resorbable.

Alloplastic materials are most often made of different formulations of calcium phosphate in the forms of HA, TCP, or combinations of these, also called *biphasic calcium phosphates*. There have been big advances in the biologic performance of these materials because the ideal surface characteristics for the osteogenic cells are better understood and technical production methods have improved. So far, it has not been possible to mimic the surface of natural bone mineral, but the currently available alloplasts are already valuable alternatives for patients and clinicians who hesitate to use bone substitute materials of natural origin.

References

1. Mastrogiacomo M, Scaglione S, Martinetti R, et al. Role of scaffold internal structure on in vivo bone formation in macroporous calcium phosphate bioceramics. Biomaterials 2006;27:3230–3237.
2. Eggli PS, Müller W, Schenk RK. Porous hydroxyapatite and tricalcium phosphate cylinders with two different pore size ranges implanted in the cancellous bone of rabbits. A comparative histomorphometric and histologic study of bone ingrowth and implant substitution. Clin Orthop Relat Res 1988;232:127–138.
3. Yamada S, Heymann D, Bouler JM, Daculci G. Osteoclastic resorption of calcium phosphate ceramics with different hydroxyapatite/β-tricalcium phosphate ratios. Biomaterials 1997;18:1037–1041.
4. Ong JL, Hoppe CA, Cardenas HL, et al. Osteoblast precursor cell activity on HA surfaces of different treatments. J Biomed Mater Res 1998;39:176–183.
5. Berube P, Yang Y, Carnes DL, Stover RE, Boland EJ, Ong JL. The effect of sputtered calcium phosphate coatings of different crystallinity on osteoblast differentiation. J Periodontol 2005;76:1697–1709.

6. Rohanizadeh R, Padrines M, Bouler JM, Couchourel D, Fortun Y, Daculsi G. Apatite precipitation after incubation of biphasic calcium-phosphate ceramic in various solutions: Influence of seed species and proteins. J Biomed Mater Res 1998;42:530–539.
7. Jensen SS, Yeo A, Dard M, Hunziker E, Schenk R, Buser D. Evaluation of a novel biphasic calcium phosphate in standardized bone defects. A histologic and histomorphometric study in the mandibles of minipigs. Clin Oral Implants Res 2007;18:752–760.
8. Jensen SS, Bornstein MM, Dard M, Bosshardt D, Buser D. Comparative study of biphasic calcium phosphates with different HA/TCP ratios in mandibular bone defects. A long-term histomorphometric study in minipigs. J Biomed Mater Res B Appl Biomater 2009;90B:171–181.
9. Buser D, Martin W, Belser UC. Optimizing esthetics for implant restorations in the anterior maxilla: Anatomic and surgical considerations. Int J Oral Maxillofac Implants 2004;19(suppl):43–61.
10. Buser D, Chen ST, Weber HP, Belser UC. Early implant placement following single-tooth extraction in the esthetic zone: Biologic rationale and surgical procedures. Int J Periodontics Restorative Dent 2008;28:441–451.
11. Buser D, Hoffmann B, Bernard JP, Lussi A, Mettler D, Schenk RK. Evaluation of filling materials in membrane-protected bone defects. A comparative histomorphometric study in the mandibles of miniature pigs. Clin Oral Implants Res 1998;9:137–150.
12. Jensen SS, Broggini N, Weibrich G, Hjørting-Hansen E, Schenk R, Buser D. Bone regeneration in standardized bone defects with autografts or bone substitutes in combination with platelet concentrate: A histologic and histomorphometric study in the mandibles of minipigs. Int J Oral Maxillofac Implants 2005;20:703–712.
13. Jensen SS, Broggini N, Hjørting-Hansen E, Schenk R, Buser D. Bone healing and graft resorption of autograft, anorganic bovine bone and β-tricalcium phosphate. A histologic and histomorphometric study in the mandibles of minipigs. Clin Oral Implants Res 2006;17:237–243.
14. Hönig J, Merten HA. Das Göttinger Miniatureschwein (GMS) als Versuchstier in der humanmedizinischen osteologischen Grundlagenforschung. Z Zahnärztl Implantol 1993;2:244–254.
15. Pearce AI, Richards RG, Milz S, Schneider E, Pearce SG. Animal models for implant biomaterial research in bone: A review. Eur Cells Mater 2007;13:1–10.
16. Schmitz J, Hollinger J. The critical size defect as an experimental model for craniomandibular nonjunction. Clin Orthop 1986;205:299–304.
17. Burchardt H. The biology of bone graft repair. Clin Orthop Rel Res 1983;174:28–42.
18. Pallesen L, Schou S, Aaboe M, Hjørting-Hansen E, Nattestad A, Melsen F. Influence of particle size on the early stages of bone regeneration: A histologic and stereologic study in rabbit calvarium. Int J Oral Maxillofac Implants 2002;17:498–506.
19. Stenderup K, Justesen J, Clausen C, Kassem M. Aging is associated with decreased maximal life span and accelerated senescence of bone marrow stromal cells. Bone 2003;33:919–926.
20. Pinholt EM, Solheim E, Talsnes O, Larsen TB, Bang G, Kirkeby OJ. Revascularization of calvarial, mandibular, tibial, and iliac bone grafts in rats. Ann Plast Surg 1994;33:193–197.
21. De Marco AC, Jardini MA, Lima LP. Revascularization of autogenous block grafts with or without an e-PTFE membrane. Int J Oral Maxillofac Implants 2005;20:867–874.
22. Gordh M, Alberius P, Lindberg L, Johnell O. Bone graft incorporation after cortical perforations of the host bed. Otolaryngol Head Neck Surg 1997;117:664–670.
23. Widmark G, Andersson B, Ivanoff CJ. Mandibular bone graft in the anterior maxilla for single-tooth implants. Int J Oral Maxillofac Surg 1997;26:106–109.
24. Johansson B, Grepe A, Wannfors K, Hirsch JM. A clinical study of changes in the volume of bone grafts in the atrophic maxilla. Dentomaxillofac Radiol 2001;30:157–161.
25. Gordh M, Alberius P. Some basic factors essential to autogeneic nonvascularized onlay bone grafting to the craniofacial skeleton. Scand J Plast Reconstr Surg Hand Surg 1999;32:129–146.
26. Springer ING, Terheyden H, Geiss S, Härle F, Hedderich J, Acil Y. Particulated bone grafts—Effectiveness of bone cell supply. Clin Oral Implants Res 2004;15:205–212.
27. Chiapasco M, Abati S, Romeo E, Vogel G. Clinical outcome of autogenous bone blocks or guided bone regeneration with e-PTFE membranes for the reconstruction of narrow edentulous ridges. Clin Oral Implants Res 1999;10:278–288.
28. Peleg M, Garg AK, Misch CM, Mazor Z. Maxillary sinus and ridge augmentations using surface-derived autogenous bone graft. J Oral Maxillofac Surg 2004;62:1535–1544.
29. Artzi Z, Kozlovsky A, Nemcovsky CE, Weinreb M. The amount of newly formed bone in sinus grafting procedures depends on tissue depth as well as the type and residual amount of the grafted material. J Clin Periodontol 2005;32:193–199.
30. Zaffe D, D'Avenia F. A novel bone scraper for intraoral harvesting. A device for filling small bone defects. Clin Oral Implants Res 2007;18:525–533.
31. Kainulainen VS, Kainulainen TJ, Oikarinen KS, Carmicheal RP, Sandor GKB. Performance of six bone collectors designed for implant surgery. Clin Oral Implants Res 2006;17:282–287.
32. Young MPJ, Korachi M, Carter DH, Worthington H, Drucker DB. Microbial analysis of bone collected during implant surgery: A clinical and laboratory study. Clin Oral Implants Res 2001;12:95–103.
33. Etcheson AW, Miley D, Gillespie J. Osseous coagulum collected in bone traps: Potential for bacterial contamination and methods for decontamination. J Oral Implantol 2007;33:109–115.

34. Pradel W, Tenbieg P, Lauer G. Influence of harvesting technique and donor site location on in vitro growth of osteoblastlike cells from facial bone. Int J Oral Maxillofac Implants 2005;20:860–866.
35. Hjørting-Hansen E. Bone grafting to the jaws with special reference to reconstructive preprosthetic surgery. A historical review. Mund Kiefer Gesichtschir 2002;6:6–14.
36. Summers BN, Eisenstein SM. Donor site pain from the ileum. A complication of lumbar spine fusion. J Bone Joint Surg Br 1989;71:677–680.
37. Tomford WW. Bone allografts: Past, present and future. Cell Tissue Banking 2000;1:105–109.
38. Lyford RH, Mills MP, Knapp CI, Scheyer ED, Mellonig JT. Clinical evaluation of freeze-dried block allografts for alveolar ridge augmentation: A case series. Int J Periodontics Restorative Dent 2003;23:417–425.
39. Block MS, Degen M. Horizontal ridge augmentation using human mineralized particulate bone: Preliminary results. J Oral Maxillofac Surg 2004;62:67–72.
40. Reddi AH, Wientroub S, Muthukumaran N. Biologic principles of bone induction. Orthop Clin North Am 1987;18:207–212.
41. Schwartz Z, Mellonig JT, Carnes DL Jr, et al. Ability of commercial demineralized freeze-dried bone allograft to induce new bone formation. J Periodontol 1996;67:918–926.
42. Boyan BD, Ranly DM, McMillan J, Sunwoo M, Roche K, Schwartz Z. Osteoinductive ability of human allograft formulations. J Periodontol 2006;77:1555–1563.
43. Jensen SS, Aaboe M, Pinholt EM, Hjørting-Hansen E, Melsen F, Ruyter IE. Tissue reaction and material characteristics of four bone substitutes. Int J Oral Maxillofac Implants 1996;11:55–66.
44. Piecuch JF, Ponichtera A, Nikoukari H. Long-term evaluation of porous hydroxyapatite blocks for alveolar ridge augmentation. Int J Oral Maxillofac Surg 1990;19:147–150.
45. Hjørting-Hansen E, Worsaae N, Lemons JE. Histologic response after implantation of porous hydroxylapatite ceramic in humans. Int J Oral Maxillofac Implants 1990;5:255–263.
46. Ewers R. Maxilla sinus grafting with marine algae derived bone forming material: A clinical report of long-term results. J Oral Maxillofac Surg 2005;63:1712–1723.
47. Thorwarth M, Wehrhan F, Srour S, et al. Evaluation of substitutes for bone: Comparison of microradiographic and histological assessments. Br J Oral Maxillofac Surg 2007;45:41–47.
48. Schwartz Z, Weesner T, van Dijk S, et al. Ability of deproteinized cancellous bovine bone to induce new bone formation. J Periodontol 2000;71:1258–1269.
49. Wenz B, Oesch B, Horst M. Analysis of the risk of transmitting bovine spongiform encephalopathy through bone grafts derived from bovine bone. Biomaterials 2001;22:1599–1606.
50. Mellonig JT. Donor selection, testing, and inactivation of the HIV virus in freeze-dried bone allografts. Pract Periodontics Aesthet Dent 1995;7:13–22.
51. Taylor JC, Cuff SE, Leger JPL, Morra A, Anderson GI. In vitro osteoblast resorption of bone substitute biomaterials used for implant site augmentation: A pilot study. Int J Oral Maxillofac Implants 2002; 17:321–330.
52. Piattelli M, Favero GA, Scarano A, Orsini G, Piattelli A. Bone reactions to anorganic bovine bone (Bio-Oss) used in sinus augmentation procedures: A histologic long-term report of 20 cases in humans. Int J Oral Maxillofac Implants 1999;14:835–840.
53. Hämmerle CHF, Chiantella GC, Karring T, Lang NP. The effect of a deproteinized bovine bone mineral on bone regeneration around titanium dental implants. Clin Oral Implants Res 1998;9:151–162.
54. Wilson CJ, Clegg RE, Leavesley DI, Pearce MJ. Mediation of biomaterial-cell interactions by adsorbed proteins: A review. Tissue Eng 2005;11:1–18.
55. Buser D, Schenk RK, Steinemann S, Fiorellini JP, Fox CH, Stich H. Influence of surface characteristics on bone integration of titanium implants: A histomorphometric study in miniature pigs. J Biomed Mater Res 1991;25:889–902.
56. Buser D, Broggini N, Wieland M, et al. Enhanced bone apposition to a chemically modified SLA titanium surface. J Dent Res 2004;83:529–533.
57. Bagno A, Di Bello C. Surface treatments and roughness properties of Ti-based biomaterials. J Mater Sci Mater Med 2004;15:935–949.
58. Bohner M. Calcium orthophosphates in medicine: From ceramics to calcium phosphate cements. Injury 2000;31(suppl 4):37–47.
59. von Arx T, Cochran DL, Hermann JS, Schenk RK, Higginbottom FL, Buser D. Lateral ridge augmentation and implant placement: An experimental study evaluating implant osseointegration in different augmentation materials in the canine mandible. Int J Oral Maxillofac Implants 2001;16:343–354.
60. LeGeros RZ, Lin S, Rohanizadeh R, Mijares D, LeGeros JP. Biphasic calcium phosphate bioceramics: Preparation, properties and applications. J Mater Sci Mater Med 2003;14:201–209.
61. Vitale-Brovarone C, Verné E, Robiglio L, Martinasso G, Canuto RA, Muzio G. Biocompatible glass-ceramic for bone substitution. J Mater Sci Mater Med 2008;19:471–478.
62. Götz W, Gerber T, Michel B, Lossdörfer S, Henkel KO, Heinemann F. Immunohistochemical characterization of nanocrystalline hydroxyapatite silica gel (NanoBone) osteogenesis: A study on biopsies from human jaws. Clin Oral Implants Res 2008;19:1016–1026.

CHAPTER 5

Intraoral Bone Harvesting

Thomas von Arx

An important diagnostic factor in patient evaluation for dental implant placement is the amount of bone available at the desired implant location. Insertion of an endosteal implant requires sufficient bone volume for complete bone coverage to obtain optimal function and esthetics. In many instances, alveolar resorption following extraction, trauma, or pathologic conditions has resulted in a ridge form with inadequate height or width for implant placement.

Traditionally, autogenous bone grafts are considered the gold standard for reconstruction of deficient bone volumes.[1] In their early application, bone grafts were primarily measured by their ability to withstand mechanical stress. Today, bone grafts are viewed as biologic structures and are used for contouring, expanding, or changing the three-dimensional configuration of the alveolar process in patients with insufficient bone volume or osseous defects.

Although autogenous bone grafts do not produce adverse reactions, biologic properties and biocompatibility are still key factors in their use. In the past two decades, autogenous bone grafts have been challenged by bone-replacing materials, that is, bone substitutes (see chapter 4). However, autogenous bone grafts still constitute the best bone grafting system for the human body because they have biologic and mechanical properties that are unparalleled by bone substitutes. Drawbacks include the fact that the procedure for harvesting autogenous bone grafts is associated with additional surgery, costs, morbidity, and sequelae.

The professional using bone grafts should be adept in harvesting, placing, and assessing the final outcome of the bone graft. A careful evaluation of the host site is the primary step in determining the need for and extent of the grafting procedure and what type of bone graft is required. The second step includes a thorough clinical and radiographic assessment of possible donor sites to determine which is most appropriate in terms of bone quality and quantity.

Intraoral bone harvesting usually can be accomplished under local anesthesia (with or without sedation) in a routine dental office setting or on a hospital outpatient basis. This option helps not only to minimize the patient's costs for procedures that are frequently not covered by insurance but also to lessen the patient's perception of the complexity of the procedure.[2] The advantages of intraoral donor sites are their convenient surgical access and the close proximity of donor and recipient sites, both of which reduce operative time. The disadvantages of intraoral donor sites include

Box 5-1 Characteristics of bone grafts

Cortical bone grafts
- Have compact architecture
- Are less likely to be revascularized, to be incorporated, and to become viable than cancellous bone grafts
- Require proper fixation
- Are used primarily in areas with mechanical stress
- Have high risk of sequestration in contaminated area

Cancellous bone grafts
- Have spongy, trabecular architecture
- Are excellent for achieving fusion
- Result in fast and complete revascularization
- Result in new bone formation (regeneration, remodeling, and substitution)
- Can be used in clean-contaminated wounds

the limited amount of bone available and possible complications, such as donor site morbidity, infection, or neurosensory disturbances.

Intraorally harvested bone grafts have been used for a variety of surgical procedures, including periodontal surgery, grafting of cystic defects, reconstruction of alveolar clefts, maxillofacial orthognathic surgery, and malar augmentation. This chapter will focus on intraoral bone graft harvesting in conjunction with guided bone regeneration and implant dentistry.

Types of Bone Grafts

Autogenous bone grafts can be characterized by their biologic effect, their composition, or their embryologic origin. However, the embryologic aspect has lost importance with regard to choice and usage of autogenous bone grafts. Bone graft healing is now believed to be primarily determined by the degree of revascularization that takes place.[3] The less compact the bone graft, the more rapid the revascularization and healing. The more compact the bone graft, the less the chance of complete and rapid revascularization. The degree of revascularization is also related to the stimuli in surrounding tissue that allow vessels to start budding into the grafts.

Bone blocks, particulate bone, bone chips, and bone slurry are the four types of nonvascularized bone grafts. The characteristics of cortical and cancellous bone are summarized in Box 5-1.

Block grafts

Autogenous block grafts can be monocortical, corticocancellous (Fig 5-1a), or bicortical. These types of grafts are usually harvested from the mandible (symphysis or ramus). In implant dentistry, intraorally harvested block grafts are mainly used for lateral ridge augmentation prior to implant placement in a staged approach (Fig 5-1b). Other indications

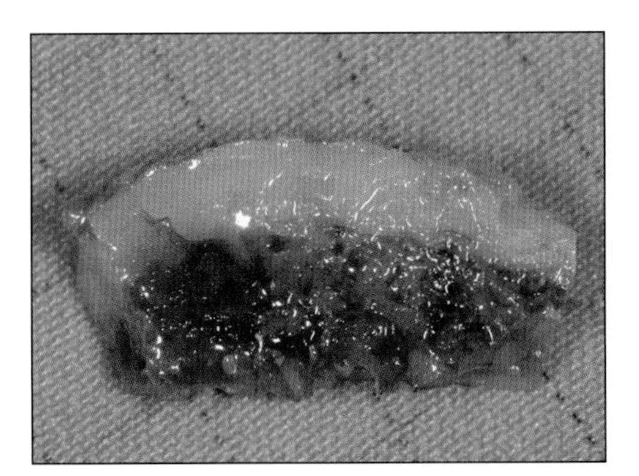

Fig 5-1a Corticocancellous block graft (length 15 mm; depth 6 mm) that was harvested in the mandibular symphysis.

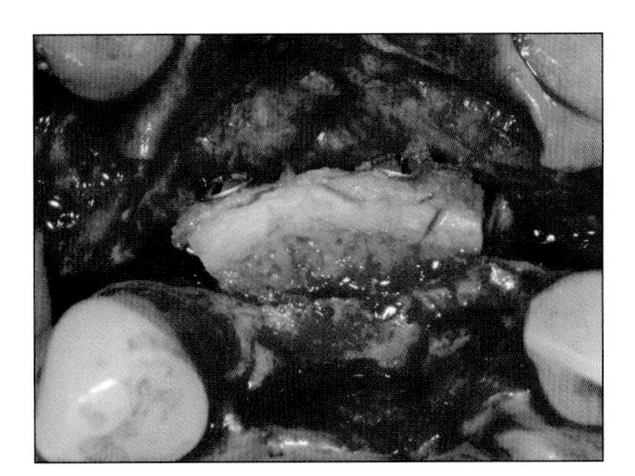

Fig 5-1b Autogenous block graft positioned and secured with two fixation screws for lateral ridge augmentation in the right anterior maxilla.

include vertical or combined lateral and vertical ridge augmentation. Simultaneous application of block grafts and implant placement is not common because of the limitations of block graft revascularization.

Block grafts must be secured with proper fixation to the host site. It is recommended that the necessary holes for the graft's fixation screws be drilled after block graft mobilization but before removal from the donor location to prevent fracture of the block. This requires detailed examination of the defect site so that the fixation points can be predicted.[4]

Veneer grafts

These grafts are mainly composed of cortical bone, are thinner than block grafts, and are harvested from the retromolar area in the mandible. Veneer grafts can also be prepared in the zygomaticomaxillary buttress (as described later in the chapter). Similar to block grafts, veneer grafts should be stabilized with screw fixation. Veneer grafts are mainly indicated for contour augmentation, for example, in the esthetic zone.

Particulate bone

Particulate bone is formed by dividing larger bone grafts or bone blocks into smaller particles (of 1 to 2 mm) by means of a bone mill or rongeurs[4,5] (Fig 5-2). The particles are usually applied in an area where there is no need for mechanical strength, such as in voids between block grafts and the recipient bed, in peri-implant bone defects, or in sinus floor elevation procedures. Particulate bone may also be used with a bone substitute to form a composite graft.

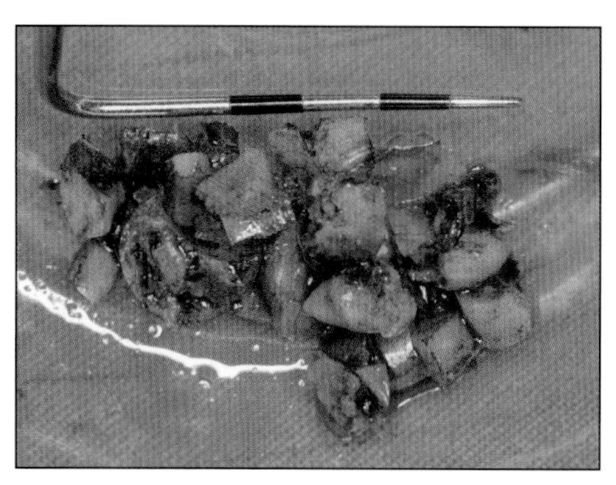

Fig 5-2a Large bone particles harvested with trephines in the mandibular symphysis (particle size of 3 to 6 mm).

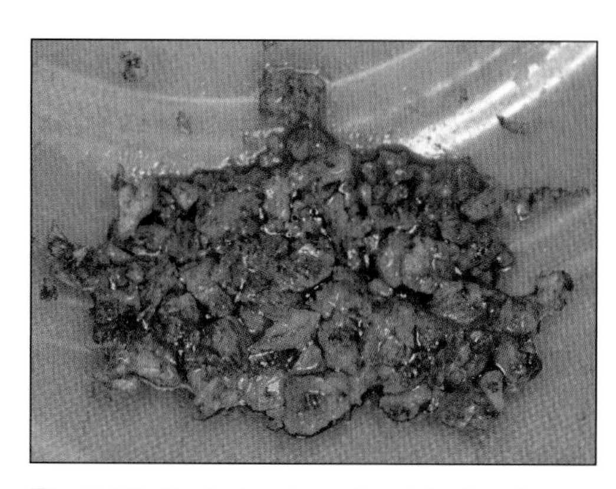

Fig 5-2b Particulate bone (particle size of 1 to 2 mm) following grinding of the larger bone grafts with a bone mill.

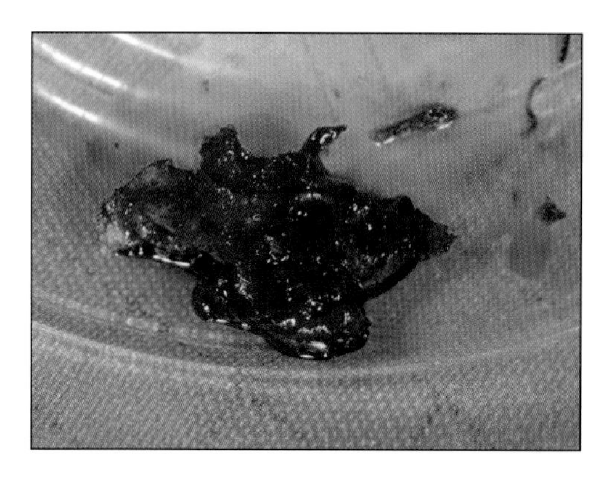

Fig 5-3 Bone chips (shavings) obtained from cortical bone surfaces utilizing a handheld bone scraper.

Bone chips

The differences between particulate bone and bone chips are the harvesting technique and the size of the particles. Bone chips (250 µm to 1 mm) are smaller than particulate bone (Fig 5-3). They are normally harvested with scrapers or chisels from cortical bone surfaces and less frequently with surgical curettes or spoons from cancellous bone compartments.

Again, bone chips do not provide mechanical strength but yield a large surface-volume ratio to enhance bone deposition (osteoconductivity). If they are of cancellous origin, they will promote new bone formation (osteoinduction and osteogenesis) to a markedly greater degree than will cortical chips. It has been shown that unmilled spongy bone chips offer greater amounts of viable osteoblasts than does milled cortical bone or drill sludge.[6,7]

Bone chips planed off the cortical surface form narrow, ribbonlike shavings. The shavings are collected without the use of suction, greatly decreasing the chance of graft contamination and avoiding graft desiccation. The potential for cell survival is also enhanced by the minimal cutting temperatures generated with a handheld instrument.[2] As the bone is harvested, blood from the cut bone surface is passively collected and mixed with the bone to form a moldable matrix. This matrix has a mortarlike consistency that enables it to be easily handled and positioned. It can be molded with any flat surface instrument. The high porosity enables the graft to be revascularized much more rapidly than cortical blocks, similar to particulate preparations. Success rates are likely so high because of the high surface area of the bone graft.[2]

Bone slurry

Bone dust or slurry is typically obtained during drilling of cortical or corticocancellous bone, for example, during preparation of the implant bed. Bone slurry is a mixture of small debris of bone in the range of 100 to 250 μm. The histologic composition of bone collected with a bone trap was shown to be affected by pore size.[8] Savant and coworkers[9] determined the amount of bone harvested from implant bed preparations using an inline bone collector. The mean volume was 0.195 mL from a site approximately 4 × 13 mm.

The technique of collecting bone slurry using bone collectors has recently been questioned because such bone debris is always contaminated by bacteria.[10,11] The other concern is the quality of the bone dust. Studies have shown that less osteogenic cell proliferation and differentiation take place in bone slurry than in cortical bone chips or cancellous bone.[6,7,12] For both reasons—that is, risk of bacterial contamination and reduced osteogenic potential—bone slurry or bone drill dust is considered a less ideal grafting material and should be used with caution.[9]

Harvesting Techniques

Intraoral autogenous bone grafts can be harvested with handheld instruments or with machine-driven (rotating or oscillating) instruments.

Handheld instruments

Handheld instruments commonly used for bone harvesting include chisels (or osteotomes) and bone scrapers. The former have a long history of use in maxillofacial bone surgery, whereas the latter have recently been introduced for bone grafting in conjunction with implant dentistry.

Chisels, with either a flat or curved working end, are available in different sizes (Fig 5-4). They can be used with a pushing action (shoveling technique) or with a mallet (carving technique). Caution must be exercised when the mallet is used because of applied forces and risk of injury to adjacent anatomic structures. Chisels are best used to harvest larger cortical bone chips or to collect spongy bone from the cancellous bone compartment once the cortex has been removed. Similarly, surgical curettes or spoons can be used to collect spongy bone.

In contrast, bone scrapers have been developed to harvest small to medium bone chips (shavings) from cortical bone surfaces (Fig 5-5). Abundant bone surfaces are

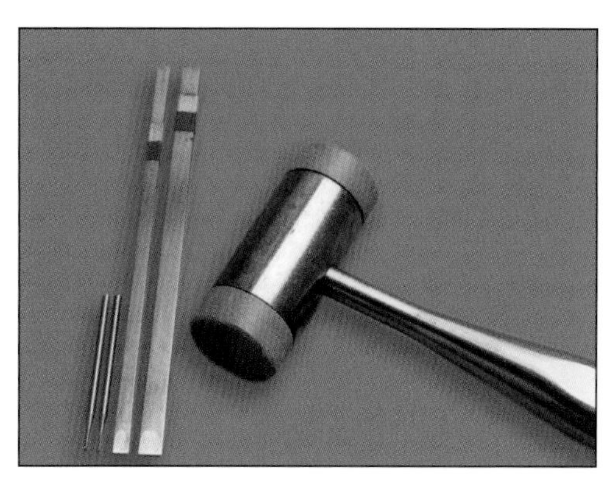

Fig 5-4 *(left to right)* Round and fissure burs; chisels with sharp, straight working ends in two sizes (4 and 6 mm); and a mallet.

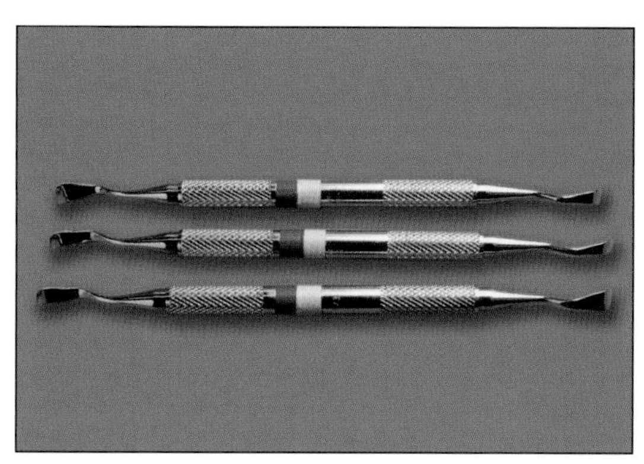

Fig 5-5 Handheld bone scrapers in various double-ended configurations (*top to bottom*: 3 and 5 mm, 4 and 5 mm, and 4 and 6 mm).

available as donor sites in the maxillofacial region, such as the posterior mandibular body, the anterior and lateral walls of the maxilla, and the zygomaticomaxillary buttress. Bone scrapers are either disposable (they have an extremely sharp blade, and the bone chips are directly collected in a protective compartment) or they can be sterilized for reuse but must be resharpened accordingly.

Collected bone chips have been measured at up to 5 mm in length and about 100 µm in thickness.[13] Histologic analysis of cortical bone chips collected with a handheld instrument has shown that most chips contain living cells, and haversian canals with living osteoblasts and stromal cells can occasionally be observed inside the chips. The mean viability of osteocytes ranges from 45% to 70%.[13] In one study,[2] the volume of a surface-derived autogenous bone graft harvested with a handheld instrument was reported to range from 1 to 5 mL, and no nerve injuries, dental injuries, or tears of the sinus membrane were noted. In that study, all donor sites (lateral aspect of mandibular body, anterior maxillary wall, zygomaticomaxillary buttress, and tuberosity) healed without complications.

Rotating instruments

This group of instruments includes burs, trephines, and saw disks. A traditional and easy method of block graft harvesting is the use of a small round bur to outline the size of the block. Drill holes are subsequently connected with a fissure bur.[14] This technique is relatively straightforward and allows the shape of the bone block to be customized. Disadvantages of rotating instruments include the loss of bone during cutting (determined by the diameter of the burs), possible impingement on adjacent soft tissue (laceration or burns), and restricted access to the surgical site (positioning of the handpiece). Attention must be paid to adequate cooling to prevent overheating of the bone structure.

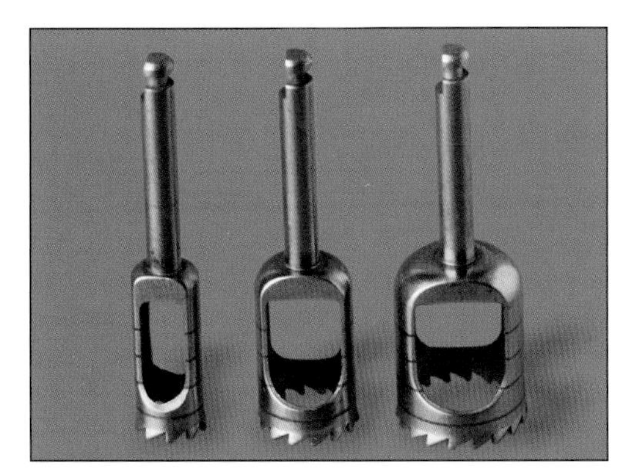

Fig 5-6a Bone trephines with three different diameters (*left to right*: 4, 6, and 8 mm) and depth markings.

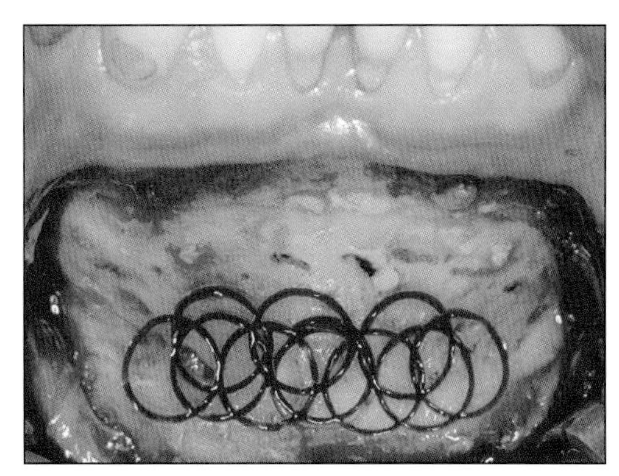

Fig 5-6b Overlapped drilling of the trephines for ease of bone graft removal.

Bone trephines (Fig 5-6a) can be used for procurement of bone cylinder blocks with a defined diameter. Because of the size of trephines, access can be problematic (positioning of the handpiece), and cooling of the instrument is paramount to avoid bone necrosis. The trephine technique has also been recommended for cases in which particulate bone is needed.[4,14] Drilling with the trephines is overlapped for ease of bone graft removal (Fig 5-6b). These grafts are subsequently particulated with a bone mill.

Saw disks have also been developed for bone block cutting.[15] When such a device is used, it is of the utmost importance to avoid damage to adjacent soft tissues, and positioning of the disk can be problematic when access is restricted. Because of the fine cutting lines that are created, the removal of the bone block can be challenging.

Oscillating instruments

Oscillating instruments used for bone harvesting include motor-driven or piezoelectric instruments. The former use a special handpiece with a helically reciprocating motion that is converted to a smooth linear movement. Various inserts are available for bone cutting and shaping. The instruments are claimed to be minimally invasive to adjacent soft tissues. However, this technique has not gained wide acceptance for bone harvesting.

In contrast, piezoelectric surgery has dramatically changed the approach to intraoral bone harvesting in the last decade. Piezoelectric surgery systems use a modulated ultrasonic frequency (29 kHz) that permits precise and safe cutting of hard tissues. Bone cuts are accurate and controlled tactilely (Figs 5-7a to 5-7c), and surgical access in the deep oral cavity is easier (Fig 5-7d) than it is when surgical burs are used.[16–18] A variety of inserts allow bone cutting for block harvesting, bone splitting, and bone preparation or bone scraping for chip harvesting (Fig 5-7e).

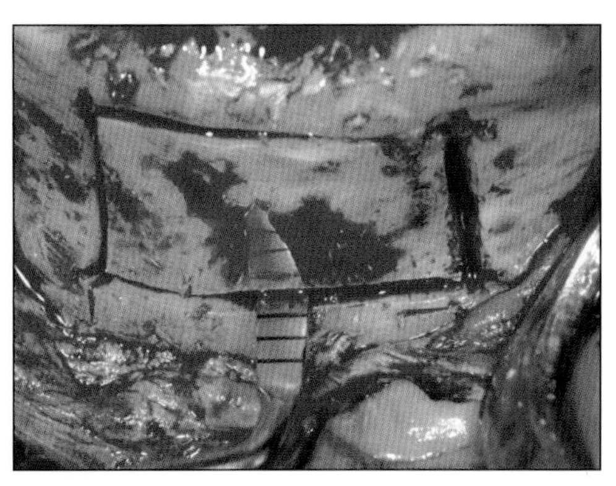

Fig 5-7a Precise and fast bone cutting with piezoelectric surgery. The depth of cuts can be easily controlled using the markings on the inserts.

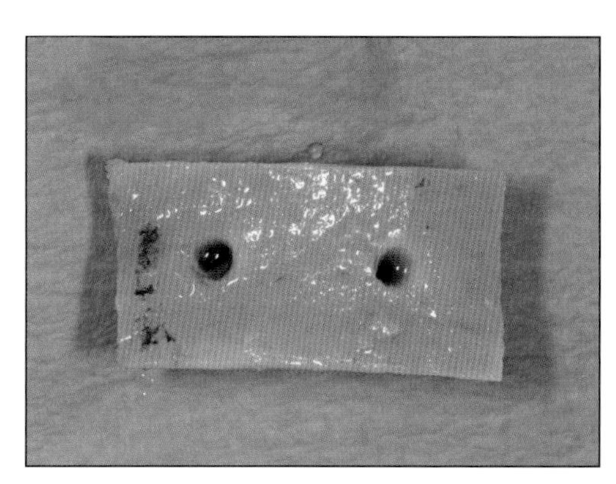

Fig 5-7b Bone block harvested from the symphysis and prepared using piezoelectric surgery.

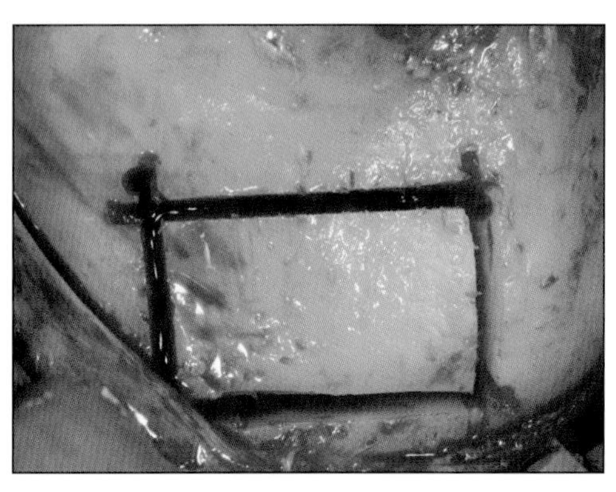

Fig 5-7c Special attention must be paid to the corners when piezoelectric surgery is used for cutting bone blocks.

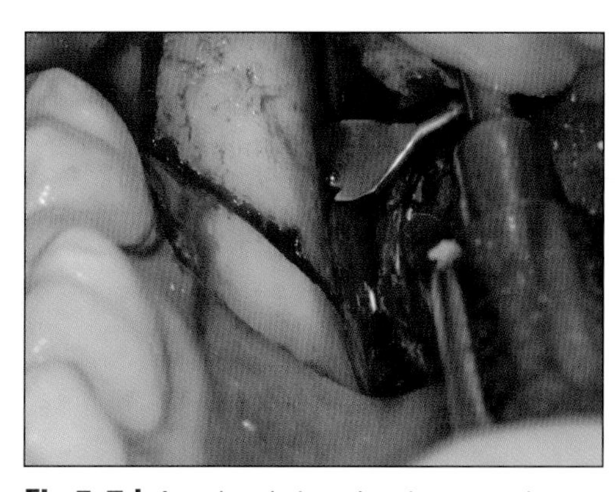

Fig 5-7d Angulated piezoelectric surgery inserts used to simplify the inferior horizontal bone cut when surgical access is limited, such as in the ramus area.

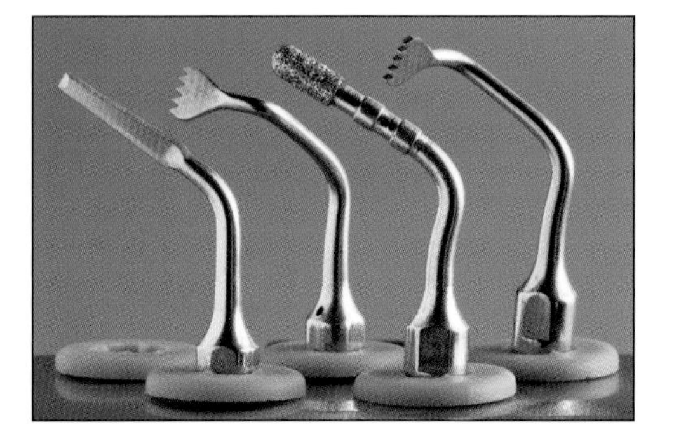

Fig 5-7e Selection of inserts to be mounted on a piezoelectric surgery handpiece.

The device causes little or no soft tissue trauma during intraoral bone harvesting because nerves, vessels, and mucosa are not injured by the microvibrations. The surgical site remains virtually blood-free because of the physical phenomenon of cavitation. Present scientific data demonstrate that bone in defects created with an ultrasonic device regenerates similarly to or even better than bone in defects made with rotary instruments.[19–21]

Infection Control

Oral surgery is considered a clean-contaminated operative procedure because the intraoral surgical access inevitably entails contamination of the surgical wound with the facultative pathogenic mixed flora of the oral cavity.[22] The efficacy of prophylactic antibiotic administration in reconstructive surgery with autogenous bone grafts is largely unstudied, and most oral and maxillofacial surgeons prescribe prolonged antibiotic administration for 5 to 10 days after these procedures.

In a randomized clinical trial, Lindeboom and van den Akker[22] showed that the administration of 2 g of penicillin (phenethicillin) orally 1 hour preoperatively prevented infection of the retromolar donor site for block grafts, whereas 30% of patients with placebo developed an infection. In a subsequent study, the same group evaluated two different antibiotics for infection control (a single oral dose of 600 mg of clindamycin or 2 g of penicillin [phenethicillin] 1 hour preoperatively).[23] Block-shaped bone grafts were obtained from the retromolar area. Infection at the donor site occurred in 3 of 75 patients (4%) in both groups. No side effects were reported for the single antibiotic prophylactic administration.

In a study by Lindeboom and coworkers,[24] infection rates following a single dose of clindamycin (600 mg administered orally 1 hour preoperatively) were compared to rates following a 24-hour clindamycin regimen (600 mg administered orally 1 hour preoperatively and 300 mg administered orally every 6 hours postoperatively for 24 hours). No significant difference was found between the two regimens (6.4% versus 3.2% infection rate at donor sites). All three of the studies appear to support the efficacy of single-dose, preoperative antibiotic administration for bone block harvesting procedures.

Intraoral Donor Sites

Intraoral donor sites include the maxilla, mandible, and zygoma. The criteria for donor site selection should be based on the following factors: the type and volume of bone needed (extension of defect), the access and anatomy of the donor site, the time required for the harvesting procedure, the costs, the surgical risks and possible sequelae, and the compliance of the patient.[25]

If only a small amount of bone chips is required, grafts can usually be harvested with the use of bone scrapers in the vicinity of the implant site. In the anterior maxilla (esthetic zone), the anterior nasal spine (Fig 5-8) and the canine fossa (Fig 5-9) are additional donor sites for harvesting cortical bone chips. If a palatal flap has been reflected, bone chips can also be collected from the palatal cortex (Fig 5-10). In the posterior maxillary zone, typical donor sites include the tuberosity[26] and the zygomaticomaxillary buttress. The use of the cortical surface as a source of graft material greatly increases the number of intraoral sites available for harvesting bone.

Many intraoral sites are accessed through relatively small incisions in the subperiosteal plane that are developed into mucoperiosteal flaps that can be raised eas-

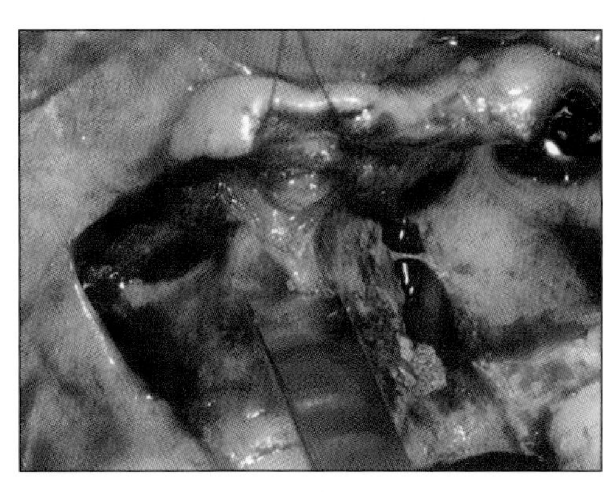

Fig 5-8 Chisel with a straight working end used to harvest bone chips from the anterior nasal spine.

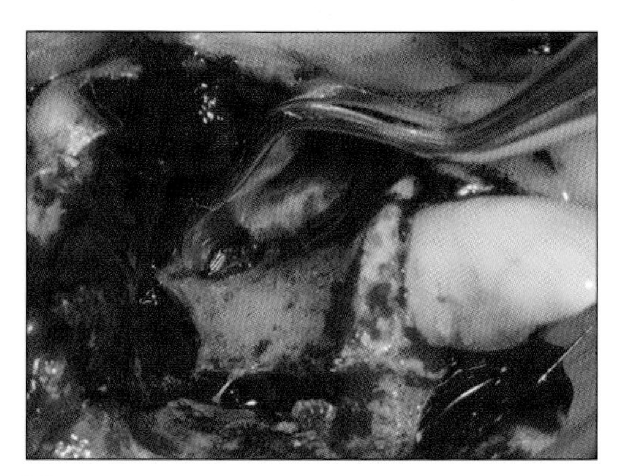

Fig 5-9 Bone chips harvested with a bone scraper from the cortical surface of the canine fossa area lateral to the piriform aperture.

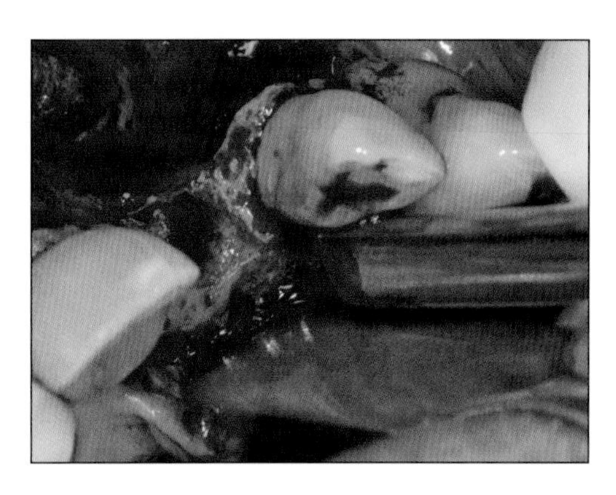

Fig 5-10 Chisel with a curved working end used to carve bone chips from the anterior palatal cortex.

ily and safely to expose large surfaces of bone. Such sites are not constrained by concerns of deeper elements, such as tooth roots and neurovascular structures. Furthermore, patient morbidity is minimized if only a small thickness of bone is removed from the donor bone surface.[2]

The zygomaticomaxillary buttress has recently generated interest for the harvesting of bone grafts using an intraoral approach. However, only limited information is available about this donor site, including case reports,[27–30] one ex vivo study,[31] and one clinical study.[32] Advantages of the zygoma donor site include good access and visibility, the convex surface morphology of the graft, the presence of adequate volume to reconstruct an osseous defect of up to two teeth, and low postsurgical morbidity. Future clinical studies are needed to evaluate this promising intraoral donor site. Recent case reports[29,30] have pointed to the beneficial effect of using piezoelectric surgery for bone harvesting in the zygoma region because of a reduction in the risk of sinus membrane perforation.

Smaller cortical bone blocks have also been harvested from the lingual aspect of the mandible, for example through the removal of mandibular tori. No donor site complications have been reported.[33,34] However, when larger block grafts are needed, common intraoral donor sites include the symphysis (chin area) and the ramus (retromolar area).

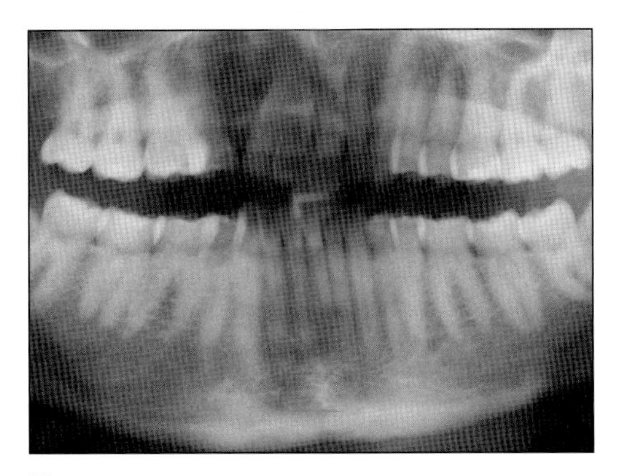

Fig 5-11a A panoramic radiograph of a 30-year-old patient used to assess the mandibular symphysis for bone harvesting.

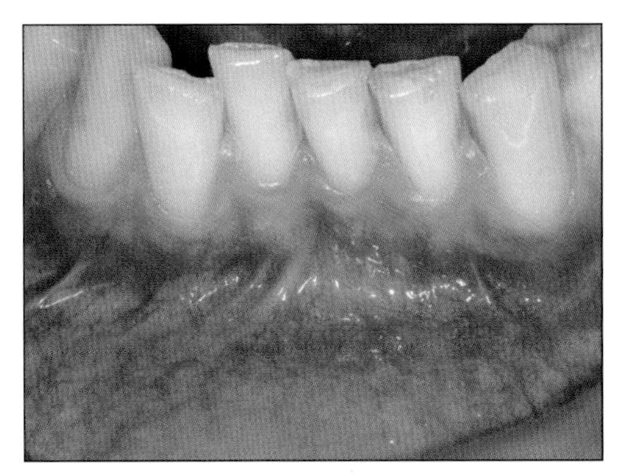

Fig 5-11b The clinical appearance of the anterior mandible shows short attached gingiva but a relatively high vestibule.

Symphysis (chin area)

Symphysis graft procedures are being performed in clinical practice more frequently than ever before. Convenient surgical access, the proximity of donor and recipient sites, the availability of larger quantities of cortical and cancellous bone in comparison with other intraoral donor sites, minimal resorption, and the avoidance of hospitalization are the main advantages of this procedure.

A radiographic and clinical examination of the symphysis is necessary to determine whether enough hard tissue exists to supply the deficient ridge (Figs 5-11a and 5-11b). The symphysis can provide adequate bone to augment an area that had been occupied by up to six teeth.[35] However, it will never offer a quantity sufficient to augment an entire arch.

The amount of bone graft material present in the mandibular symphysis has been quantified by water displacement volumetry.[36] The mean volume, including bilateral bone blocks, was 4.8 mL (range of 3.3 to 6.5 mL). The average block size measured 21.0 × 10.0 × 7.0 mm.

These dimensions can be confirmed with data from anatomical studies. The mean distance from the mental foramen to the mandibular midline has been reported to be 24 mm.[37,38] The mean height of the mandible from its lower border to the apices of the mandibular incisors has been calculated to be 20.0 mm.[39,40] With a safety margin of 5.0 mm around the bone graft, separating it from the adjacent anatomical landmarks, the mean length of a unilateral block graft would be 19.0 mm and the mean height would be 10.0 mm. With regard to the depth of the graft, the mean cortical thickness in the anterior mandible ranges from 1.3 to 2.4 mm (becoming thicker from the superior to the inferior aspects), and the mean trabecular bone thickness ranges from 3.3 to 6.8 mm (being greatest in the lower third of the mandible).[41,42] A comparison revealed that chin block bone grafts contain 69.3% bone, while chin particulate bone grafts contain 62.6% bone.[43]

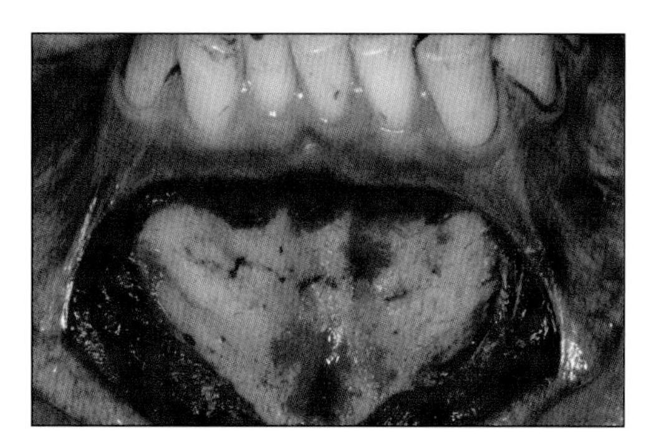

Fig 5-11c A semilunar incision is made below the mucogingival line. The incision is not extended beyond the distal aspects of the canine teeth. The approximate location of the adjacent apices has been marked with a sterile marker.

Table 5-1 Characteristics of different incision designs for symphysis harvesting procedures

Incision	Advantages	Disadvantages
Alveolar mucosa incision	Flap elevation Prevention of gingival recession Easier suturing	More bleeding Risk of dehiscence Scarring
Intrasulcular incision	Less bleeding Lower risk of dehiscence	Crestal bone loss Gingival recession More difficult suturing
Attached gingiva incision (submarginal incision)	Minimal trauma to marginal tissues Easier suturing	Scarring Risk of dehiscence

When the incision design for symphysis graft procedures is planned, the following clinical findings should be assessed: the periodontal status (probing depth, level of gingival margin, and calculated clinical attachment level), the risk of root fenestration, the amount of attached gingiva, the presence of restoration margins at the gingival level, the depth of the vestibule, and the mentalis posture.

Three different types of incision have been described for symphysis graft procedures[44]: an incision in the alveolar mucosa, a submarginal incision of attached gingiva, and an intrasulcular incision of the attachment apparatus. A vestibular approach below the mucogingival junction permits easier access but produces more soft tissue bleeding and intraoral scar formation (Fig 5-11c). With the intrasulcular incision, the anatomy of the papillae makes reapproximation of the wound edges less than ideal[45] and poses a greater risk for facial gingival recession than other incision designs.[46] Some of the complications of the intrasulcular incision can be avoided through the use of the attached gingiva (submarginal) incision. However, caution must be exercised when a submarginal incision is used in patients with limited width of attached gingiva.

The characteristics of the different incision techniques are summarized in Table 5-1. With regard to the use of distal vertical or oblique relieving incisions, limiting the distal extent of incisions within the canine areas has considerably reduced the incidence of mental nerve paresthesia.[14,47]

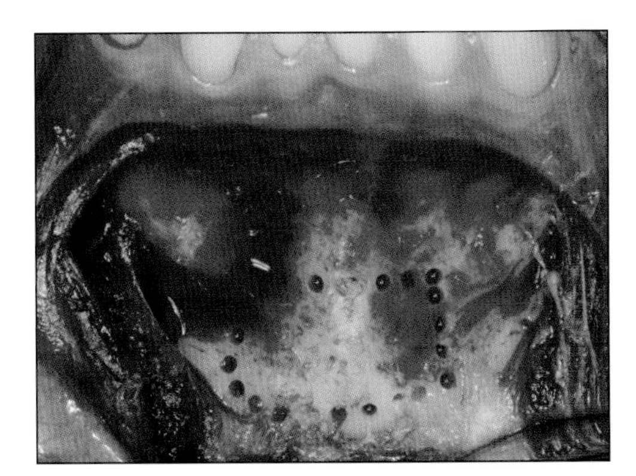

Fig 5-11d A small round bur has been used to outline the dimensions of the desired block graft.

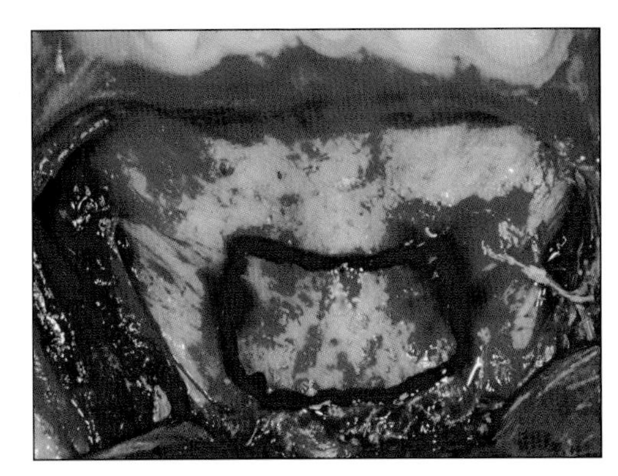

Fig 5-11e Drill holes have been connected by means of a fissure bur to complete the bone cutting.

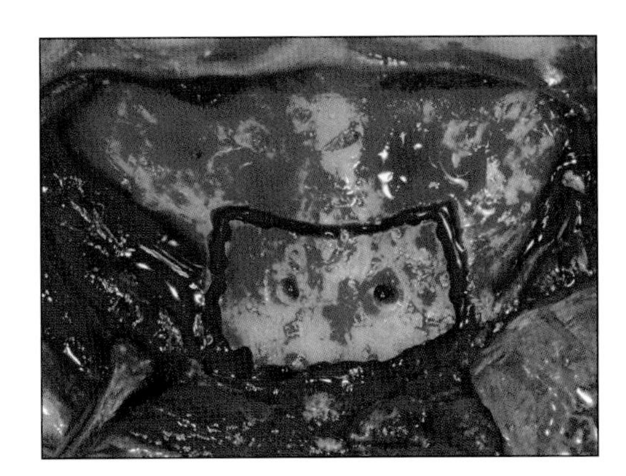

Fig 5-11f Following mobilization of the block graft, two holes have been drilled using special twist drills.

Technique

A full mucoperiosteal flap is elevated to expose the symphysis. Wet gauze (2 × 2 cm) can be applied with finger pressure to aid in the elevation of the flap. Complete "degloving" of the mandible and of the mentalis muscle should be avoided to prevent chin ptosis resulting from loss of muscular tone or labial mental fold irregularities.[48] A sterile marker is used to indicate the level of the apices of the mandibular anterior teeth and to outline the shape of the graft. In case of a block graft harvesting procedure, bone cutting is performed under copious irrigation with sterile saline at 4°C (Figs 5-11d and 5-11e). The maximum depth of bone cutting should not exceed 5 to 7 mm to leave the lingual cortex intact.

The block is mobilized with a flat chisel, preferably placed within the vertical bone cuts; inserting the chisel within the upper and lower cuts is not recommended because it may damage adjacent roots or the inferior border of the mandible. The bone block is levered by means of the chisels to disrupt the cancellous connection. If mobilization of the block is difficult, it is important to redefine the borders with the chisel, piezo insert, or bur, paying special attention to the corners. The block is not removed until the holes for the fixation screws have been drilled (Fig 5-11f).

Following removal of the bone block, additional cancellous bone may be harvested from the cancellous compartment. However, minimization of cancellous bone har-

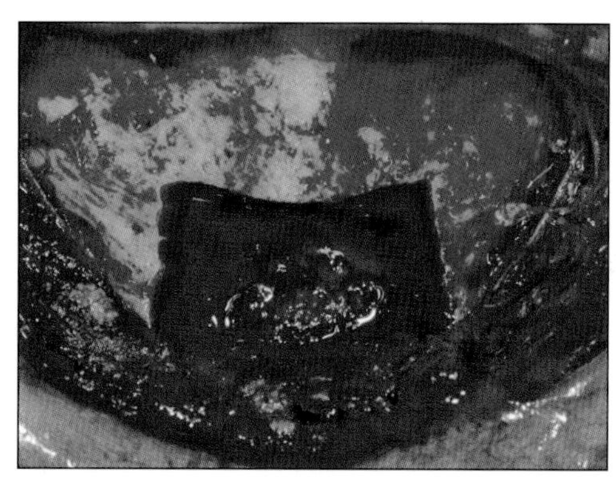

Fig 5-11g The symphyseal donor site is shown after removal of the block graft.

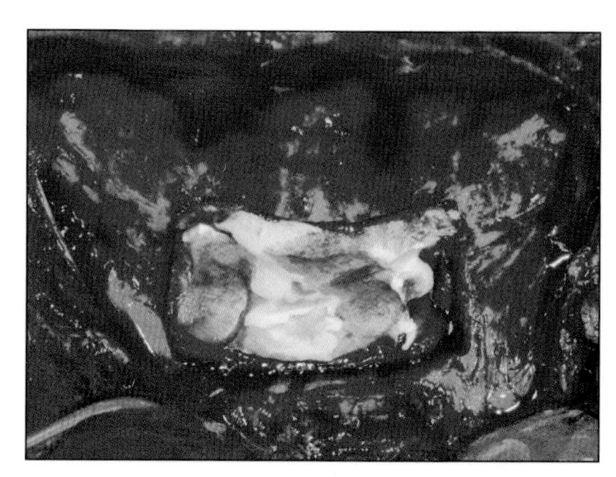

Fig 5-11h The bone defect of the donor site is packed with collagen fleece.

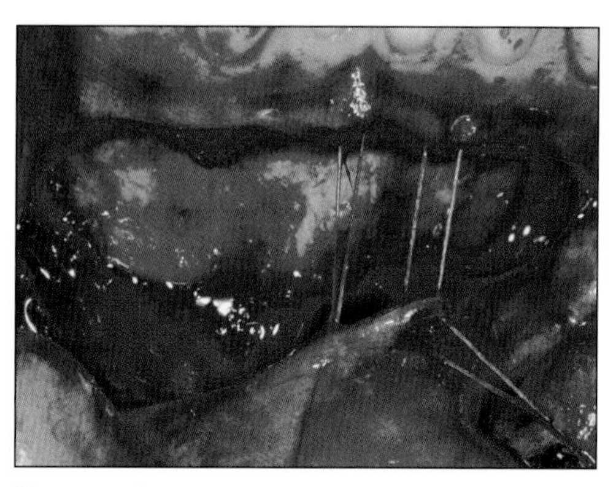

Fig 5-11i A resorbable suture material is used for this type of wound closure.

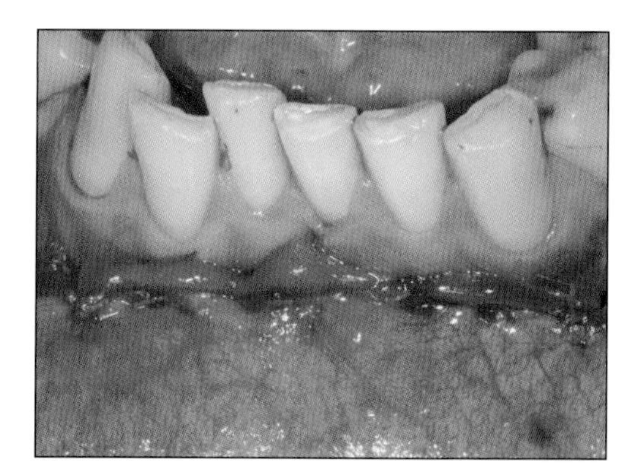

Fig 5-11j Watertight wound closure is accomplished with multiple horizontally placed mattress sutures.

vesting and the avoidance of deep cutting are highly recommended because postoperative paresthesia is the possible result if these limits are exceeded.[4] Once the bone graft has been harvested, the donor site can be filled with a hemostatic agent (collagen fleece) or with a bone substitute with or without a resorbable membrane (Figs 5-11g and 5-11h). The donor site is sutured either with horizontal mattress sutures (Figs 5-11i and 5-11j) or with a two-layer technique that consists of internal (periosteum and muscle layers) and external (mucosa) suturing. Careful and tension-free wound closure is important to avoid dehiscence of wound margins.

Swelling and tension can be controlled by one-time steroid therapy, extraoral pressure dressing (tape), and cold application for 2 to 3 days. A postoperative radiograph should be taken to assess the baseline situation at the donor and recipient sites (Fig 5-11k). During follow-up sessions, the healing is further monitored (Figs 5-11l and 5-11m).

Complications

Ptosis of the chin and lip incompetence are worrisome complications of surgery in the mandibular symphyseal region. The mentalis muscle controls the posture of the chin.

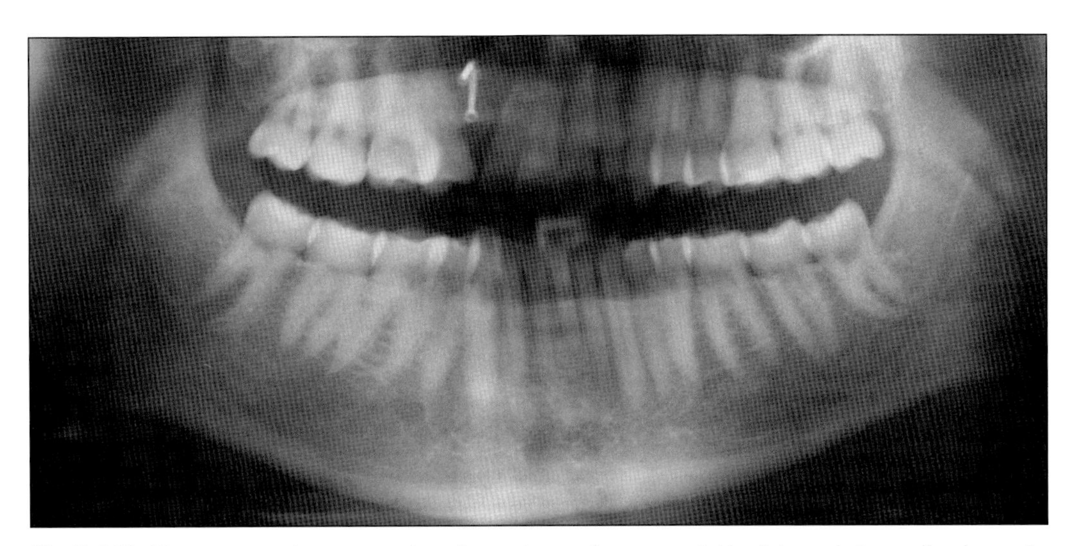

Fig 5-11k The postoperative panoramic radiograph reveals an acceptable distance between the donor site defect and the adjacent anatomic structures (apices, mental foramina, and inferior border of mandible).

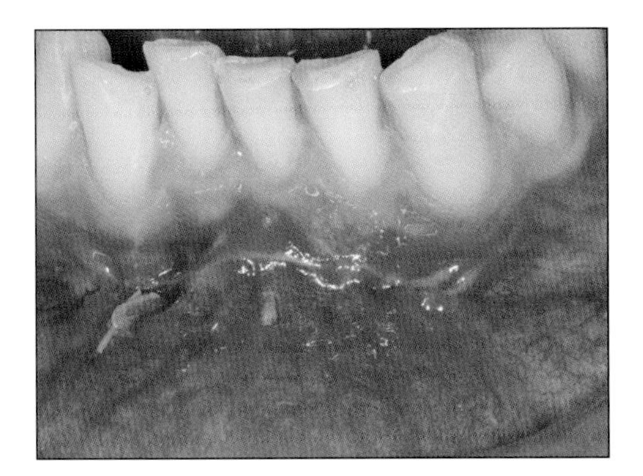

Fig 5-11l Four weeks after surgery, a scar is visible in the vestibule.

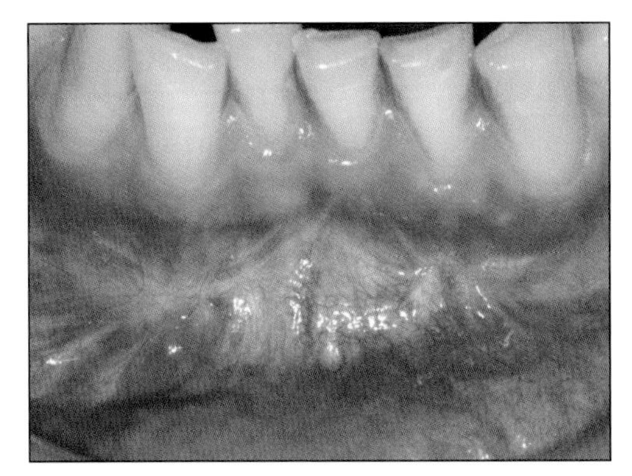

Fig 5-11m At the 14-month follow-up, resolution of the scar is nearly complete.

Muscle fibers originate from an oval area of bone, opposite the roots of the incisors, on the anterior surface of the mandibular symphysis. The fibers of the mentalis muscle fan out in three basic directions and penetrate the integument of the skin. There is always a risk of chin ptosis when the origin of the mentalis muscle is stripped from bone.[49] When surgery is performed in the chin region, it is best to avoid a complete degloving.[50]

Ramus (retromolar area)

Indications for the mandibular ramus as a donor site include localized moderate to severe alveolar atrophy or a bone defect involving a one- to four-tooth edentulous span.[51] The bone harvested from this area is well suited for use as a veneer graft to gain additional ridge width. The anatomical proximity makes the ramus the site of choice for augmentation of the thin posterior mandible.[51] The anatomical limits of the ramus include the coronoid process, the molar teeth, the mandibular canal, and the width of the posterior mandible. Grafts may also be taken from the buccal aspects of the most distal molars when the thickness of the buccal plate, or linea obliqua, allows it.[52]

A panoramic radiograph is essential for evaluating the posterior mandible as a donor site. Nkenke and coworkers[53] calculated a mean bone height of 11 mm (range of 7 to 15 mm) above the mandibular canal by assessing panoramic radiographs. The same authors also intraoperatively measured the width of the retromolar area, which ranged from 10 to 17 mm (average of 14 mm). Similar measurements were reported previously.[54] However, anatomical trials have shown that the mandibular base is, on average, 5 mm smaller than the alveolar shelf.[54] If the mandibular canal is radiographically positioned close or superior to the external oblique ridge, or if the ramus is less than 10 mm wide, other donor sites should be considered.[51]

To fully appreciate the posterior mandibular donor site, it is important to differentiate the mandibular body from the mandibular ramus.[55] The mandibular body, or the buccal shelf, is the more anterior harvest site located lateral to the first and second mandibular molars. It allows harvesting of up to 25 mm of monocortical bone without affecting the viability of the existing teeth.[55] The mandibular ramus is the proximal extension of this harvest site. The mandibular ramus harvest site is at its thickest at the junction of the ramus and body.

The following mean volumes of block grafts from the ramus have been reported: 0.9 cm^3 for grafts harvested with round and fissure burs in a straight handpiece,[47] 1.15 cm^3 for grafts obtained with piezoelectric surgery,[52] and 1.7 cm^3 for grafts harvested by means of diamond saws. The morphology of block grafts obtained from the ramus was found to be more cortical, while the morphology of grafts from the symphysis was more corticocancellous.[47,52,56]

Technique

An incision similar to that used for removal of an impacted mandibular third molar is made. The incision starts 1 cm lateral and superior to the retromolar pad, continues anteriorly, and makes a 45-degree turn through the lateral third of the retromolar pad. If teeth are present, the incision proceeds anteriorly around the facial sulcus of the teeth. Capelli[57] described three different incision designs for surgical access to the mandibular ramus area: *(1)* an intrasulcular incision starting from the distal line angle of the second premolar and extending posteriorly lateral to the retromolar pad and medial to the external oblique ridge; *(2)* a submarginal incision along the mucogingival line, with posterior extension similar to that of the intrasulcular incision; and *(3)* a crestal incision in edentulous ridges or when implants are planned in the same edentulous crest.

A full-thickness mucoperiosteal flap is elevated to expose the lateral body of the mandible, the retromolar area of bone, and the external oblique ridge of the ascending ramus.[58] Bone grafts can be harvested with drills, trephines, or piezoelectric surgery. The use of a piezoelectric surgical device for bone harvesting in the ramus area is an interesting option to further reduce soft tissue trauma when the site is accessed because it minimizes damage to the neurovascular bundle and simplifies the lower horizontal bone cut through the use of angulated inserts.[52]

Box 5-2 Surgical sequelae and complications of bone harvesting

Normal surgical sequelae	Minor complications	Severe complications
• Swelling • Ecchymosis or bruising • Pain (less than 1 week)	• Hematoma • Wound dehiscence	• Profuse and continuous bleeding • Infection • Altered sensitivity (teeth, mucosa, or skin)

The block graft is gently detached with a chisel to prevent damage to the underlying lingual nerve. A mallet should not be used, and the chisel should not be placed into the lingual cut). If the screw hole is being drilled in situ, the drilling must be performed cautiously to avoid damage to the inferior alveolar nerve. Alternatively, the screw hole can be prepared extraorally. The block is lifted carefully to ensure that the inferior alveolar nerve is not trapped within the graft.

Access to the ramus and visibility may be limited in patients with restricted jaw opening or temporomandibular joint dysfunction. To increase acceptance of the procedure by the patient, the harvesting procedure for retromolar grafts can be performed in conjunction with removal of a mandibular third molar.[48,59] Compared to harvesting from the chin bone, the suggestion of harvesting from the retromolar region was accepted with significantly greater frequency when the third molar was removed as part of the procedure.[48] Care should be exercised when the tooth is removed after graft harvesting because the removal of a large portion of the cortex can structurally weaken the jaw in this area. The patient must be informed about the potential weakness and the consequent predisposition to fracture in this area.

Management of the retromolar donor site is similar to management in the chin area. Harvesting of additional cancellous bone with blunt instruments should be performed with care to avoid damage to the neurovascular bundle. A hemostatic agent can be placed in the donor site, and wound closure is accomplished in a single-layer technique of multiple interrupted sutures.

Surgical Sequelae

A significant number of studies have evaluated temporary and permanent complications following bone harvesting in the symphysis or ramus. With all clinical studies, comparison must be made with caution because of differences in the study designs, the number of treated patients, the follow-up periods, the methods of assessment, and, in particular, the definitions of complications (Box 5-2). Nevertheless, the reported data show that the symphysis donor site has a tendency for more frequent and more severe complications than the ramus donor site (Table 5-2).

Table 5-2 Sequelae of bone harvesting

Author	Study type	Site	N	Evaluation time point	Sequela					
					Other	Wound dehiscence	Hematoma	Infection	Altered tooth sensitivity	Altered skin sensation
Misch et al[60]	Prosp	Symphysis	11	Postop 4 mo	NA NA	27.3% (3/11) NA	NA NA	NA NA	0% (0/11) 0% (0/11)	0% (0/11) 0% (0/11)
Raghoebar et al[61]	Retrosp, comp	Symphysis	12	Postop 3 mo	NA NA	NA NA	NA NA	NA NA	0% (0/12) 0% (0/12)	0% (0/12) 0% (0/12)
		Ramus	7	Postop 3 mo	NA NA	NA NA	NA NA	NA NA	0% (0/7) 0% (0/7)	0% (0/7) 0% (0/7)
Misch[47]	Prosp, comp	Symphysis	31	Postop 6 mo	NA NA	VI, 10.7% (3/28) SI, 0% (0/3) NA	NA NA	VI, 7.1% (2/28) SI, 0% (0/3) NA	29.0% (9/31) 0% (0/31)	9.7% (3/31) 0% (0/31)
		Ramus	19	Postop 6 mo	NA NA	0% (0/19) NA	NA NA	0% (0/19) NA	0% (0/19) 0% (0/19)	0% (0/19) 0% (0/19)
Widmark et al[62]	Prosp	Symphysis	9	Postop 4 mo	NA NA	0% (0/9) NA	NA NA	NA NA	NA NA	22.2% (2/9) 0% (0/9)
von Arx and Kurt[63]	Retrosp, comp	Symphysis	15	Postop 6 mo	NA NA	20% (3/15) NA	13.3% (2/15) NA	NA NA	33.3% (5/15) 13.3% (2/15)	0% (0/15) 0% (0/15)
		Ramus	13 P, 15 S	Postop 6 mo	NA NA	0% (0/15) NA	6.7% (1/15) NA	NA NA	0% (0/15) 0% (0/15)	6.7% (1/15) 0% (0/15)
Hunt and Jovanovic[4]	Retrosp	Symphysis	44	Postop 6 mo	NA NA	NA NA	NA NA	NA NA	13.6% (6/44) 6.8% (3/44)	6.8% (3/44) 0% (0/44)
Bedrossian et al[55]	Prosp	Ramus	63	Postop 4 mo	NA NA	NA NA	NA NA	0% (0/63) NA	NA NA	3.2% (2/63) 0% (0/63)
Nkenke et al[64]	Prosp	Symphysis	20	Postop 12 mo	NA NA	NA NA	NA NA	NA NA	21.6% (38/176 T) 11.4% (20/176 T)	40% (8/20) 10% (2/20)

N = number of patients (unless otherwise noted); P = patients; S = sites; T = teeth; Prosp = prospective; Retrosp = retrospective; Comp = comparative; Postop = postoperatively; Subj = subjectively; Obj = objectively; NA = parameter not mentioned in study; VI = vestibular incision; SI = sulcular incision.

Table 5-2 *(cont)* Sequelae of bone harvesting

Author	Study type	Site	N	Evaluation time point	Sequela: Other	Wound dehiscence	Hematoma	Infection	Altered tooth sensitivity	Altered skin sensation
Raghoebar et al[65]	Retrosp	Symphysis	21	Postop	42.9% (9/21)*	4.8% (1/21)	NA	NA	Subj: 19% (4/21)†	Subj: 42.9% (9/21); Obj: 0% (0/21)
				1–3 y	NA	NA	NA	NA	0% (0/21)	Subj: 33.3% (7/21); Obj: 0% (0/21)
Sethi and Kaus[66]	Prosp, comp	Symphysis	27	Postop	NA	7.4% (2/27)	NA	NA	3.7% (1/27)	3.7% (1/27)
				3–6 mo	NA	NA	NA	NA	0% (0/27)	0% (0/27)
		Ramus	33	Postop	NA	NA	NA	3% (1/33)‡	0% (0/33)	Buccal nerve: 3% (1/33)
				3–6 mo§	NA	NA	NA	NA	0% (0/33)	Buccal nerve: 3% (1/33)§
Cotter et al[49]	Retrosp	Symphysis (lower border)	15	Postop	NA	NA	NA	NA	Subj: 13.3% (2/15)	Subj: 40% (6/15)
				6 mo	33% (5/15)‖	NA	NA	NA	Subj: 6.7% (1/15)	Subj: 6.7% (1/15)
Nkenke et al[53]	Prosp	Ramus	20	Postop	NA	NA	0% (0/20)	NA	0% (0/20)	0% (0/20)
				12 mo¶	NA	NA	NA	NA	0% (0/20)	0% (0/20)
Proussaefs et al[67]	Prosp	Ramus	8	Postop	25% (2/8)#	NA	NA	NA	NA	NA
Clavero and Lundgren[68]	Retrosp, comp	Symphysis	29	Postop	40% (approx)*	NA	NA	0% (0/29)	NA	75.9% (22/29)
				18 mo	NA	NA	NA	NA	NA	51.7% (15/29)
		Ramus	24	Postop	10% (approx)*	NA	NA	0% (0/24)	NA	20.8% (5/24)
				18 mo	NA	NA	NA	NA	NA	4.2% (1/24)
Joshi[69]	Prosp	Symphysis	27	1 wk	NA	NA	NA	NA	18.5% (5/27)	7.4% (2/27)
				12 mo	NA	NA	NA	NA	7.4% (2/27)	

N = number of patients (unless otherwise noted); P = patients; S = sites; T = teeth; Prosp = prospective; Retrosp = retrospective; Comp = comparative; Postop = postoperatively; Subj = subjectively; Obj = objectively; NA = parameter not mentioned in study; VI = vestibular incision; SI = sulcular incision.

*Prolonged pain (> 1 week).

†Teeth reacted to cold.

‡Infection of the graft material, which was collected from the bone trap and used to fill the defect at the donor site.

§The patient that experienced altered skin sensation of the buccal nerve was followed for 18 months.

‖Subjective contour change.

¶Only followed when sequelae were found.

#Persistant pain.

Table 5-2 continues on next page.

Table 5-2 *(cont)* **Sequelae of bone harvesting**

Author	Study type	Site	N	Evaluation time point	Sequela: Other	Wound dehiscence	Hematoma	Infection	Altered tooth sensitivity	Altered skin sensation
Lindeboom et al[24]	Prosp, comp, randomized**	Symphysis	58	8 wk	NA	NA	NA	5.2% (3/58)	NA	NA
		Ramus	66	8 wk	NA	NA	NA	4.5% (3/66)	NA	NA
Proussaefs and Lozada[70]	Prosp	Symphysis	3	Postop	NA	33% (1/3)	NA	NA	NA	NA
		Ramus	9	Postop	22% (2/9)#	NA	NA	NA	NA	NA
von Arx et al[14]	Prosp	Symphysis	30	Postop	NA	NA	NA	NA	43.3% (13/30 P) 18.6% (30/161 T)	3.3% (1/30)
				12 mo	NA	NA	NA	NA	3.3% (1/30 P) 0.6% (1/161 T)	0% (0/30)
Raghoebar et al[48]	Prosp, comp	Symphysis	15	Postop	33% (5/15)*	NA	0% (0/15)	0% (0/15)	Subj: 13.3% (2/15) Obj: 0% (0/15)	Subj: 40% (6/15) Obj: 6.7% (1/15)
				12 mo	NA	NA	NA	NA	0% (0/15)	Subj: 13.3% (2/15) Obj: 0% (0/15)
		Ramus	15	Postop	20% (3/15)	NA	0% (0/15)	0% (0/15)	0% (0/15)	Subj: 6.7% (1/15) Obj: 0% (0/15)
				12 mo	NA	NA	NA	NA	0% (0/15)	0% (0/15)
		Ramus and third molar removal	15	Postop	20% (3/15)	NA	0% (0/15)	6.7% (1/15)††	0% (0/15)	Subj: 6.7% (1/15) Obj: 0% (0/15)
			12 mo	NA	NA	NA	NA	0% (0/15)	0% (0/15)	
Happe[52]	Prosp	Ramus	40 P, 45 S	Postop	NA	2.5% (1/40)	NA	2.5% (1/40)	NA	2.5% (1/40)
				4 mo	NA	NA	NA	NA	NA	0% (0/40)
von Arx et al[71]	Prosp	Symphysis	20	6 mo	NA	NA	NA	NA	25% (5/20 P) 11.4% (12/105 T)	NA

N = number of patients (unless otherwise noted); P = patients; S = sites; T = teeth; Prosp = prospective; Retrosp = retrospective; Comp = comparative; Postop = postoperatively; Subj = subjectively; Obj = objectively; NA = parameter not mentioned in study; VI = vestibular incision; SI = sulcular incision.

*Prolonged pain (>1 week).

#Persistant pain.

**Randomization related to antibiotic prophylaxis or placebo (no data given for individual regimen at each donor site).

††Delayed socket healing.

Wound dehiscence

Several studies[47,60,63,65,66] have documented that the risk of wound dehiscence is up to 27% in the symphysis when an alveolar mucosa incision is used. Measures to avoid wound dehiscences include use of a two-layer suturing technique or mattress sutures to evert wound margins, placement of an extraoral pressure dressing, administration of anti-inflammatory medication, and postsurgical application of cold. In patients with a shallow vestibule or tense mentalis posture, use of an intrasulcular incision along the mandibular anterior teeth is advocated. In ramus donor sites, the risk of wound dehiscence is negligible.

Prolonged postoperative pain

Data from multiple studies[48,60,65,67,68,70] demonstrate that the percentage of patients experiencing prolonged pain is greater in symphysis sites (up to 43%) than in ramus sites (up to 25%). This finding may be explained by the fact that surgical trauma (and therefore postsurgical swelling) is greater in symphysis donor sites than in ramus donor sites. Measures to prevent prolonged postoperative pain are similar to those mentioned to prevent incision dehiscence and further include an atraumatic surgical approach (sharp incision and blunt dissection to avoid severing of the periosteum during flap elevation).

Hematoma

Bone harvesting in the mandibular ramus and symphyseal areas carries some, although minimal, risk of postsurgical hematoma.[48,53,61] Bleeding sources include the cancellous compartment, the rupture of large vessels (inferior alveolar artery), or the dissection of muscles (mentalis muscle). Identification of bleeding sites and adequate hemorrhage control should aim at minimizing the hazard of postsurgical hematomas.

Infection

Postsurgical infections of symphysis or ramus donor sites are rare.[22–24,47,48,52,55,66,68] The use of single-dose antibiotics administered at least 1 hour before surgery has been recommended to avoid an infection at the donor site.[22–24]

Ptosis of chin

Visible alteration of the chin contour appears to occur only rarely, although patients still might perceive and complain of such a change.[4,48,60,65,68,69] The change might also be associated with a perception of altered skin sensitivity in the chin area. Preservation of the mentalis muscle attachment to the underlying bone through the periosteal complex is mandatory. Contour changes have not been reported for ramus donor sites.[68] Patients may also be less concerned about a facial contour change in the ramus than in the symphyseal area.

Altered skin sensation

At the symphysis donor site, temporary paresthesia of the mental nerve is frequent.[4,14,48,49,62,64,65,68,69] Often, postsurgical paresthesia reported in the chin region cannot be confirmed with objective tests and probably results from neuropraxia to the mandibular incisive nerve or terminal branches of the mental nerve.[48,65] Fortunately, the majority of patients who report altered skin sensitivity fully recover over time. However, in some cases, a permanent (12-months or longer) change in sensitivity has been reported.[64,66,68] Whenever possible, the incision line should be limited to the distal aspect of the canines to avoid damage to the mental nerve. It can further be speculated that damage to the mandibular incisive nerve when bone is cut for block removal might also retrogradely affect the mental nerve.

Permanently altered skin sensitivity has been reported following bone harvesting from the symphysis.[48,49,64,65,68] In contrast, altered skin sensation after bone harvesting in the ramus area is a rare sequela.[47,48,52,53,55,61,66,68]

Altered pulpal sensitivity

Similar to altered skin sensation, changes of pulpal sensitivity are frequently observed following bone harvesting in the symphysis.[4,14,47,61,64–66,69] Although most authors have reported that a minimum safety distance of 5 mm was observed between the upper horizontal bone cut and the apices of the adjacent teeth, this measure does not predictably prevent altered tooth sensitivity. Interestingly, a large number of teeth regain their pulpal sensitivity over time.[4,14,47,48,64–66,69] This observation has been associated with anastomoses of neurovascular structures entering the lingual aspect of the mandible with supply to the anterior mandibular teeth.[72,73]

Some authors also have noted that, although patients complained subjectively about altered tooth sensation, the same teeth responded normally to cold testing.[48] In a few cases, permanent (12-month or more) changes in the sensitivity of the anterior mandibular teeth have been observed following block harvesting in the symphysis.[14,64,69] With regard to the ramus donor site, altered pulpal sensitivity of adjacent or ipsilateral teeth has not been reported.[47,48,53,61]

Conclusion

The use of intraorally harvested autogenous bone grafts is still an important aspect of guided bone regeneration techniques. The advantages comprise the biologic characteristics and tissue compatibility of autografts and the convenient surgical access and close proximity of intraoral donor and recipient sites.

The selection of donor site depends on the type of graft (eg, bone block versus bone chips) and the volume of bone needed. Although the harvesting of bone chips is relatively straightforward and can be performed in nearly all maxillary and mandibular areas, block grafts are procured mainly from the symphysis and the ramus. The mandibular ramus has some advantages over the mandibular symphysis as a donor site. These include minimal patient concern for altered facial contour, a lower incidence of incision dehiscence, decreased complaints of postoperative sensory disturbance, and the proximity to posterior mandibular recipient sites. In contrast, the symphysis offers better access, the potential for thicker grafts, and a greater cancellous component.

References

1. Habal MB, Reddi A. Introduction to bone grafting. In: Habal MB, Reddi A (eds). Bone Grafts and Bone Substitutes. Philadelphia: Saunders, 1992:3–5.
2. Peleg M, Garg AK, Misch CM, Mazor Z. Maxillary sinus and ridge augmentations using a surface-derived autogenous bone graft. J Oral Maxillofac Surg 2004;62:1535–1544.
3. Pinholt EM, Solheim E, Talsnes O, Larsen TB, Bang G, Kirkeby OJ. Revascularization of calvarial, mandibular, tibial and iliac bone grafts in rats. Ann Plast Surg 1994;33:193–197.
4. Hunt DR, Jovanovic SA. Autogenous bone harvesting: A chin graft technique for particulate and monocortical bone blocks. Int J Periodontics Restorative Dent 1999;19:165–173.
5. Wood RM, Moore DL. Grafting of the maxillary sinus with intraorally harvested autogenous bone prior to implant placement. Int J Oral Maxillofac Implants 1988;3:209–214.
6. Springer ING, Terheyden H, Geiss S, Härle F, Hedderich J, Acil Y. Particulated bone grafts—Effectiveness of bone cell supply. Clin Oral Implants Res 2004;15:205–212.
7. Gruber R, Baron M, Busenlechner D, Kandler B, Fürst G, Watzek G. Proliferation and osteogenic differentiation of cells from cortical bone cylinders, bone particles from mill, and drilling dust. J Oral Maxillofac Surg 2005;63:238–243.
8. Young MPJ, Worthington HV, Lloyd RE, Drucker DB, Sloan P, Carter DH. Bone collected during dental implant surgery: A clinical and histological study. Clin Oral Implants Res 2002;13:298–303.
9. Savant TD, Smith KS, Sullivan SM, Owen WL. Bone volume collected from dental implant sites during osteotomy. J Oral Maxillofac Surg 2001;59:905–907.
10. Kürkcü M, Öz IA, Köksal F, Benlidayi E, Günesli A. Microbial analysis of the autogenous bone collected by bone filter during oral surgery: A clinical study. J Oral Maxillofac Surg 2005;63:1593–1598.
11. Graziani F, Cei S, Ivanovski S, La Ferla F, Gabriele M. A systematic review of the effectiveness of bone collectors. Int J Oral Maxillofac Implants 2007;22:729–735.
12. Pradel W, Tenbieg P, Lauer G. Influence of harvesting technique and donor site location on in vitro growth of osteoblastlike cells from facial bone. Int J Oral Maxillofac Implants 2005;20:860–866.
13. Zaffe D, d'Avenia F. A novel bone scraper for intraoral harvesting: A device for filling small bone defects. Clin Oral Implants Res 2007;18:525–533.
14. von Arx T, Häfliger J, Chappuis V. Neurosensory disturbances following bone harvesting in the symphysis: A prospective clinical study. Clin Oral Implants Res 2005;16:432–439.
15. Khoury F. Augmentation of the sinus floor with mandibular bone block and simultaneous implantation: A 6-year clinical investigation. Int J Oral Maxillofac Implants 1999;14:557–564.
16. Vercellotti T, de Paoli S, Nevins M. The piezoelectric bony window osteotomy and sinus membrane elevation: Introduction of a new technique for simplification of the sinus augmentation procedure. Int J Periodontics Restorative Dent 2001;21:561–567.

17. Stübinger S, Kuttenberger J, Filippi A, Sader R, Zeilhofer HF. Intraoral piezosurgery: Preliminary results of a new technique. J Oral Maxillofac Surg 2005; 63:1283–1287.
18. Sohn DS, Ahn MR, Lee WH, Yeo DS, Lim SY. Piezoelectric osteotomy for intraoral harvesting of bone blocks. Int J Periodontics Restorative Dent 2007;27: 127–131.
19. Horton JE, Tarpley TM, Jacoway JR. Clinical applications of ultrasonic instrumentation in the surgical removal of bone. Oral Surg Oral Med Oral Pathol 1981;51:236–242.
20. Chiriac G, Herten M, Schwarz F, Rothamel D, Becker J. Autogenous bone chips: Influence of a new piezoelectric device (piezoelectric surgery) on chip morphology, cell viability and differentiation. J Clin Periodontol 2005;9:994–999.
21. Vercellotti T, Nevins ML, Kim DM, et al. Osseous response following resective therapy with piezoelectric surgery. Int J Periodontics Restorative Dent 2005;25:543–549.
22. Lindeboom JAH, van den Akker HP. A prospective placebo-controlled double-blind trial of antibiotic prophylaxis in intraoral bone grafting procedures: A pilot study. Oral Surg Oral Med Oral Pathol Oral Radiol Endod 2003;96:669–672.
23. Lindeboom JA, Frenken JW, Tuk JG, Kroon FH. A randomized prospective controlled trial of antibiotic prophylaxis in intraoral bone-grafting procedures: Preoperative single-dose penicillin versus preoperative single-dose clindamycin. Int J Oral Maxillofac Surg 2006;35:433–436.
24. Lindeboom JAH, Tuk JGC, Kroon FHM, van den Akker HP. A randomized prospective controlled trial of antibiotic prophylaxis in intraoral bone grafting procedures: Single-dose clindamycin versus 24-hour clindamycin prophylaxis. Mund Kiefer Gesichtschir 2005;9:384–388.
25. Chiapasco M, Abati S, Romeo E, Vogel G. Clinical outcome of autogenous bone blocks or guided bone regeneration with e-PTFE membranes for the reconstruction of narrow edentulous ridges. Clin Oral Implants Res 1999;10:278–288.
26. ten Bruggenkate CM, Kraaijenhagen HA, van der Kwast WAM, Krekeler G, Oostenbeek HS. Autogenous maxillary bone grafts in conjunction with placement of ITI endosseous implants. A preliminary report. Int J Oral Maxillofac Surg 1992;21:81–84.
27. Kainulainen VT, Sandor GKB, Oikarinen KS, Clokie CML. Zygomatic bone: An additional donor site for alveolar bone reconstruction. Technical note. Int J Oral Maxillofac Implants 2002;17:723–728.
28. Stübinger S, Robertson A, Zimmerer KS, Leiggener C, Sader R, Kunz C. Piezoelectric harvesting of an autogenous bone graft from the zygomaticomaxillary region: Case report. Int J Periodontics Restorative Dent 2006;26:453–457.
29. Bormann KH, Kokemüller H, Rücker M, Gellrich NC. New methods and techniques for biologically adequate jaw crest augmentation. Minimally invasive, precise bone transplantation using grafts from the zygomatic crest [in German]. Implantologie 2007; 15:253–261.
30. Gellrich NC, Held U, Schön R, Pailing T, Schramm A, Bormann KH. Alveolar zygomatic buttress: A new donor site for limited preimplant augmentation procedures. J Oral Maxillofac Surg 2007;65:275–280.
31. Kainulainen VT, Sandor GKB, Clokie CML, Keller AM, Oikarinen KS. The zygomatic bone as a potential donor site for alveolar reconstruction—A quantitative anatomic cadaver study. Int J Oral Maxillofac Surg 2004;33:786–791.
32. Kainulainen VT, Sandor GKB, Carmichael RP, Oikarinen KS. Safety of zygomatic bone harvesting: A prospective study of 32 consecutive patients with simultaneous zygomatic bone grafting and 1-stage implant placement. Int J Oral Maxillofac Implants 2005;20:245–252.
33. Neiva RF, Neiva GF, Wang HL. Utilization of mandibular tori for alveolar ridge augmentation and maxillary sinus lifting: A case report. Quintessence Int 2006;37:131–137.
34. Proussaefs P. Clinical and histologic evaluation of the use of mandibular tori as donor site for mandibular block autografts: Report of three cases. Int J Periodontics Restorative Dent 2006;26:43–51.
35. Cranin AN, Katzap M, Demirdjan E, Ley J. Autogenous bone ridge augmentation using the mandibular symphysis as a donor. J Oral Implantol 2001;27: 43–47.
36. Montazem A, Valauri DV, St-Hilaire H, Buchbinder D. The mandibular symphysis as a donor site in maxillofacial bone grafting: A quantitative anatomic study. J Oral Maxillofac Surg 2000;58:1368–1371.
37. Cutright B, Ouillopa N, Schubert W. An anthropometric analysis of the key foramina for maxillofacial surgery. J Oral Maxillofac Surg 2003;61:354–357.
38. Agthong S, Huanmanop T, Chentanez V. Anatomical variations of the supraorbital, infraorbital, and mental foramina related to gender and side. J Oral Maxillofac Surg 2005;63:800–804.
39. de Andrade E, Otomo-Corgel J, Pucher J, Ranganath KA, St George N. The intraosseous course of the mandibular incisive nerve in the mandibular symphysis. Int J Periodontics Restorative Dent 2001; 21:591–597.
40. Jacobs R, Mraiwa N, van Steenberghe D, Gijbels F, Quirynen M. Appearance, location, course, and morphology of the mandibular incisive canal: An assessment on spiral CT scan. Dentomaxillofac Radiol 2002;31:322–327.
41. Mraiwa N, Jacobs R, Moerman P, Lambrichts I, van Steenberghe D, Quirynen M. Presence and course of the incisive canal in the human mandibular interforaminal region: Two-dimensional imaging versus anatomical observations. Surg Radiol Anat 2003; 25:416–423.
42. Park HD, Min CK, Kwak HH, Youn KH, Choi SH, Kim HJ. Topography of the outer mandibular symphyseal region with reference to the autogenous bone graft. Int J Oral Maxillofac Surg 2004;33:781–785.
43. Lorenzetti M, Mozzati M, Campanino PP, Valente G. Bone augmentation of the inferior floor of the maxillary sinus with autogenous bone or composite bone grafts: A histologic-histomorphometric preliminary report. Int J Oral Maxillofac Implants 1998; 13:69–76.

44. Gapski R, Wang HL, Misch CE. Management of incision design in symphysis graft procedures: A review of the literature. J Oral Implantology 2001;27:134–142.
45. Kramper BJ, Kaminski EJ, Osetek EM, Heuer MA. A comparative study of the wound healing of three types of flap design used in periapical surgery. J Endod 1984;10:17–25.
46. von Arx T, Vinzens-Majaniemi T, Bürgin W, Jensen SS. Changes of periodontal parameters following apical surgery: A prospective clinical study of three incision techniques. Int Endod J 2007;40:959–969.
47. Misch CM. Comparison of intraoral donor sites for onlay grafting prior to implant placement. Int J Oral Maxillofac Implants 1997;12:767–776.
48. Raghoebar GM, Meijndert L, Kalk WWI, Vissink A. Morbidity of mandibular bone harvesting: A comparative study. Int J Oral Maxillofac Implants 2007;22:359–365.
49. Cotter CJ, Maher A, Gallagher C, Sleeman D. Mandibular lower border: Donor site of choice for alveolar grafting. Br J Oral Maxillofac Surg 2002;40:429–432.
50. Rubens BC, West RA. Ptosis of the chin and lip incompetence: Consequences of lost mentalis muscle support. J Oral Maxillofac Surg 1989;47:359–366.
51. Misch CM. Use of the mandibular ramus as a donor site for onlay bone grafting. J Oral Implantol 2000;26:42–49.
52. Happe A. Use of a piezoelectric surgical device to harvest bone grafts from the mandibular ramus: Report of 40 cases. Int J Periodontics Restorative Dent 2007;27:241–249.
53. Nkenke E, Radespiel-Tröger M, Wiltfang J, Schultze-Mosgau S, Winkler G, Neukam FW. Morbidity of harvesting of retromolar bone grafts: A prospective study. Clin Oral Implants Res 2002;13:514–521.
54. Smith BR, Rajchel JL, Waite DE, Read L. Mandibular anatomy as it relates to rigid fixation of the sagittal ramus split osteotomy. J Oral Maxillofac Surg 1991;49:222–226.
55. Bedrossian E, Tawfilis A, Alijanian A. Veneer grafting: A technique for augmentation of the resorbed alveolus prior to implant placement. A clinical report. Int J Oral Maxillofac Implants 2000;15:853–858.
56. Khoury F, Happe A. Zur Diagnostik und Methodik von intraoralen Knochenentnahmen. Z Zahnärztl Implantol 1999;15:167–176.
57. Capelli M. Autogenous bone graft from the mandibular ramus: A technique for bone augmentation. Int J Periodontics Restorative Dent 2003;23:277–285.
58. Crawford EA. The use of ramus bone cores for maxillary sinus bone grafting: A surgical technique. J Oral Implantol 2001;27:82–88.
59. Misch CM. The harvest of ramus bone in conjunction with third molar removal for onlay grafting before placement of dental implants. J Oral Maxillofac Surg 1999;57:1376–1379.
60. Misch CM, Misch CE, Resnik RR, Ismail YH. Reconstruction of maxillary alveolar defects with mandibular symphysis grafts for dental implants: A preliminary procedural report. Int J Oral Maxillofac Implants 1992;7:360–366.
61. Raghoebar GM, Batenburg RHK, Vissink A, Reintsema H. Augmentation of localized defects of the anterior maxillary ridge with autogenous bone before insertion of implants. J Oral Maxillofac Surg 1996;54:1180–1185.
62. Widmark G, Andersson B, Ivanoff CJ. Mandibular bone graft in the anterior maxilla for single-tooth implants. Presentation of a surgical method. Int J Oral Maxillofac Surg 1997;26:106–109.
63. von Arx T, Kurt B. Intraoral bone harvesting for autotransplantation [in German]. Schweiz Monatsschr Zahnmed 1998;108:447–453.
64. Nkenke E, Schultze-Mosgau S, Radespiel-Tröger M, Kloss F, Neukam FW. Morbidity of harvesting of chin grafts: A prospective study. Clin Oral Implants Res 2001;12:495–502.
65. Raghoebar GM, Louwerse C, Kalk WWI, Vissink A. Morbidity of chin bone harvesting. Clin Oral Implants Res 2001;12:503–507.
66. Sethi A, Kaus T. Ridge augmentation using mandibular block bone grafts: Preliminary results of an ongoing prospective study. Int J Oral Maxillofac Implants 2001;16:378–388.
67. Proussaefs P, Lozada J, Kleinman A, Rohrer MD. The use of ramus autogenous block grafts for vertical alveolar ridge augmentation and implant placement: A pilot study. Int J Oral Maxillofac Implants 2002;17:238–248.
68. Clavero J, Lundgren S. Ramus or chin grafts for maxillary sinus inlay and local onlay augmentation: Comparison of donor site morbidity and complications. Clin Implant Dent Relat Res 2003;5:154–160.
69. Joshi A. An investigation of post-operative morbidity following chin graft surgery. Br Dent J 2004;196:215–218.
70. Proussaefs P, Lozada J. The use of intraorally harvested autogenous block grafts for vertical alveolar ridge augmentation: A human study. Int J Periodontics Restorative Dent 2005;25:351–363.
71. von Arx T, Chappuis V, Winzap-Kälin C, Bornstein MM. Laser Doppler flowmetry for assessment of anterior mandibular teeth in conjunction with bone harvesting in the symphysis: A clinical pilot study. Int J Oral Maxillofac Implants 2007;22:383–389.
72. Liang X, Jacobs R, Lambrichts I, Vandewalle G. Lingual foramina on the mandibular midline revisited: A macroanatomical study. Clin Anat 2007;20:246–251.
73. Stein P, Brueckner J, Milliner M. Sensory innervation of mandibular teeth by the nerve to the mylohyoid: Implications in local anesthesia. Clin Anat 2007;20:591–595.

CHAPTER 6

Implant Placement with Simultaneous Guided Bone Regeneration: Selection of Biomaterials and Surgical Principles

Daniel Buser

Today, more and more implants are placed with simultaneous guided bone regeneration (GBR) procedures that use barrier membranes combined with bone grafts, bone substitutes, or both. The use of the GBR technique has helped clinicians to provide patients with successful treatment outcomes despite the presence of localized bone defects at implant sites. The primary objective of a GBR procedure is the achievement of successful bone regeneration in the defect area with high predictability and low risk of complications. Secondary objectives are to obtain successful outcomes with the least number of surgical interventions, low morbidity for patients, and reduced healing periods. This chapter presents the decision criteria for use of a simultaneous GBR procedure, the biologic rationale for the selection of appropriate biomaterials, and the step-by-step surgical procedures for implant placement with a simultaneous GBR procedure. The main emphasis will be on crestal dehiscence and apical fenestration defects, whereas implant placement in postextraction sites is discussed in detail in chapter 7.

Decision Criteria for a Simultaneous GBR Procedure

Localized bone defects in implant patients are common clinical situations, and the clinician has the choice to use the GBR procedure with either a simultaneous or a staged approach. Considering the aforementioned treatment objectives, implant placement with a simultaneous GBR procedure is preferred whenever possible in order to limit the number of surgical interventions to one surgery with an open flap procedure. The clinician has to use his or her clinical experience in making this important decision, which is often based on a gut feeling. However, the clinician can use the following criteria to aid in the decision-making process:

- The implant must be placed in a correct three-dimensional position from both a functional and an esthetic point of view.
- It must be possible to achieve primary implant stability in this specific position.
- The peri-implant bone defect must have a favorable defect morphology to allow predictable bone regeneration of the defect area.

Placement of the implant in the correct three-dimensional position is most important for an optimal functional and esthetic treatment outcome. This principle was introduced in implant dentistry in the mid-1990s and is often called *restoration-driven implant placement*.[1,2] The correct three-dimensional implant positioning—in particular in esthetic implant sites—is much better understood today.

Good primary implant stability is an important prerequisite for osseointegration, as described in the 1960s and 1970s.[3–5] Having an immobilized implant is important during the initial healing period to allow the deposition of new bone onto the implant surface by osteoblasts.[6]

Finally, the morphology of the peri-implant bone defect is an important determinant of whether simultaneous procedures are possible. Schenk et al[7] found that new bone formation mainly depends on the surface area of exposed bone and its marrow cavity because angiogenic and osteogenic cells are mainly responsible for new bone formation in the defect area, and these cells reside in the marrow cavity.

The healing potential for new bone formation in an implant site with a peri-implant bone defect depends on general and local factors. The relevant general factors are the age and health status of the patient. As a rule, a young, healthy patient has better healing potential in a defect site than does a patient older than 70 years, who might be additionally compromised by health problems such as diabetes and osteoporosis, typical diseases in this age category, or by medications such as anticoagulation therapy or bisphosphonates. These factors cannot be changed by the clinician, but they must be considered during preoperative examination and will influence the decision about which surgical approach is most appropriate in a given clinical situation.

The most important local factor is the ratio between the surface area of exposed bone and the defect volume to be regenerated. A well-established method used to differentiate various clinical situations is the counting of bone walls that can contribute to new bone formation. This method has been adopted from periodontal regeneration.[8] The rule of thumb is easy: The more bone walls available in a defect area, the better the healing potential in a given defect site. One-wall defects present a much more demanding clinical situation than do two- or three-wall defects (Fig 6-1).

A direct comparison between a one-wall and a two-wall defect may illustrate the difference in healing potential for a simultaneous GBR procedure (Fig 6-2). A two-wall defect has a favorable defect morphology (see Fig 6-2a). These defects are frequently found in postextraction sites and often have a rather small mesiodistal extension at the facial bone surface. The two bone walls form a craterlike defect morphology on the facial aspect of the implant. In addition, the exposed implant surface of the correctly positioned implant is located inside the alveolar crest (see Fig 6-2b). These small defects have an excellent potential for bony regeneration within weeks because angiogenic and osteogenic cells residing in the marrow cavity of adjacent bone walls have only short distances to bridge the defect.

In contrast, one-wall defects have a much more demanding defect morphology (see Fig 6-2c). These sites are frequently seen in healed ridges at least 6 months following extraction or traumatic tooth loss. These ridges often have a reduced crest width resulting in an exposed implant surface outside the alveolar crest and a flattened, wide de-

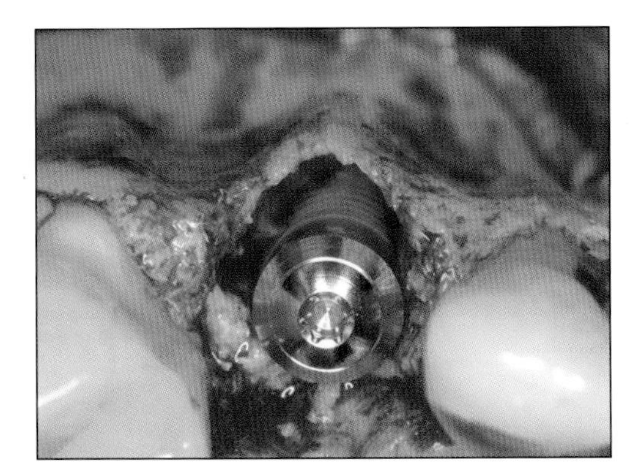

Fig 6-1a Immediate implant placement in a postextraction site has achieved a correct three-dimensional position. The resulting three-wall defect is favorable for a successful regenerative outcome.

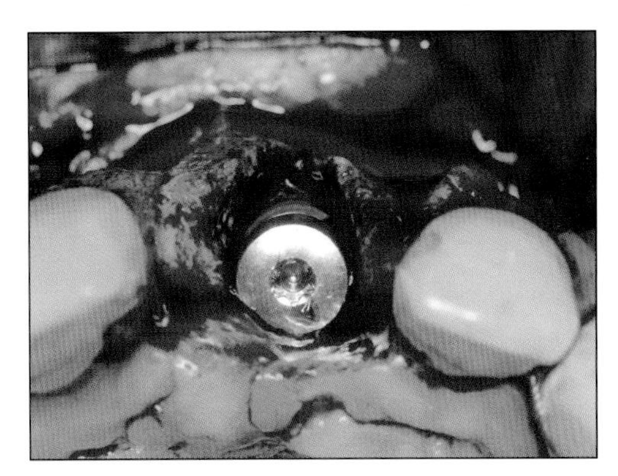

Fig 6-1b Implant placement in a postextraction site has resulted in a craterlike two-wall defect, favorable for a successful regenerative outcome.

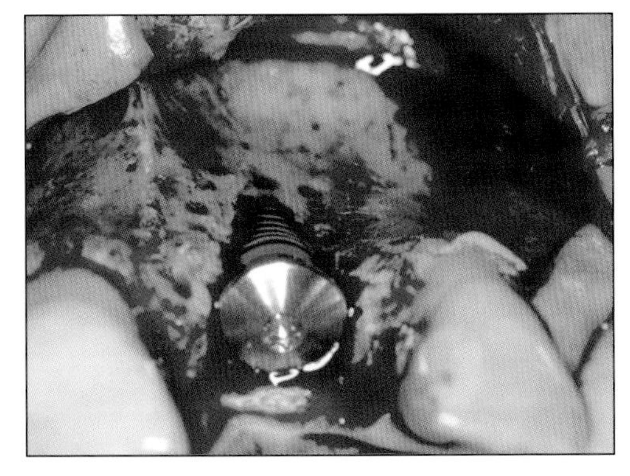

Fig 6-1c Implant placement in a healed ridge of approximately 5 mm has resulted in a borderline situation between a one-wall and a two-wall defect. The predictability of a successful regenerative outcome is reduced.

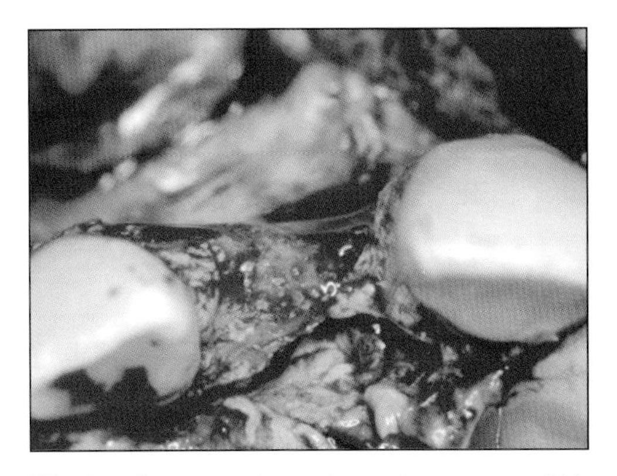

Fig 6-1d The single-tooth gap has a crest width of less than 4 mm. Implant placement would result in a one-wall defect with the exposed implant surface outside the alveolar crest. A staged approach is advisable.

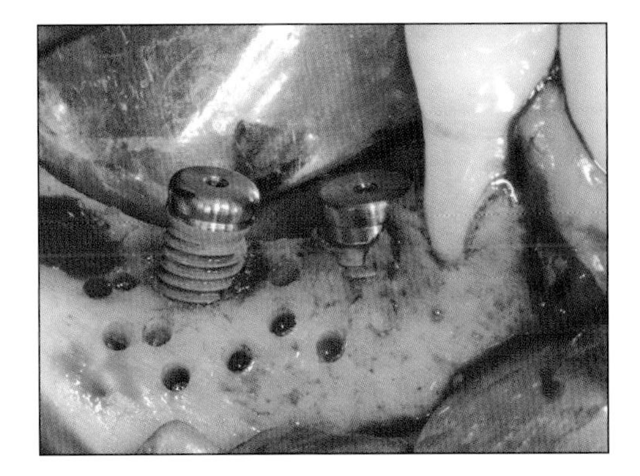

Fig 6-1e A vertical bone defect is present following implant placement in the posterior mandible. This is the most demanding clinical situation for a successful regenerative outcome.

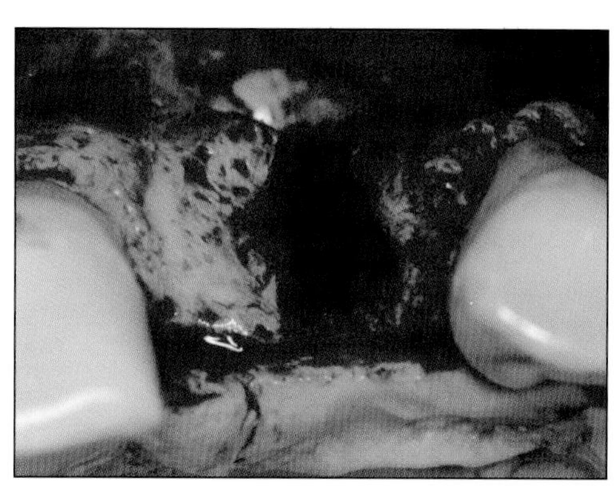

Fig 6-2a Eight weeks following tooth extraction in preparation for implant placement, the ridge shows a crest width of more than 6 mm and a residual craterlike socket defect in the alveolar crest.

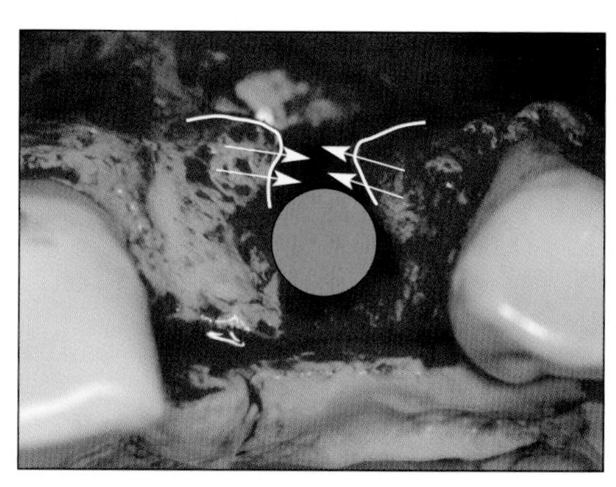

Fig 6-2b Virtual placement of a 4-mm implant indicates that implant placement will result in a craterlike two-wall defect. This defect is favorable and can be regenerated by ingrowing osteogenic cells *(arrows)* from the marrow cavity of adjacent bone walls.

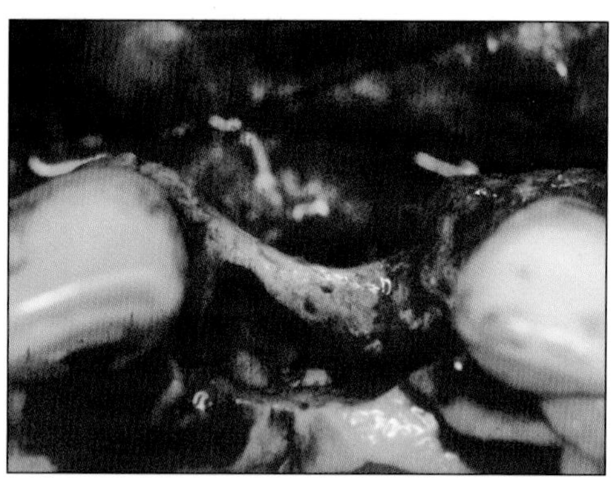

Fig 6-2c An extensive bone defect has resulted in facial flattening and a crest width of less than 4 mm.

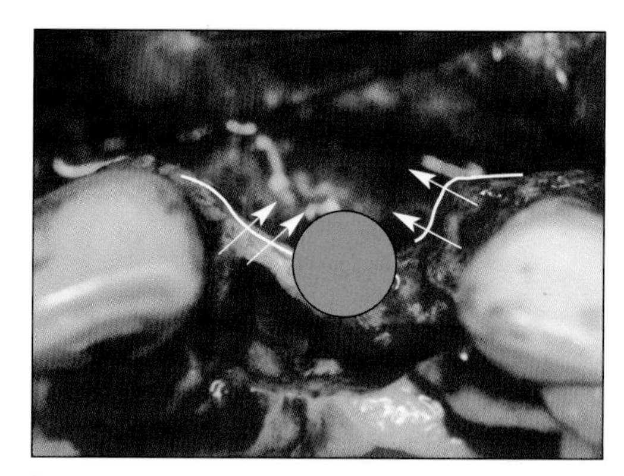

Fig 6-2d Virtual placement of a 4-mm implant indicates that implant placement will result in a wide one-wall defect. This defect is unfavorable for simultaneous implant placement because ingrowing osteogenic cells would have to bridge long distances *(arrows)* on the facial aspect of the exposed implant surface for a successful regenerative outcome.

fect. In such defects, angiogenic and osteogenic cells would have much longer distances to bridge (see Fig 6-2d). Thus, the risk for an insufficient regenerative outcome is increased. If the alveolar crest measures less than 5 mm, a staged approach is strongly recommended; first a block graft and GBR are used for horizontal ridge augmentation, and then the implant is placed in a second surgical intervention (see chapter 8).

A second local factor is the structure of the bone wall in the defect area. If the exposed surface area is cortical bone, multiple perforations of the cortical plate with a small round bur are strongly recommended. Experimental studies have shown that these perforations improve the healing in a membrane-protected defect.[9,10] These drill holes open the marrow cavity and stimulate bleeding in the defect area. If the exposed bone surface is bleeding, as in extraction socket defects, such drill holes are not necessary.

The healing potential of a defect site can be influenced by the clinician through a third factor: the selection of an appropriate bone filler to augment the peri-implant defect. Originally, bone fillers were primarily used as support to prevent membrane collapse.[11,12] Later, it was recognized that the osteogenic and osteoconductive properties of the applied bone fillers could also stimulate new bone formation in a membrane-protected defect.[13] These aspects are discussed in the next section.

Selection of Appropriate Biomaterials

The selection of appropriate biomaterials plays an important role in the treatment outcome of GBR procedures (see Fig 1-3). Biomaterials used for GBR include the implant itself, the barrier membrane, and the bone filler. In daily routine, it is strongly recommended that surgeons use only biomaterials that are *(1)* scientifically well documented in preclinical and clinical studies and *(2)* characterized by properties that help to achieve the previously defined primary and secondary treatment objectives.

Implant type and implant surface

Today, screw-type titanium implants with a modern microrough surface are clearly preferred in daily practice. Threaded implants offer better primary implant stability than do nonthreaded implants. Modern microrough titanium surfaces offer a faster and more intense bone apposition during healing. These modern surfaces were developed in the past 20 years and have more or less replaced the standard implant surfaces of the 1980s—the machined and the titanium plasma-sprayed surfaces.

In the 1990s, sandblasted or grit-blasted surfaces with or without acid etching were examined in experimental studies and initiated a paradigm shift towards microrough titanium surfaces in implant dentistry.[14–17] These surfaces included, among others, the SLA (Straumann), the TiOblast (Astra Tech), and the Osseotite (Biomet 3i) surfaces. With various production techniques, the topographies of these titanium surfaces were improved to make them more osteophilic for osteoblasts during initial wound healing.[6] These microrough surfaces helped to reduce conventional healing periods, which had previously measured 3 to 6 months in implant dentistry.

Today, early loading protocols are well documented after 6 and 8 weeks of healing in standard sites without bone augmentation procedures.[18–21] In the past 5 years, chemical means have been used in attempts to improve implant surface chemistry. A typical example is the chemically modified SLA surface (SLActive, Straumann), which has showed promising results in numerous experimental studies.[22–25] Based on these convincing results in preclinical studies, screw-type chemically modified SLA implants are routinely used by the author's group in implant patients undergoing GBR procedures.

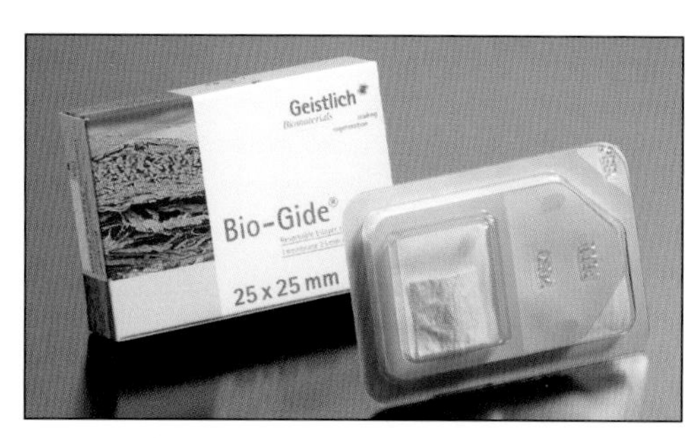

Fig 6-3a Non-cross-linked collagen membrane made of pork skin (Bio-Gide).

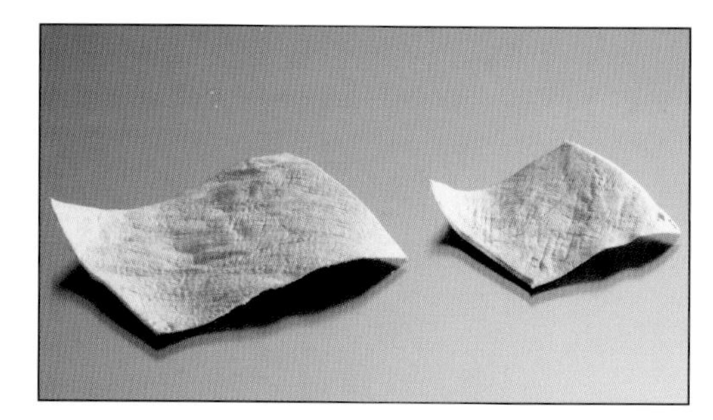

Fig 6-3b This collagen membrane is available in two sizes: 30 × 40 mm and 25 × 25 mm.

Box 6-1 Advantages and disadvantages of non–cross-linked, porcine-derived collagen membranes

Advantages

- Hydrophilic properties allow easy handling during surgery.
- This membrane does not require a second surgical procedure for membrane removal.
- In case of a soft tissue dehiscence, the membrane is not susceptible to infection.

Disadvantages

- The duration of the barrier function is rather short because the membrane is resorbed within 4 to 8 weeks.
- The membrane is soft and requires a bone filler for support to avoid collapse.

Barrier membranes

Today, bioresorbable collagen membranes dominate GBR procedures in daily practice. One of the best documented collagen membranes is a porcine-derived, non–cross-linked collagen membrane (Bio-Gide, Geistlich).[26–32] This membrane (Fig 6-3) is preferred by our group for the majority of clinical situations because it offers several clinical advantages (Box 6-1).

First, the membrane is hydrophilic and easy for the clinician to handle during surgery. When soaked in blood, the membrane becomes soft and easily adaptable to the local bone anatomy. A double-layer technique helps to improve membrane stability.[33] Therefore, the routine use of fixation pins or tacks for the stabilization of non–cross-linked collagen membranes is not required. Second, a second open flap procedure is not required for removal of the membrane because it is resorbed within a few weeks. Third, the collagen membrane offers a low risk of complications if a soft tissue dehiscence occurs during healing. Clinical studies have shown that exposed non–cross-linked collagen membranes do not cause local infection[34] because the soft tissues routinely heal by secondary wound healing without complications (Fig 6-4).

All these aspects represent significant advantages compared to the characteristics of nonresorbable, bioinert expanded polytetrafluoroethylene (ePTFE) membranes. These well-documented membranes are much more difficult to handle, always require a second surgical intervention with an open flap procedure for membrane removal, and are prone to complications because soft tissue dehiscences are common. Several clinical studies have demonstrated that early membrane exposure impairs treatment outcomes with GBR procedures.[28,35–37] As a consequence, ePTFE membranes are rarely

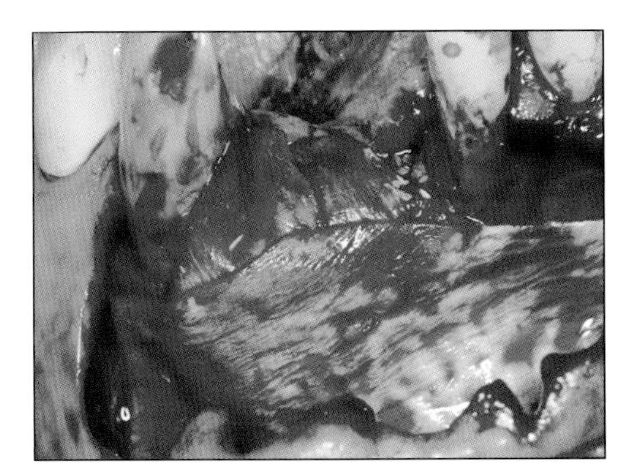

Fig 6-4a A collagen membrane is applied to the surgical site.

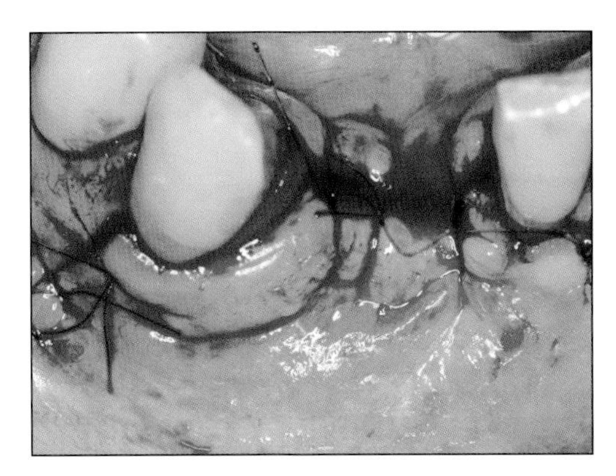

Fig 6-4b Primary wound closure is achieved with interrupted single sutures.

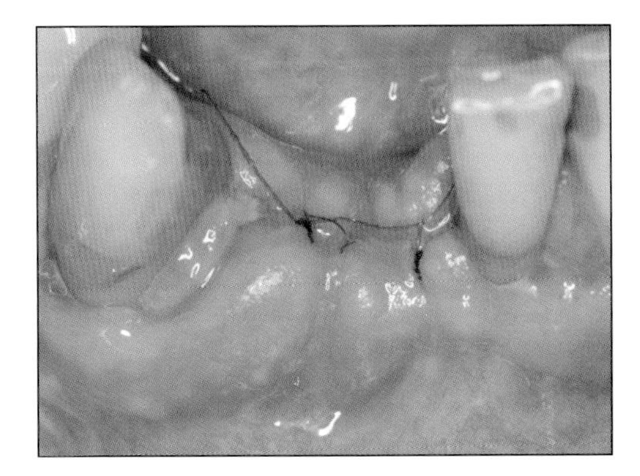

Fig 6-4c Clinical status 2 weeks after surgery. Partial necrosis of the wound margin close to the adjacent canine has caused a wound dehiscence resulting in exposure of the collagen membrane.

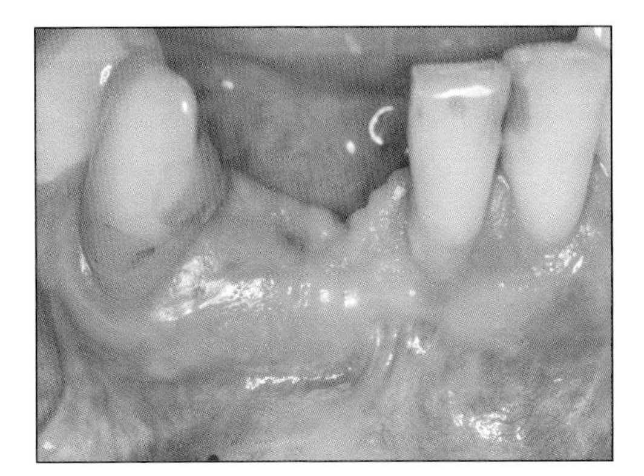

Fig 6-4d Two months later, the soft tissues have healed by secondary wound healing without development of an infectious complication at the membrane site.

used in daily routine by the author's group. Special indications for ePTFE membranes are demanding clinical situations such as defects for vertical ridge augmentation, which will be discussed in chapter 9.

Bone fillers

Bone fillers are routinely used for GBR procedures in daily practice because they improve the treatment outcome and the predictability. Bone fillers to be used in combination with barrier membranes should be able to:

- Support the membrane to avoid a membrane collapse
- Accelerate new bone formation in the membrane-protected defect
- Help maintain the created bone volume over time

The first characteristic is easy to fulfill with any type of bone filler as long as the filler has good biocompatibility. The second and third traits are more difficult. Clinicians

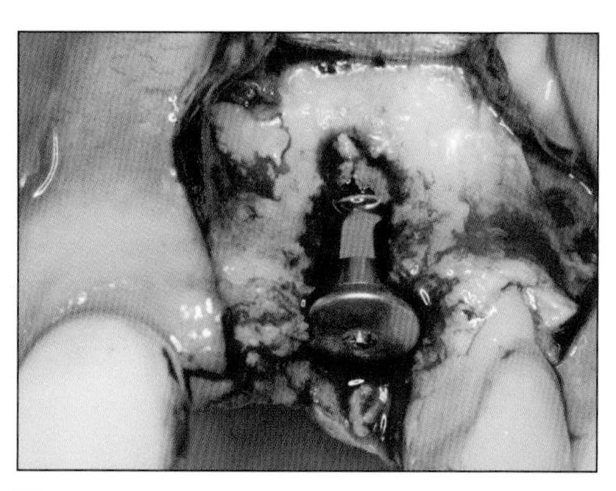

Fig 6-5a A facial peri-implant defect is present following implant placement in the area of the maxillary left canine.

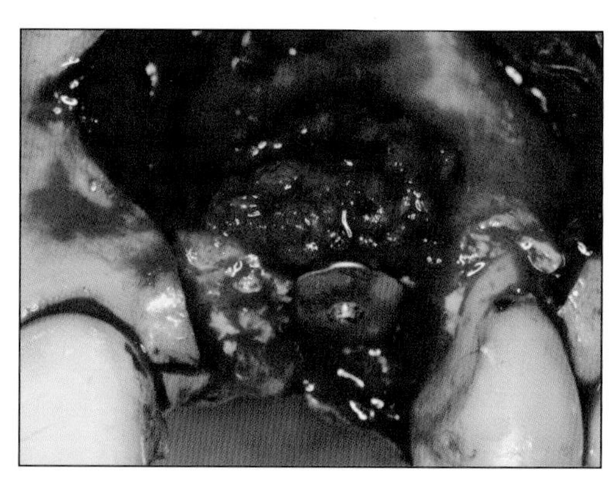

Fig 6-5b The defect is augmented with locally harvested autogenous bone chips to cover the exposed implant surface.

can choose from a large variety of available bone grafts and bone substitutes (see chapter 4). To accelerate new bone formation, the filler needs to have osteogenic properties, whereas a filler with a low substitution rate is needed to maintain the created bone volume over time. Numerous experimental studies have clearly shown that none of the available bone grafts or bone substitutes is able to fulfill both of these aspects at the same time. Thus, a combination of two fillers is recommended and was first used in 1998 by our group.

This concept of synergistically combining two bone fillers was based on observations in an experimental study by Buser et al.[13] This study showed that only autogenous bone chips are able to accelerate new bone formation in membrane-protected defects when compared to control sites with a blood clot alone. The tested bone substitutes all slowed new bone formation during initial healing. The study also showed that a hydroxyapatite-based filler was the only one with a low substitution rate. These findings have been confirmed in a number of animal studies over the past 10 years.[38–42]

Autogenous bone chips are routinely applied in the defect area. They are applied directly to the exposed implant surface to profit from the osteogenic properties of particulate autografts. These properties are discussed in detail in chapter 4, and harvesting techniques are presented in chapter 5. When used in combination with a modern microrough titanium implant surface, these autografts offer the clinician shorter healing periods because osseointegration and bone healing are both achieved more quickly. For simultaneous GBR procedures, these bone chips are routinely harvested within the same flap to avoid a second surgical site, which reduces the morbidity for the patient.

A low-substitution bone filler is applied on top of the autografts to optimize the contour of the alveolar ridge. As a first choice, deproteinized bovine bone mineral (DBBM) granules are used because they have served the author's group well in the past 15 years of clinical use (Bio-Oss, Geistlich). As an alternative, a biphasic calcium phosphate filler is used if the patient asks for a synthetic bone filler (Straumann Bone Ceramic, Straumann).

It is assumed that a low-substitution bone filler helps maintain the created volume of the alveolar ridge over time because these fillers will not be substantially resorbed

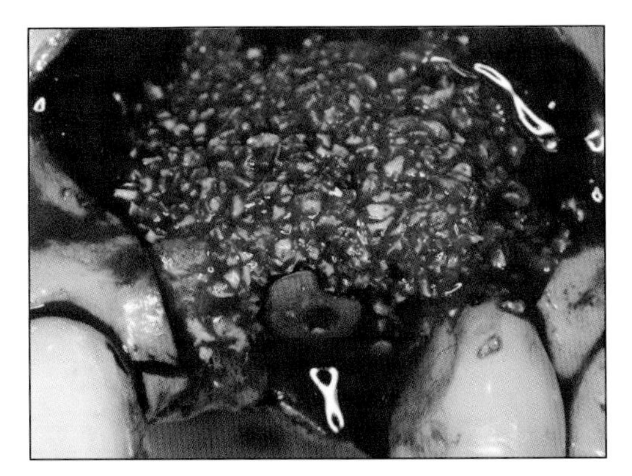

Fig 6-5c A second layer of DBBM particles is applied for contour augmentation.

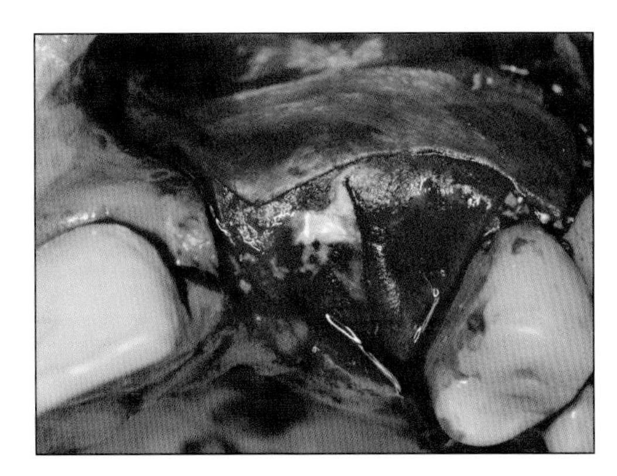

Fig 6-5d The augmentation material is covered with a collagen membrane using a double-layer technique.

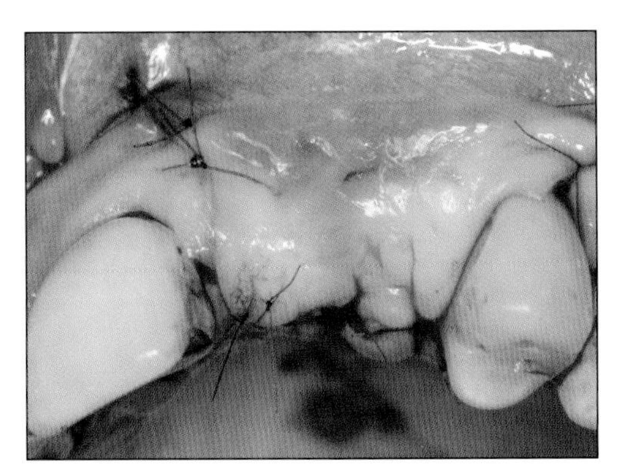

Fig 6-5e Surgery is completed with a tension-free primary wound closure.

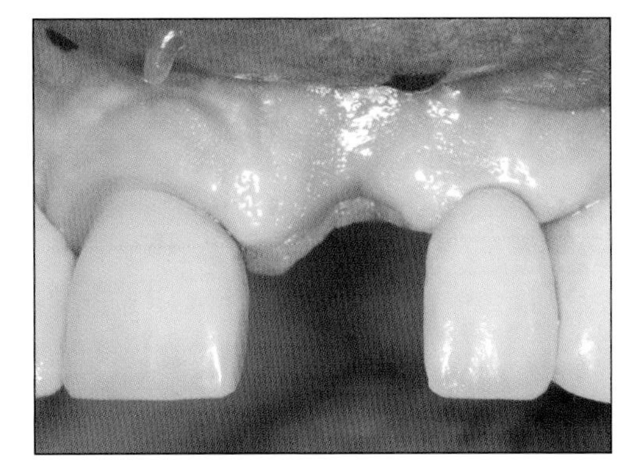

Fig 6-5f Four years later, the patient has been referred again because the maxillary left central incisor had to be removed due to a root fracture.

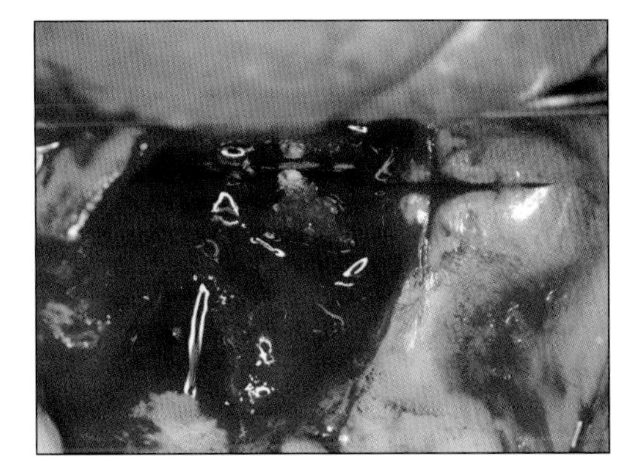

Fig 6-5g During implant surgery, a superficial biopsy specimen is harvested from the area of the left lateral incisor, where the contour augmentation had been performed 4 years earlier.

(Fig 6-5 continues on next page.)

during bone remodeling activities of the body. This has been confirmed by histologic analysis of human biopsies harvested from a few individual patients (Fig 6-5). Based on these favorable characteristics of low-substitution bone fillers, contour augmentation using two layers of different bone fillers has become a significant objective in esthetic implant dentistry because it helps to optimize esthetic outcomes of implant-supported single crowns and fixed dental prostheses (Fig 6-6).

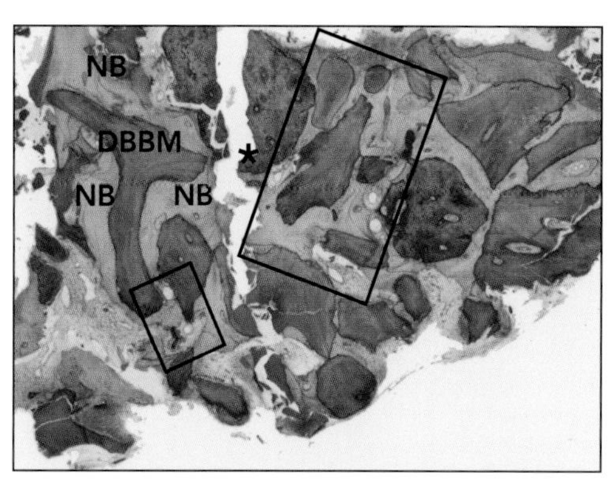

Fig 6-5h Histologic overview of the human biopsy specimen. Numerous deproteinized bovine bone mineral (DBBM) particles are visible and show good tissue integration. Newly formed bone (NB) covers part of the bone substitute surface and bridges neighboring DBBM particles. An artifactual gap *(asterisk)* is present in the center of the section (undecalcified ground section; toluidine blue stain).

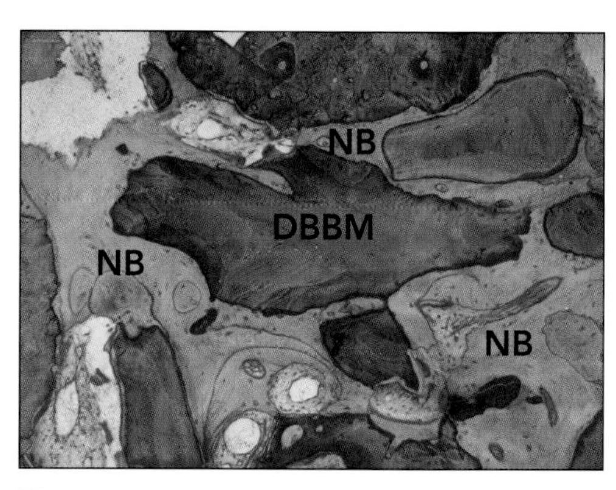

Fig 6-5i Increased magnification of area delineated by larger rectangle in Fig 6-5h. A major portion of the deproteinized bovine bone mineral (DBBM) surface is covered by newly formed bone (NB).

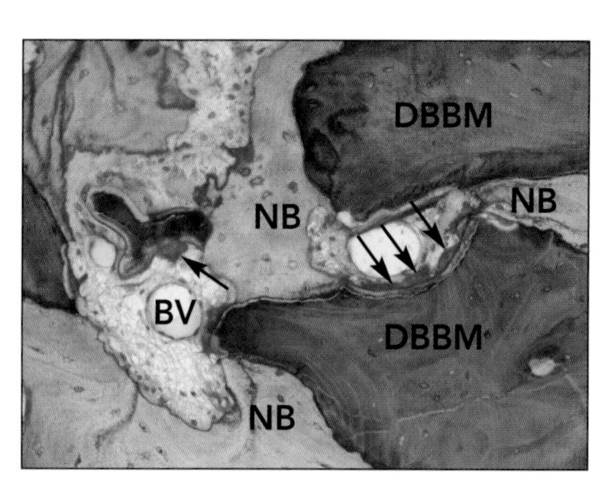

Fig 6-5j Increased magnification of area delineated by smaller rectangle in Fig 6-5h. At sites not covered by bone, osteoclast-like, multinucleated giant cells *(arrows)* are frequently seen lining the deproteinized bovine bone mineral (DBBM) surface even 4 years after augmentation. This suggests a very low substitution rate of this bone filler material. The soft tissue occupying the space between the bone matrix and the bone filler particles is rich in blood vessels (BV).

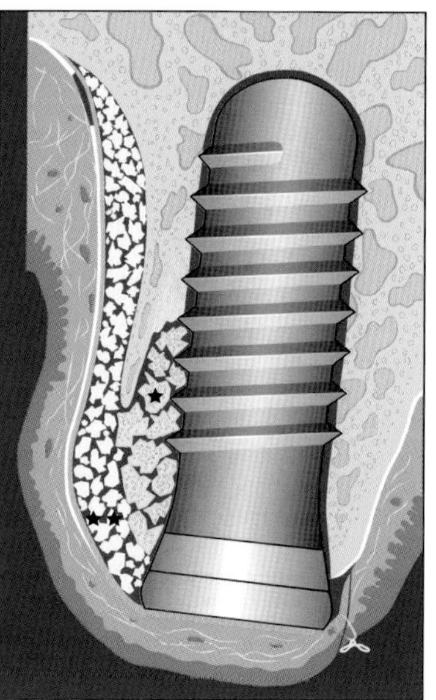

Fig 6-6 In the three-layer concept of contour augmentation, two layers of bone fillers with autogenous bone chips *(★)* cover the exposed implant surface and are augmented with a second layer of a low-substitution filler such as DBBM *(★★)*. The augmentation material is covered by a collagen membrane as a temporary barrier. The biomaterials are protected by a tension-free primary wound closure.

Surgical Principles

Surgical infrastructure and premedication

The ultimate goal of implant surgery with simultaneous GBR is a low-trauma surgical procedure. That includes not only the avoidance of unnecessary tissue damage during surgery but also the avoidance of unnecessary contamination of implant sites and applied biomaterials with intraoral and extraoral bacteria.

A low-trauma surgical procedure requires a well-trained, skilled surgeon with sufficient clinical experience. In addition, a room suitable for surgical procedures under hygienic conditions is necessary. It is recommended that the patient be covered with sterile drapes and that the surgeon and assistants wear acceptable attire. An aseptic operatory, however, is not necessary for successful implant outcomes, as demonstrated in a clinical study.[43] The availability of a competent sterile assistant and a second nonsterile assistant in the operatory is very useful for a smoothly performed surgical procedure. All surgical instruments must be sterilized properly, and a special drilling unit allowing drilling speeds between 15 and 2,000 rpm and irrigation with chilled sterile saline is highly recommended.[44]

Premedication includes a rinse of the oral cavity with chlorhexidine digluconate (0.2%) for 1 minute and the disinfection of the perioral skin prior to surgery. For male patients with planned GBR procedures, we recommend cutting beards or mustaches, if present. For anxious patients, a sedative premedication is routinely used; a benzodiazepine such as midazolam, 5.0 mg intramuscularly or 7.5 mg orally (Dormicum, Roche), is administered 30 minutes prior to surgery. All patients undergoing a simultaneous GBR procedure are prescribed perioperative antibiotic prophylaxis in the form of amoxicillin/clavulanate (Augmentin, GlaxoSmithKline), 2.0 g orally, 2 hours prior to surgery. If patients are allergic to penicillin, an alternative antibiotic medication is used.

Flap design

To optimize the treatment outcome with a simultaneous GBR procedure, tension-free primary wound closure is important to allow undisturbed submerged healing of applied biomaterials. With primary soft tissue healing, the necessary bone healing can take place underneath the intact mucosa without interference from bacteria in the oral cavity. After local augmentation of a deficient ridge, the volume of the ridge will increase. Consequently, mobilization of a full-thickness flap through the incision of the periosteum on the facial or buccal aspect is necessary if tension-free wound closure is to be achieved. This has implications for the flap design because incision of the periosteum can only be performed if the flap is released with at least one vertical incision.

The incision techniques and flap designs used follow old principles of oral surgery. These principles include, among others, creating a flap with a wide base to ensure good vascularity. A trapezoidal flap with two divergent releasing incisions was the design most often used in the past 20 years for GBR procedures. As an alternative, tri-

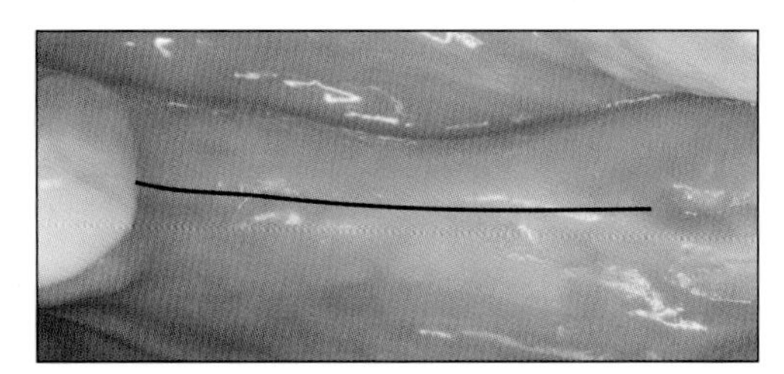

Fig 6-7a For GBR procedures with collagen membranes in mandibular sites, midcrestal incisions are routinely used.

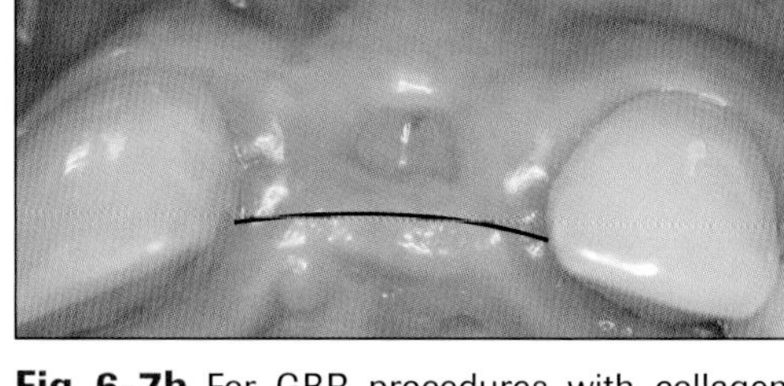

Fig 6-7b For GBR procedures with collagen membranes in maxillary sites, the incision line is positioned slightly toward the palatal aspect.

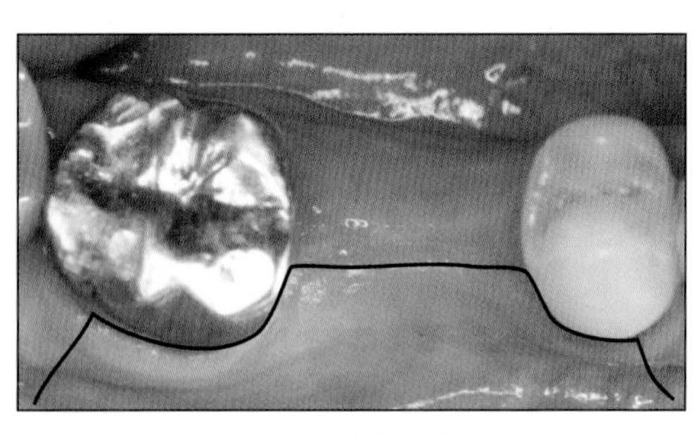

Fig 6-8 In the standard flap design in posterior mandibular GBR sites, the midcrestal incision is extended through the sulcus to the buccal aspect, where two vertical, paramedian releasing incisions are applied for a trapezoidal mucoperiosteal flap.

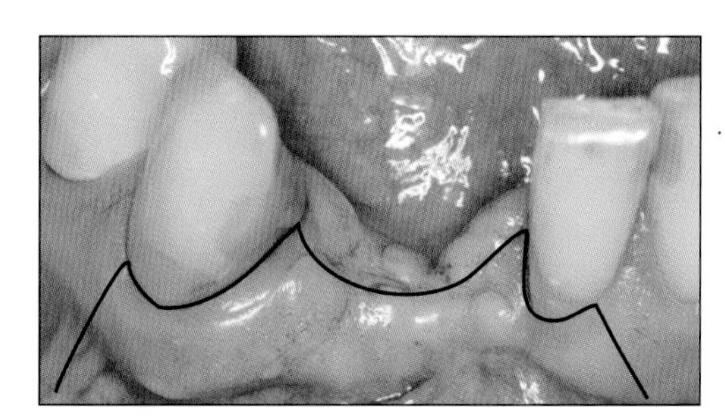

Fig 6-9 A flap design similar to that shown in Fig 6-8 is used in anterior mandibular sites with a crestal incision, a sulcular extension, and two vertical releasing incisions.

angular flap designs with only one vertical releasing incision have also been increasingly used, particularly in esthetically demanding sites.

Incision technique

When the incision line is discussed, a differentiation has to be made between the incision in the crestal area of the edentulous space and the various options for vertical or vestibular releasing incisions. In the early 1990s, lateral incisions in the crestal area were recommended when ePTFE membranes were used because midcrestal incisions often resulted in soft tissue dehiscences.[11,45] These lateral incisions were on the palatal aspects in the maxilla, whereas they were applied on the buccal aspect in the posterior mandible. These lateral incisions have been tricky for the clinician, particularly in mandibular sites. With non–cross-linked collagen membranes, a midcrestal incision can routinely be used in mandibular implant sites (Fig 6-7a). In maxillary sites, the incision line is positioned slightly toward the palatal aspect (Fig 6-7b). These incisions are much easier to apply and simplify the surgical procedure for the clinician.

In the posterior mandible, sulcular incisions at adjacent teeth are used to extend the crestal incision in the edentulous area in a mesial and distal direction (Fig 6-8). Releasing incisions in the vestibule are routinely applied. In the premolar area, the location of the mental foramen must be considered to avoid damage to the mental nerve. The same flap design is used in the anterior mandible (Fig 6-9).

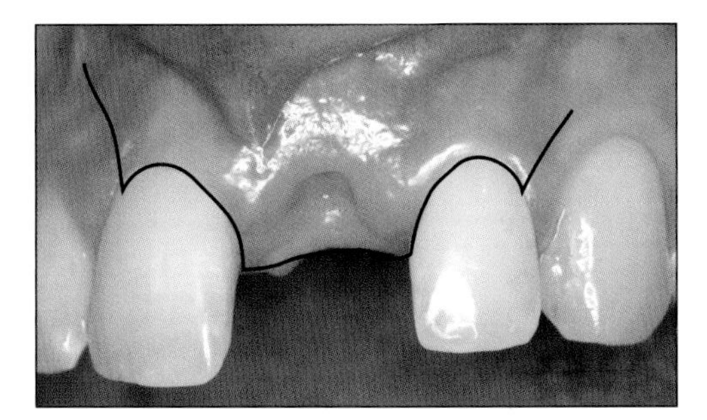

Fig 6-10a In the anterior maxilla, the typical flap design preferred by oral surgeons involves a crestal incision with a sulcular extension and two distal line angle releasing incisions that result in a trapezoidal mucoperiosteal flap.

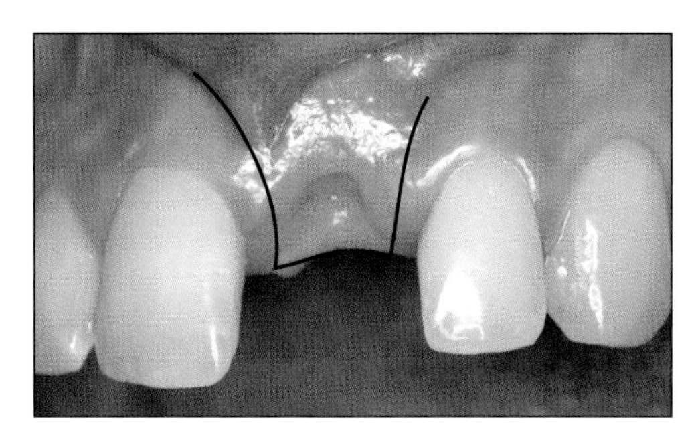

Fig 6-10b In an alternative papilla-sparing flap design often preferred by periodontists, the papillae are not elevated to avoid the exposure of approximal bone structure.

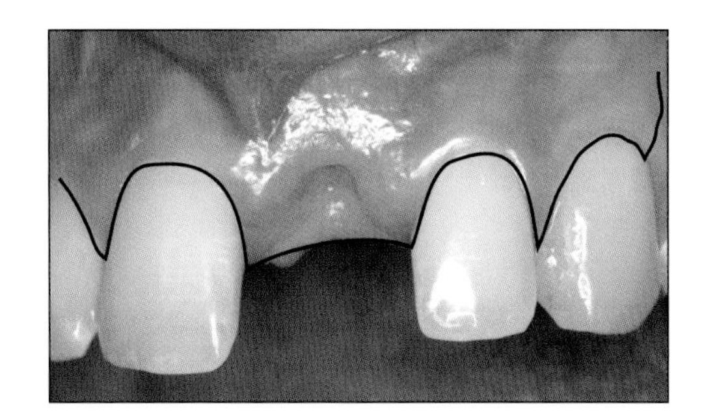

Fig 6-10c A further alternative is a triangular flap design with a crestal incision and a long intrasulcular, bilateral extension. Only one vertical releasing incision is applied, distal to the canine site, to avoid any scar lines between the canines.

In the anterior maxilla, the best incision techniques and flap designs are still a subject of controversy. Two major questions are whether *(1)* vertical releasing incisions should be applied and *(2)* the incision technique should include the papillae. The first question has already been discussed. If a contour augmentation is performed and if tension-free primary wound closure is an important part of the surgical concept, then at least one vertical releasing incision has to be applied to allow incision of the periosteum. Vertical incisions can later cause scar tissue lines, which might require an additional minor surgical procedure to remove them with either a diamond drill or a carbon dioxide laser.

The second question has been debated for many years. Oral surgeons often prefer a surgical approach that includes the papillae for the elevation of a full-thickness flap (Fig 6-10a). On the other hand, periodontists often prefer smaller flaps with a papilla-sparing incision (Fig 6-10b). Both approaches have their advantages and disadvantages. A papilla-sparing incision might cause slightly less bone resorption at approximal areas of adjacent teeth, as shown in a clinical study.[46] The disadvantage of this incision technique is a much smaller flap and two vertical scar lines in a critical area. The intrasulcular incision technique at adjacent teeth might cause more approximal bone resorption but offers a much larger flap, which improves the vascularity in the elevated flap and provides better access to the augmentation site for the application of biomaterials. The vertical releasing incisions are applied as distal line angle incisions, either at adjacent teeth or even more distantly. As an alternative, a triangular flap design with only one vertical releasing incision, distal to the canine, and an extended intrasulcular incision to the contralateral side can be used (Fig 6-10c).

This flap design offers the advantage of requiring no vertical incisions in the anterior maxilla between the canines. On the other hand, more bone surface is exposed, causing more bone resorption in these areas. In routine cases, the intrasulcular incision technique, using either a trapezoidal or a triangular flap design, is clearly preferred by our group.

Wound closure

Wound closure is also essential for a successful treatment outcome. Uneventful primary wound healing not only ensures optimal outcomes but also limits the number of postsurgical visits for the patient. This point should not be forgotten when the cost effectiveness of a procedure is discussed.

The first principle of wound closure is tension-free adaptation of the wound margins. To achieve that goal, the buccal or facial flap must be routinely released with a blade (no. 15). This must be done with caution in the premolar area of the mandible to avoid damage to the mental nerve. A second principle is to avoid too many sutures because wound healing does not take place underneath, but between, applied sutures. Therefore, an optimal distance between sutures is about 2 to 3 mm.

As suture material, a nonresorbable, monofilament, polyamide suture is preferred, with thicknesses of 4-0, 5-0, or 6-0 (Seralon, Serag Wiessner). In routine cases in the anterior maxilla, 5-0 sutures—most often interrupted single sutures—are used in the crestal area to secure the flap, whereas 6-0 interrupted single sutures are applied for the releasing incisions. In patients with extended edentulous spaces, where significant swelling must be anticipated, 4-0 sutures are used and left in place for 14 days.

Details of various clinical procedures are presented step by step in case reports in the following sections and chapters.

Surgical Procedures

Apical fenestration defects

Apical fenestration defects are routinely found in lateral incisor sites with congenitally missing teeth. These are typically healed sites with no bone defect and sufficient width in the crestal area. Fenestration defects are also found in canine or first premolar sites in the maxilla.

Case 1

A congenitally missing lateral incisor was the cause for implant therapy in a 19-year-old woman. The patient exhibited a medium smile line (Fig 6-11a). The remaining primary tooth was slightly rotated, demonstrated a completely resorbed root (Fig 6-11b), and had to be removed. The adjacent central incisor showed clearly visible root resorption of unknown etiology.

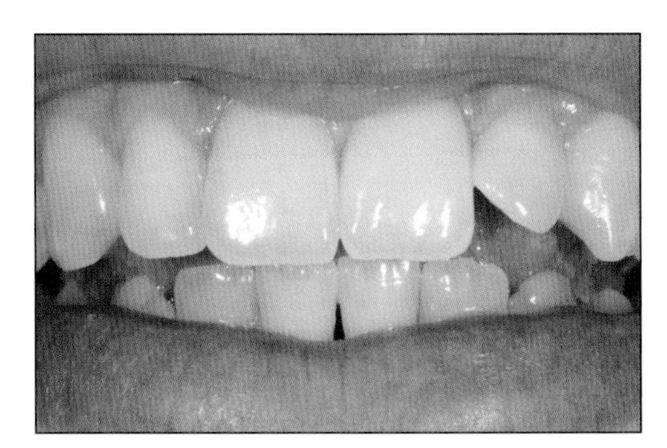

Fig 6-11a A 19-year-old woman has a remaining primary tooth that is slightly rotated and shows increased mobility.

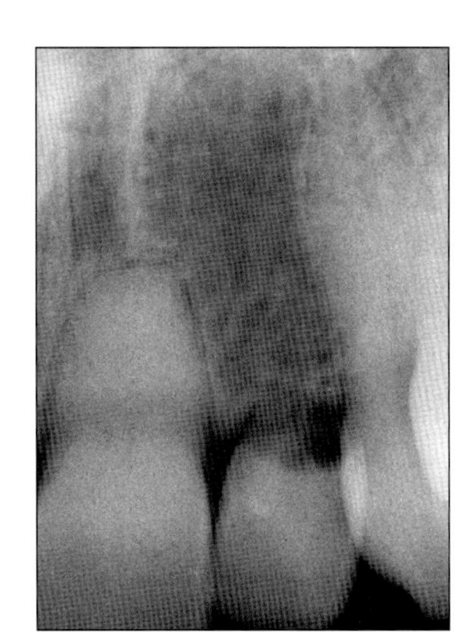

Fig 6-11b The periapical radiograph reveals complete root resorption of the primary tooth.

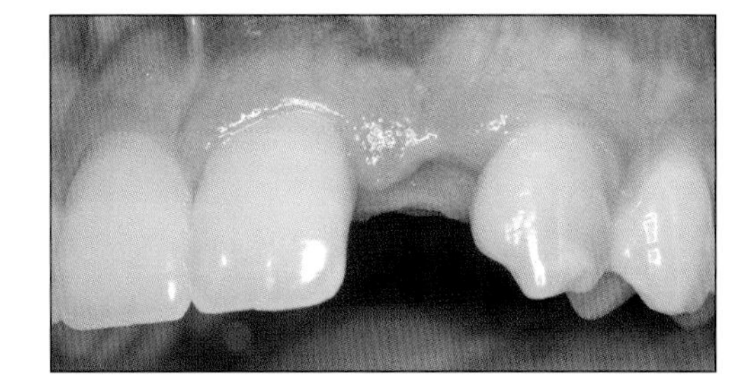

Fig 6-11c Following removal of the primary tooth and a short, soft tissue healing period, the single-tooth gap is well dimensioned for implant placement.

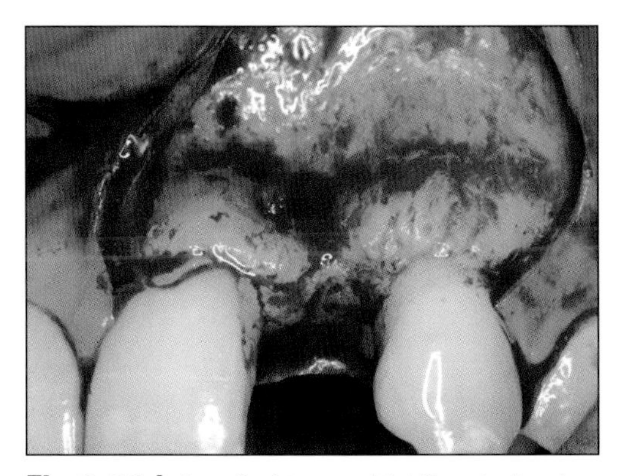

Fig 6-11d A typical trapezoidal flap design has been chosen. Following flap elevation, a significant facial undercut is clearly visible.

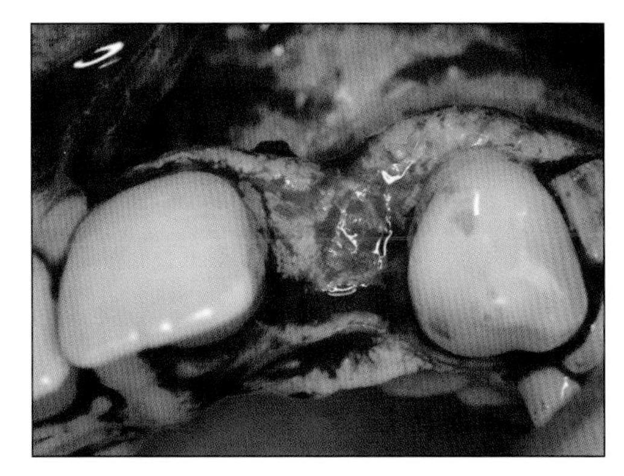

Fig 6-11e The ridge width in the crestal area measures more than 5 mm and is sufficient for implant placement.

The single-tooth gap was sufficiently spaced to insert a screw-type implant with a reduced, 3.3-mm implant diameter and a narrow-neck, 3.5-mm platform. A few weeks after extraction of the primary tooth without flap elevation, the soft tissues were sufficiently healed to allow implant placement with a simultaneous GBR procedure (Fig 6-11c). The site was opened with a typical trapezoidal full-thickness flap with a slightly palatal incision in the crestal area, an intrasulcular extension to both the mesial and distal sides, and two paramedian releasing incisions (Figs 6-11d and 6-11e).

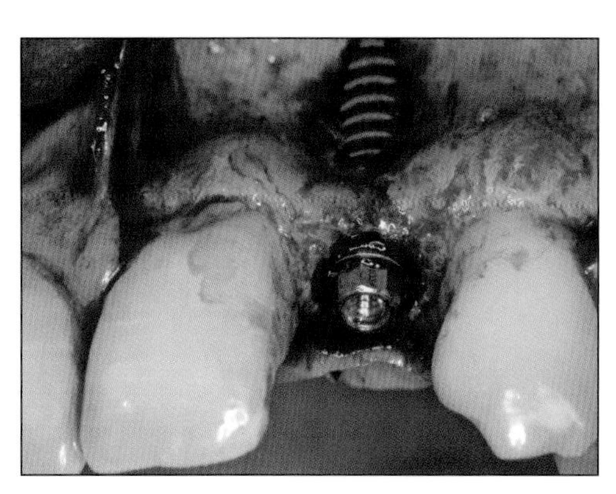

Fig 6-11f A narrow-neck implant has been placed with a correct three-dimensional position and axis, resulting in an apical fenestration defect.

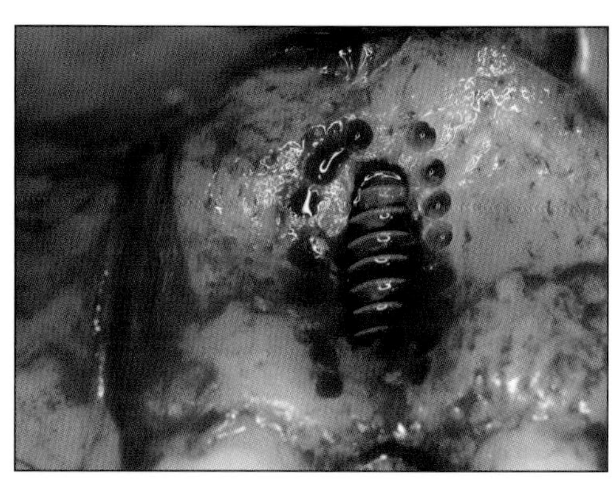

Fig 6-11g The peri-implant bone surface is cortical. Numerous drill holes are prepared to open the marrow cavity and cause bleeding in the defect area.

The crest width was sufficient to allow implant placement, but it also had a significant facial undercut. The implant bed was prepared with round burs, spiral and profile drills of increasing diameter, and copious cooling with sterile, chilled saline. This standardized low-trauma surgical approach helps to minimize trauma to the implant site.[47] The implant was inserted in a correct three-dimensional position and in an appropriate axis to allow placement of a screw-retained crown with a transocclusal access hole in the cingulum area.

This implant position and implant axis resulted, as expected, in a significant apical fenestration defect (Fig 6-11f). The surrounding bone structure was mainly cortical and required the perforation of the cortex with a small round bur to open the marrow cavity and to provoke spontaneous bleeding in the defect area (Fig 6-11g). Next, autogenous bone chips were harvested within the same flap at the nasal spine using a flat chisel, mixed with the patient's own blood, and applied to cover the exposed implant surface (Fig 6-11h). The autografts were covered with a second layer of DBBM granules to accomplish the contour augmentation (Fig 6-11i). These granules clearly overcontoured the local anatomy to serve as supporting anatomical structure for pleasing soft tissue esthetics (Fig 6-11j).

The augmentation material was covered with a collagen membrane using a double-layer technique (Figs 6-11k and 6-11l). This allowed good stabilization of the membrane serving as a temporary barrier. In addition, the membrane also helped to keep applied bone fillers in place. As a rule, collagen membranes can extend into the sulcus of adjacent teeth without causing any problems during healing. The surgery was completed with tension-free primary wound closure following the incision of the periosteum on the facial aspect. The wound margins were carefully adapted and secured in place with several interrupted single sutures (Fig 6-11m).

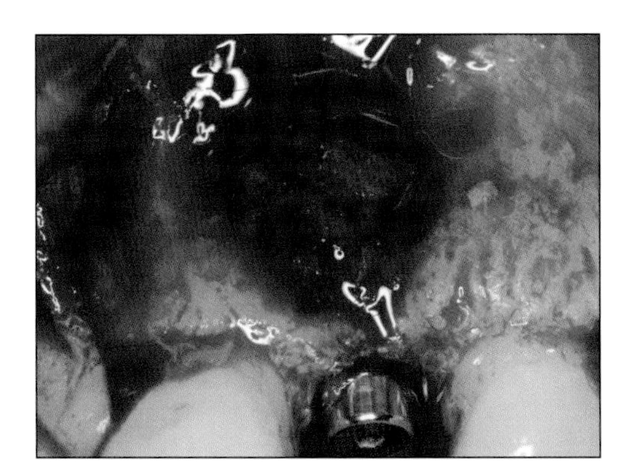

Fig 6-11h Locally harvested bone chips are applied to cover the exposed implant surface. These osteogenic autografts are supposed to speed new bone formation at the bone-implant interface.

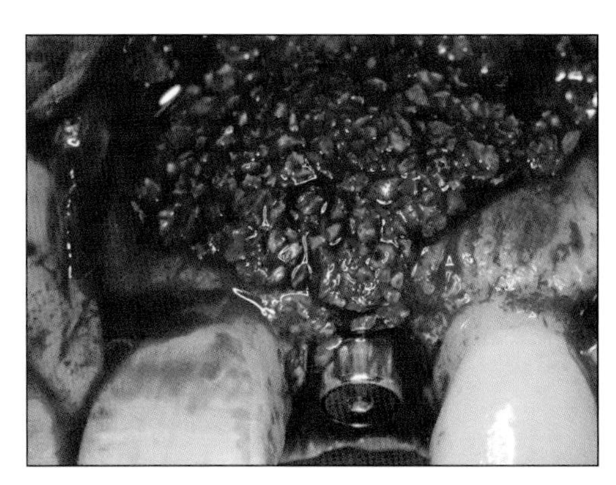

Fig 6-11i A second layer of DBBM particles is applied in the implant site. The granules are soaked in blood to facilitate application.

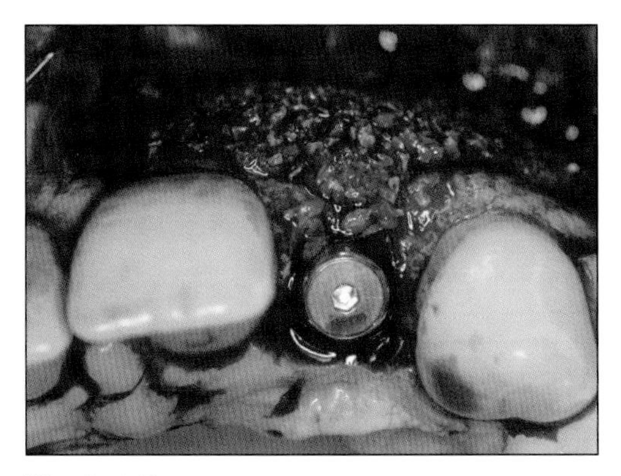

Fig 6-11j The occlusal view demonstrates the contour augmentation. The low-substitution bone filler is supposed to optimize the esthetic outcome and to provide a stable volume in the implant site.

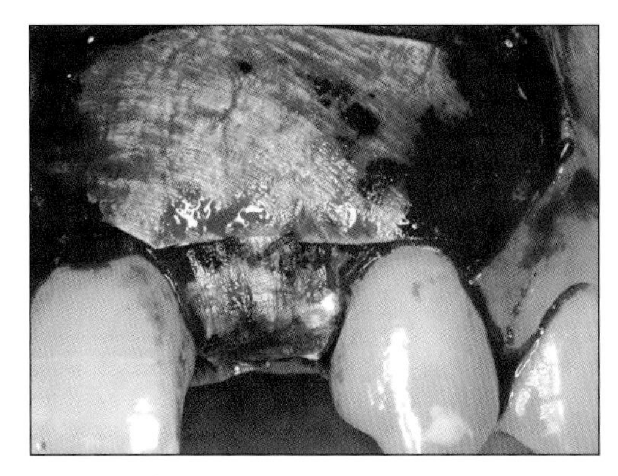

Fig 6-11k Application of a collagen membrane with a double-layer technique. The hydrophilic membrane is easy to manage as soon as it is moistened with blood.

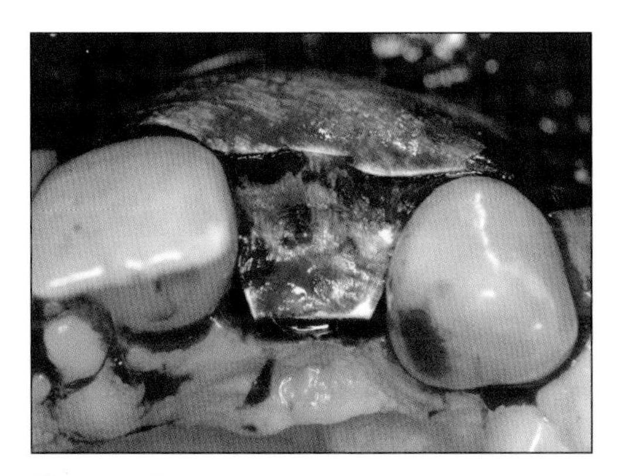

Fig 6-11l The membrane not only provides a temporary barrier function but also stabilizes the applied bone fillers.

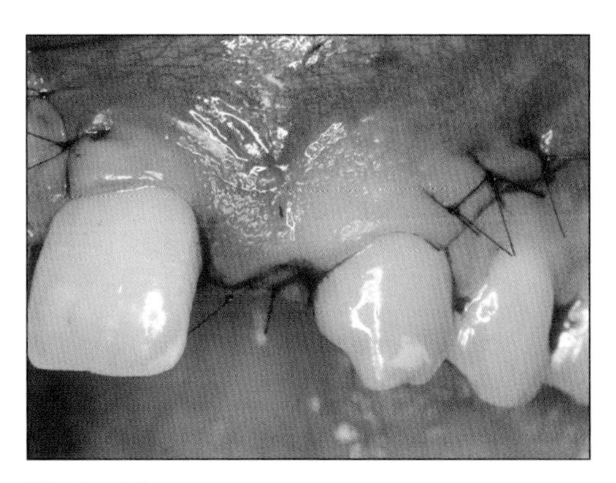

Fig 6-11m Following the release of the periosteum, tension-free primary wound closure is achieved with interrupted single sutures.

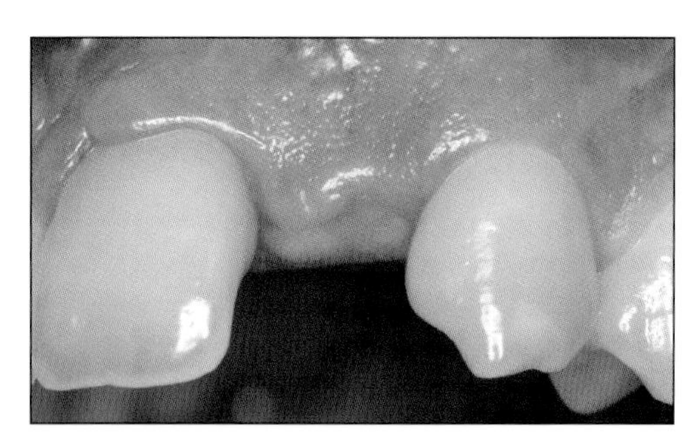

Fig 6-11n Two months later, the clinical status shows nicely healed soft tissues in the implant site. A fine scar line is still visible in the area of the mesial releasing incision.

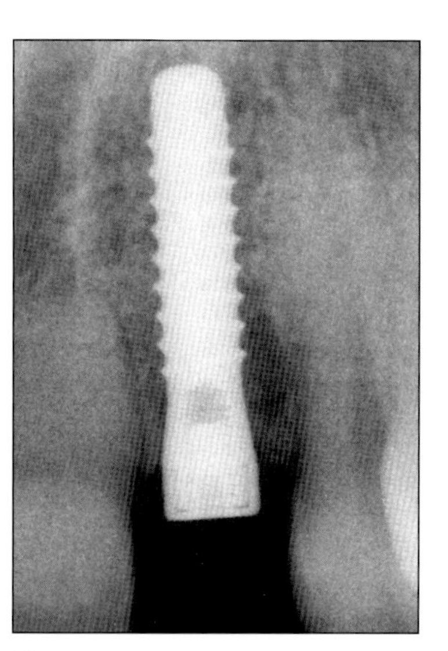

Fig 6-11o The periapical radiograph confirms good implant integration.

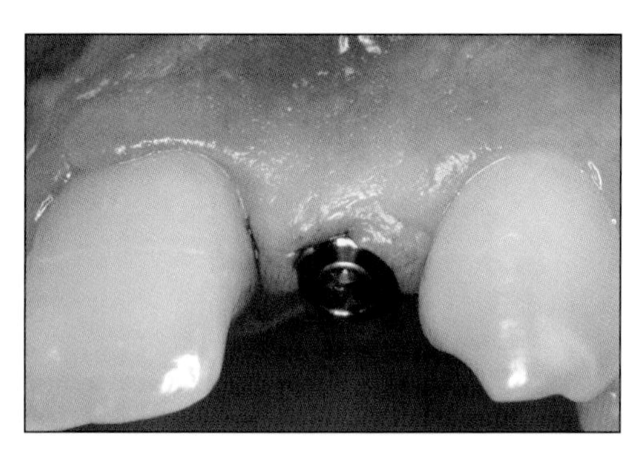

Fig 6-11p The implant site has been reopened with a small punch technique, and a longer healing cap has been placed.

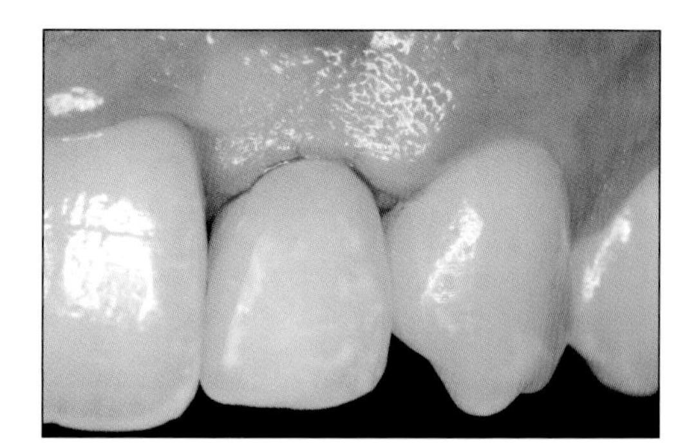

Fig 6-11q After insertion of a provisional crown, the peri-implant soft tissues are blanching and will adapt to the shape of the crown within a few days.

Following 8 weeks of uneventful healing, the clinical and radiographic examinations revealed well-healed soft tissues in the implant site and a well-integrated implant (Figs 6-11n and 6-11o). The implant was exposed with a minor punch technique using a no. 12b blade without flap mobilization (Fig 6-11p) and restored with a provisional crown for soft tissue conditioning (Fig 6-11q). A few months later, the provisional crown was restored with a metal-ceramic crown.

The 3.5-year follow-up examination demonstrated a pleasing esthetic outcome. As a result of excellent home care by the patient, peri-implant soft tissues were free of inflammation (Figs 6-11r to 6-11t). Radiographically, the narrow-neck implant was well integrated, showing typical, minor bone remodeling in the crestal area (Fig 6-11u). With these clinical and radiographic findings, the implant has an excellent long-term prognosis.

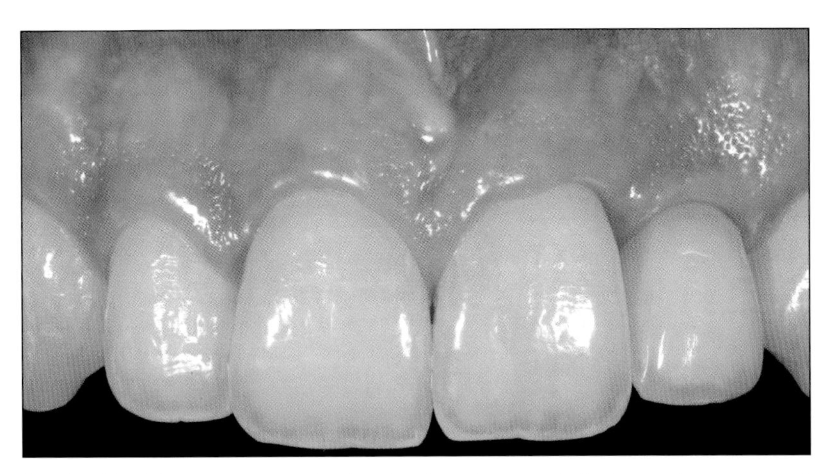

Fig 6-11r About 3.5 years following implant placement, the implant crown is well integrated within the esthetic zone. The esthetic outcome is pleasing.

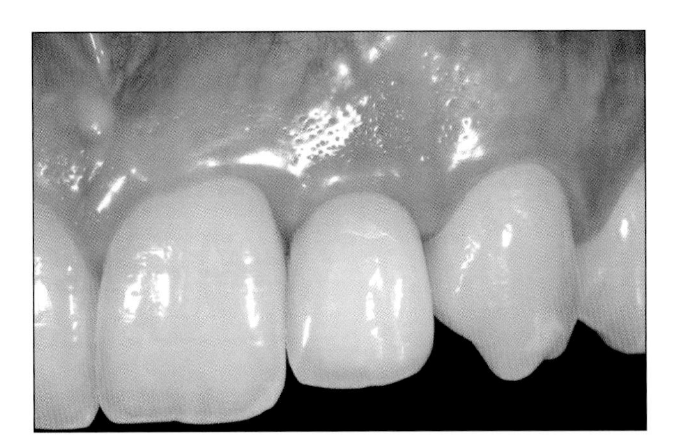

Fig 6-11s A close-up view reveals healthy peri-implant soft tissue free of visible inflammation. The facial margin of the mucosa is well positioned with a nice convexity.

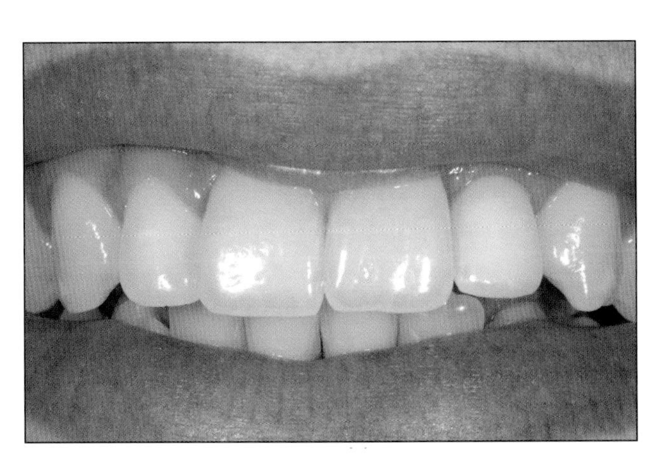

Fig 6-11t The patient's smile exhibits a pleasing esthetic outcome 3.5 years after implant placement.

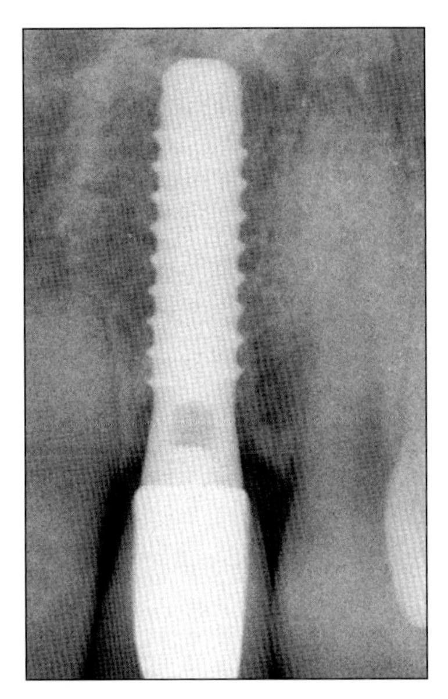

Fig 6-11u The periapical radiograph confirms a well-integrated implant with minor bone remodeling in the crestal area.

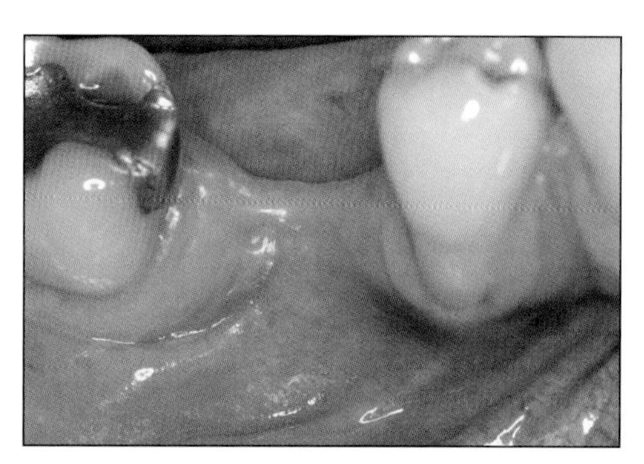

Fig 6-12a Single-tooth gap in the posterior mandible. The mandibular right first molar had been extracted several years previously. Subsequently, a buccal flattening has taken place.

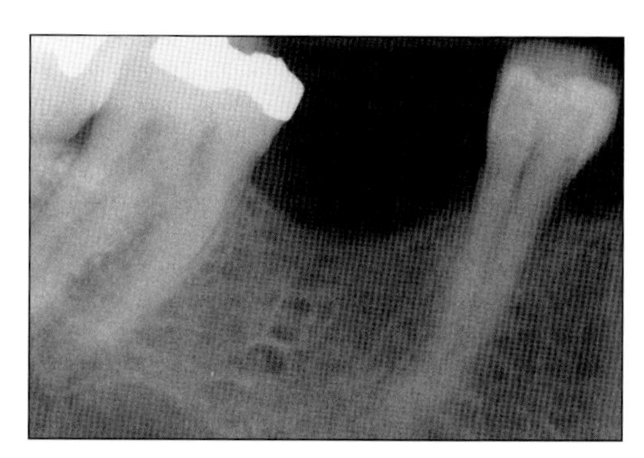

Fig 6-12b The periapical radiograph reveals normal bone structures in the edentulous space.

Crestal dehiscence defects

Crestal dehiscence defects are found in healed sites in which tooth extraction took place more than 6 months previously. These sites were frequently seen in the 1980s and even in the 1990s, when late implant placement was still the standard of care in postextraction sites. As a consequence, many implant sites had insufficient crest width when implants were placed, necessitating a simultaneous GBR procedure. Today, these crestal dehiscence defects are much less frequently encountered in daily practice because the pattern of ridge alterations following tooth extraction is well understood. Clinicians generally use more modern treatment concepts such as immediate or early implant placement (see chapter 7).

Case 2

A patient's mandibular right first molar had been extracted several years earlier. Thus, the local anatomy showed the typical buccal atrophy in the single-tooth gap (Fig 6-12a). The radiographic analysis showed that there was sufficient bone height above the mandibular canal to place a 10-mm screw-type implant (Fig 6-12b).

The site was opened with a typical trapezoidal flap to obtain sufficient access to the edentulous area in the first molar area (Fig 6-12c). Following preparation of the implant bed, the extent of the crestal bone defect on the buccal aspect was clearly visible (Fig 6-12d). To improve the predictability of new bone formation, the peri-implant bone surface was perforated with a small round bur to open the marrow cavity and to stimulate bleeding in the defect area (Fig 6-12e). In addition, the thin bone wall on the buccal aspect of the implant bed was intentionally reduced in height with a diamond drill to create a flat bottom on the buccal bone wall.

Bone chips were locally harvested from the buccal bone surface distal to the implant site with a bone scraper (Fig 6-12f) and stored in a sterile metal dish (Fig 6-12g). The implant was inserted in a correct three-dimensional position, resulting, as expected, in a two-wall defect with a flat bottom (Fig 6-12h). This defect anatomy is important to stabilize applied bone chips in a vertical direction. These chips were mixed with blood and applied to cover the exposed implant surface (Fig 6-12i).

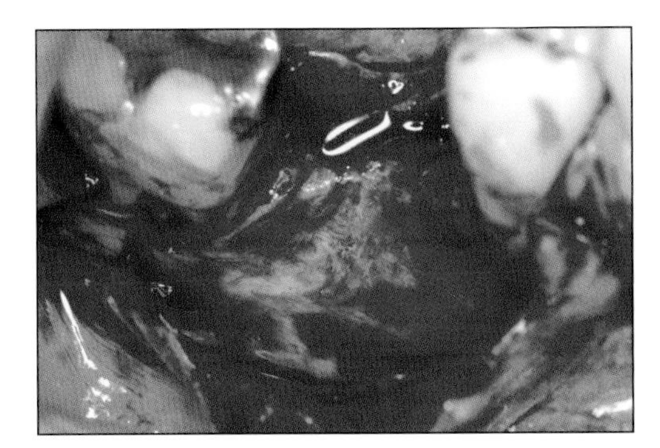

Fig 6-12c Following elevation of a trapezoidal mucoperiosteal flap with two releasing incisions, the reduced crest width is apparent.

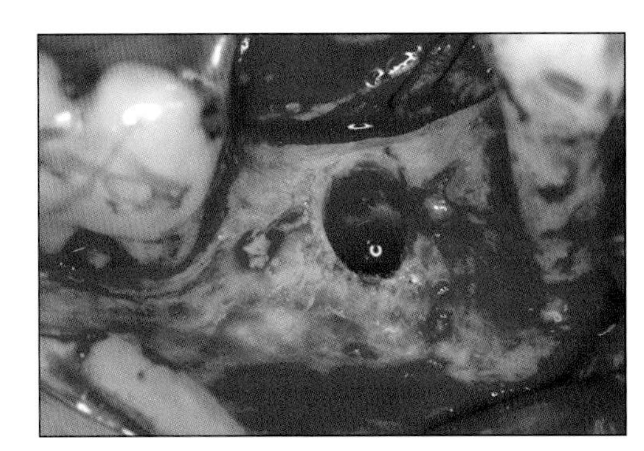

Fig 6-12d The implant bed is prepared in a correct three-dimensional position. This results in a crestal dehiscence defect.

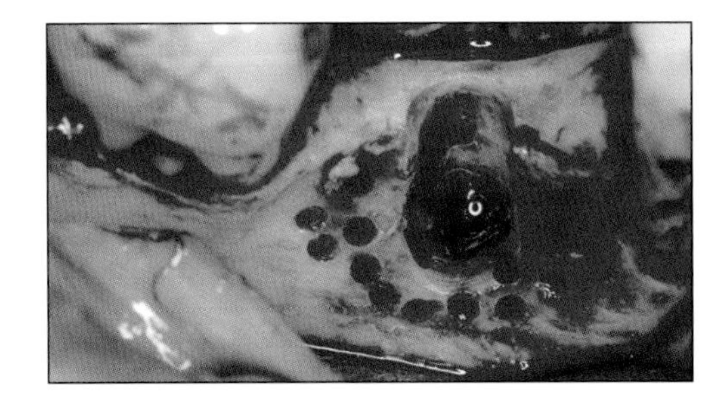

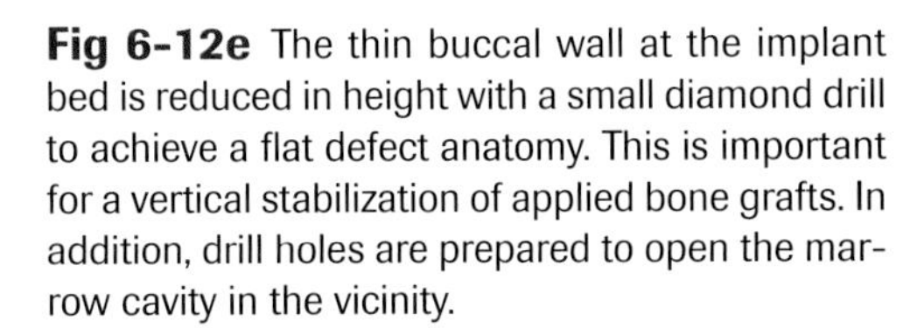

Fig 6-12e The thin buccal wall at the implant bed is reduced in height with a small diamond drill to achieve a flat defect anatomy. This is important for a vertical stabilization of applied bone grafts. In addition, drill holes are prepared to open the marrow cavity in the vicinity.

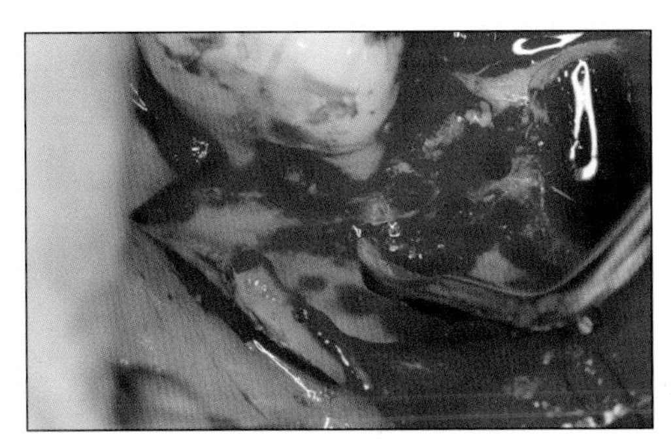

Fig 6-12f Autogenous bone chips are locally harvested with a sharp bone scraper on the facial aspect distal to the implant site.

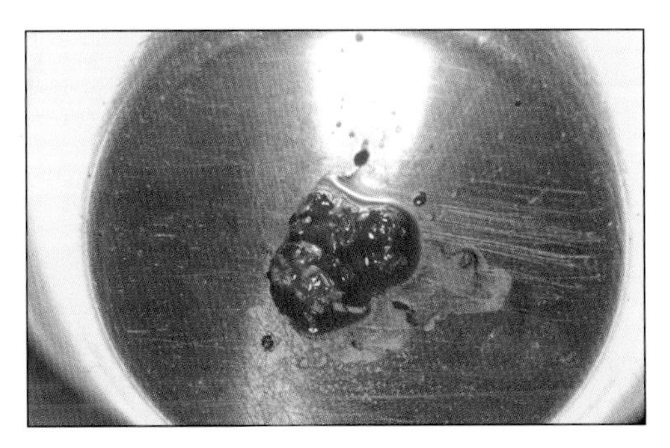

Fig 6-12g The bone chips are stored in a sterile metal dish and soaked in blood.

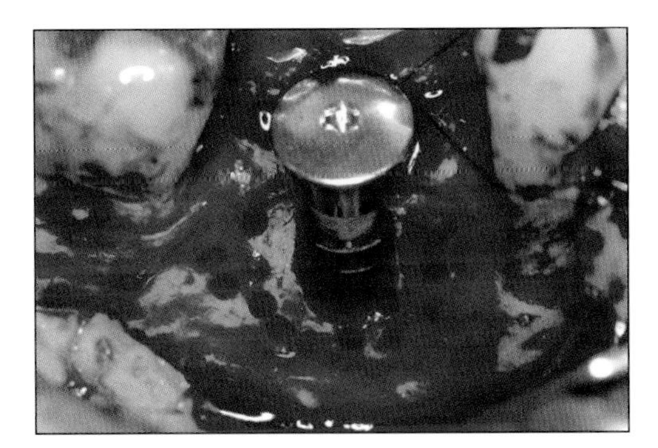

Fig 6-12h Following placement of a standard-diameter implant, the crestal dehiscence defect is apparent on the buccal aspect of the implant.

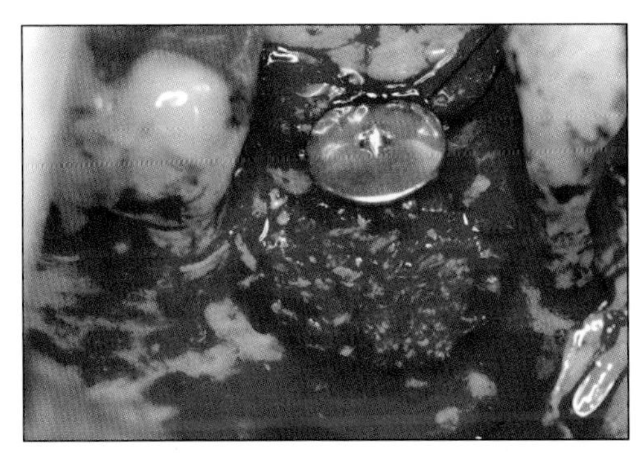

Fig 6-12i The bone defect site is augmented with locally harvested bone chips.

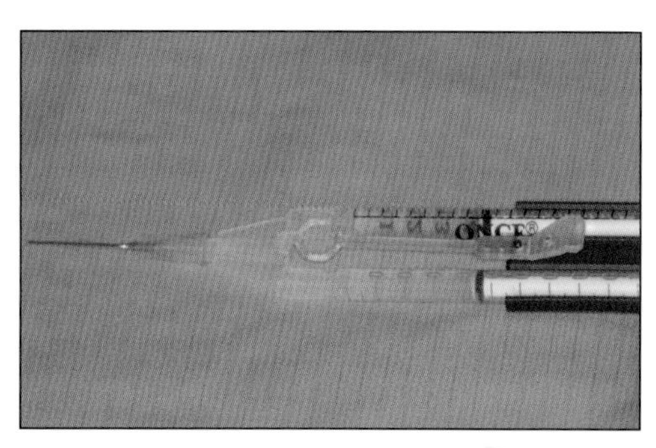

Fig 6-12j In mandibular GBR sites, fibrin sealant is often used to stabilize applied bone fillers.

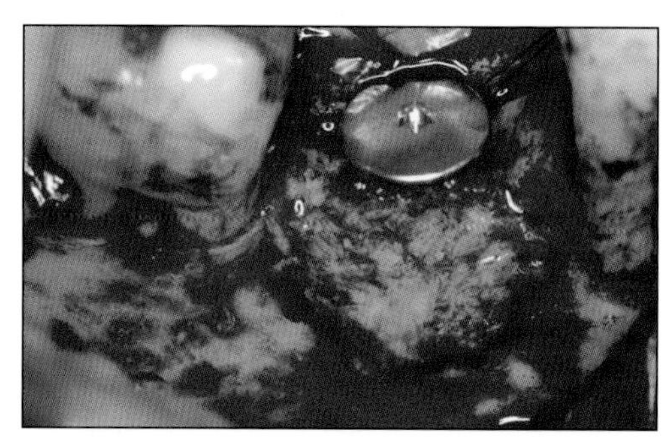

Fig 6-12k The mixture of fibrinogen and thrombin immediately causes coagulation and hence stabilizes applied bone fillers.

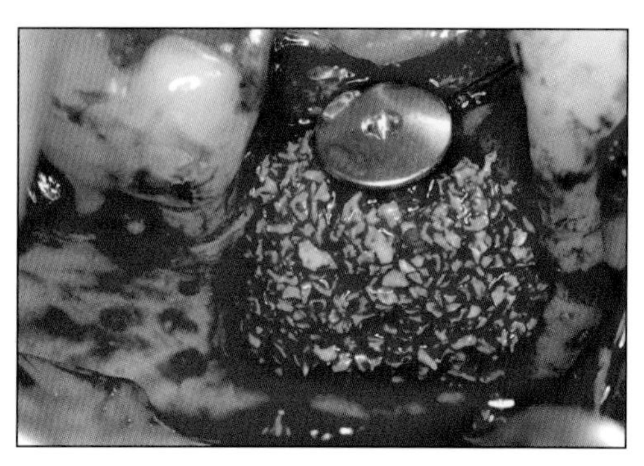

Fig 6-12l A second layer of DBBM granules is applied for contour augmentation.

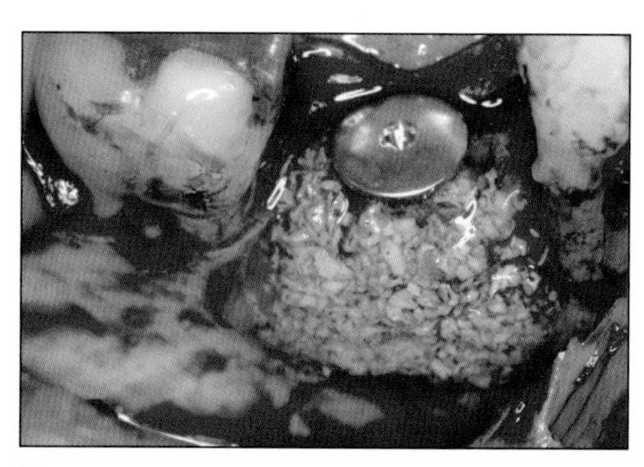

Fig 6-12m The DBBM particles are again stabilized with fibrin sealant.

In mandibular sites, gravity can be the clinician's enemy because applied chips have a tendency to slide in an apical direction. In addition to the flat bottom of the peri-implant defect, the chips can be stabilized with a fibrin sealant (Tissucol, Baxter). This two-component sealant with fibrinogen and thrombin coagulates within seconds and hence stabilizes the applied bone chips (Figs 6-12j and 6-12k). The autografts were covered with a thin layer of DBBM granules, which were again stabilized with fibrin sealant (Figs 6-12l and 6-11m).

Prior to wound closure, a collagen membrane was applied with a double-layer technique (Fig 6-12n). The mucoperiosteal flap was carefully mobilized with a superficial incision of the periosteum. The surgery was completed with tension-free primary wound closure using several interrupted single sutures (Fig 6-12o).

The surgical site was left to heal for 12 weeks, then the implant site was reopened, and the implant was restored by the referring dentist with a cemented metal-ceramic crown (Figs 6-12p and 6-12q).

The 3-year follow-up examination demonstrated a well-integrated implant that exhibited inflammation-free peri-implant soft tissues (Fig 6-12r). The periapical radiograph showed stable peri-implant bone levels in the crestal area (Fig 6-12s).

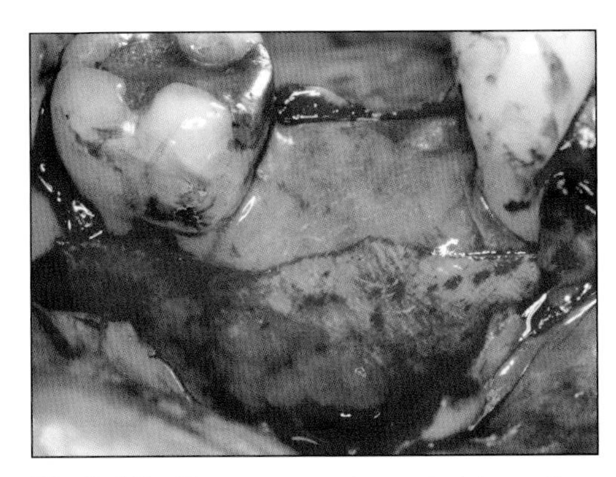

Fig 6-12n The augmentation materials are then covered with a collagen membrane applied with a double-layer technique to improve membrane stability.

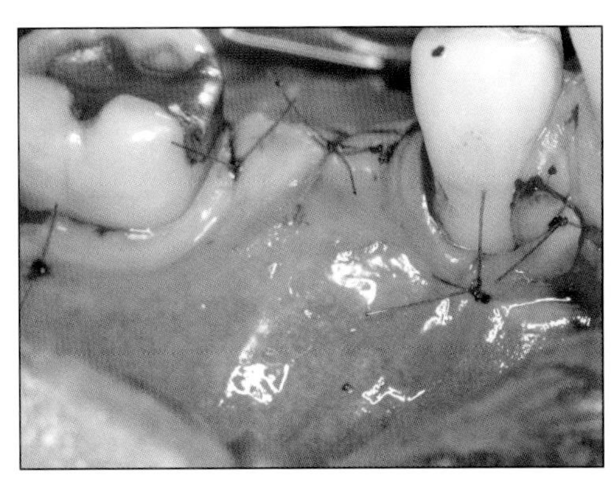

Fig 6-12o Surgery is completed with tension-free primary wound closure using interrupted single sutures.

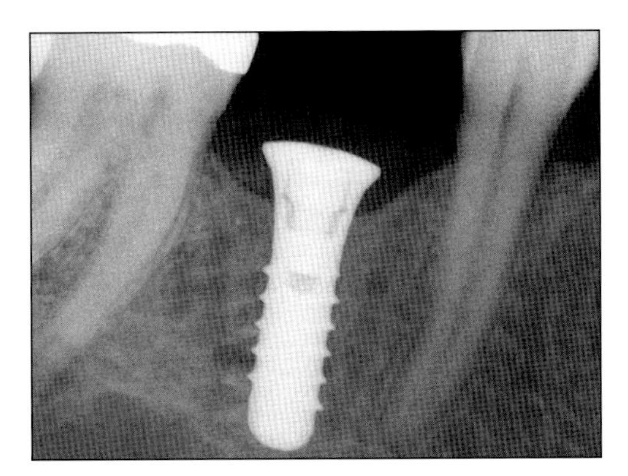

Fig 6-12p The periapical radiograph taken 12 weeks following implant placement indicates that the correctly positioned implant is well integrated and ready for restoration.

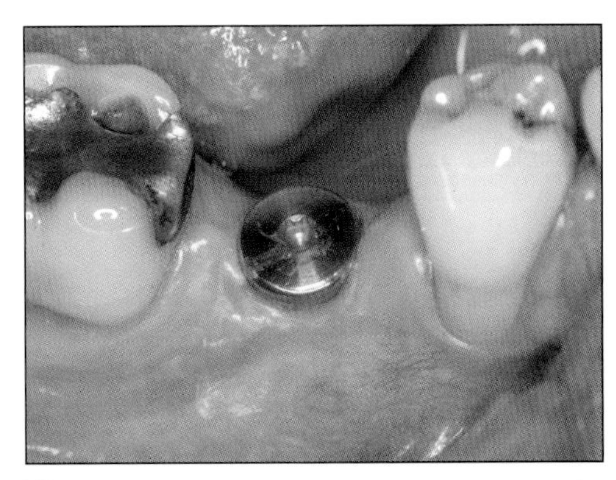

Fig 6-12q Following a reopening procedure, the implant is ready for prosthetic restoration with a cemented metal-ceramic crown.

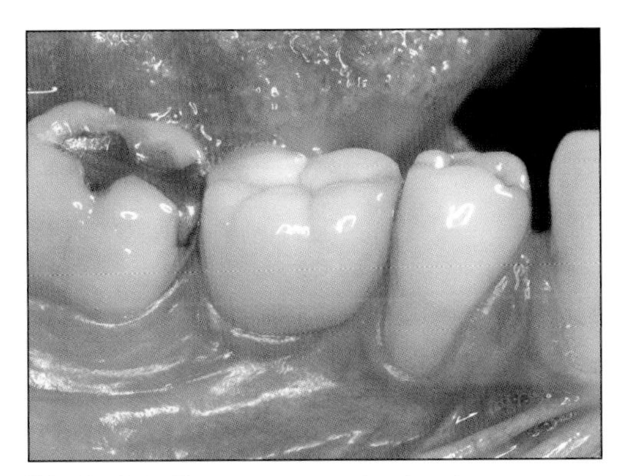

Fig 6-12r The 3-year examination demonstrates the implant-supported single crown with healthy peri-implant soft tissues.

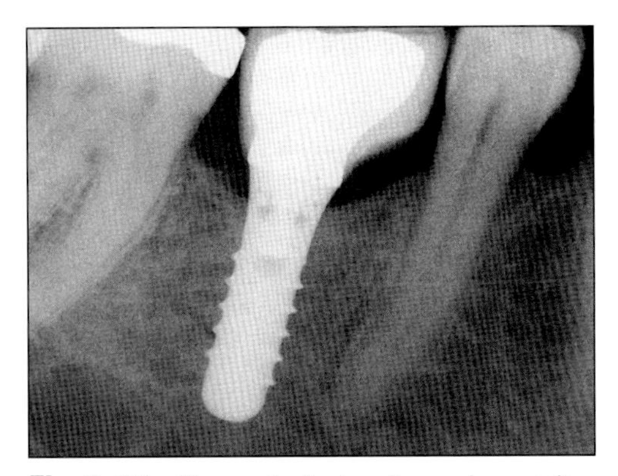

Fig 6-12s The periapical radiograph reveals a well-integrated screw-type implant without signs of peri-implant radiolucencies. The implant has an excellent long-term prognosis.

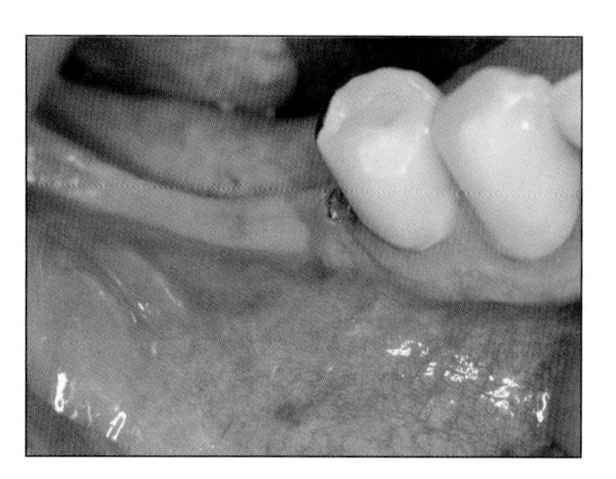

Fig 6-13a Distal-extension situation in the right side of the mandible. The most distal tooth in the arch is the first premolar with a crown. The keratinized mucosa in the edentulous area is reduced in width to a few millimeters.

Case 3

A 61-year-old man was referred to the clinic with a bilateral distal-extension situation; a first premolar was the most distal tooth on both sides of the mandible. This case report will focus on the treatment in the right mandible. The patient had been wearing a removable dental prosthesis and asked for a fixed implant-supported restoration.

The clinical examination indicated that the alveolar crest was narrow, particularly at the first molar site (Fig 6-13a). The three-dimensional radiographic examination with digital volume tomography confirmed a narrow crest in this area, less than 4 mm in width (Figs 6-13b to 6-13e), which would have required a staged approach using an initial horizontal ridge augmentation procedure with GBR to allow implant placement 5 months later. In the area of the second premolar, the crest was also flattened, but not to the same extent. This allowed implant placement with simultaneous GBR. Following intense discussions with the patient about various treatment options, the patient preferred a treatment approach with only one surgical procedure. The plan was to place just one implant, in the second premolar site, and use that implant to support a single crown with a distal cantilever unit.

The surgical procedure was very similar to that described in case 2. The incision line was slightly different because a long crestal incision line was used in the distal-extension situation, whereas the intrasulcular incision to the mesial aspect included not only the first premolar but also the canine (Fig 6-13f). This helped to bypass the mental foramen, which was clearly visualized at a safe distance by extended flap elevation during surgery (Fig 6-13g). The preparation of the implant bed resulted in a medium-sized crestal dehiscence defect, which was augmented following implant placement with the same GBR procedure described in case 2 (Figs 6-13h to 6-13o).

Eight weeks later, the implant was exposed with a small crestal incision. Following a short period of soft tissue healing, the implant was ready to be restored (Figs 6-13p and 6-13q). At the 18-month follow-up examination, the two-unit fixed dental prosthesis was successfully supported by one screw-type implant (Fig 6-13r). The periapical radiograph revealed stable bone crest levels (Fig 6-13s).

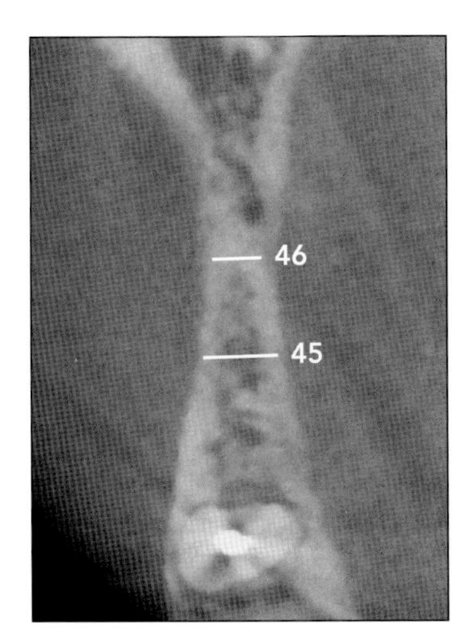

Fig 6-13b Digital volume tomography in the edentulous area. The horizontal slice shows the alveolar crest width in area 45 (mandibular right second premolar) to be roughly 5 mm and in area 46 (mandibular right first molar) to be less than 3 mm.

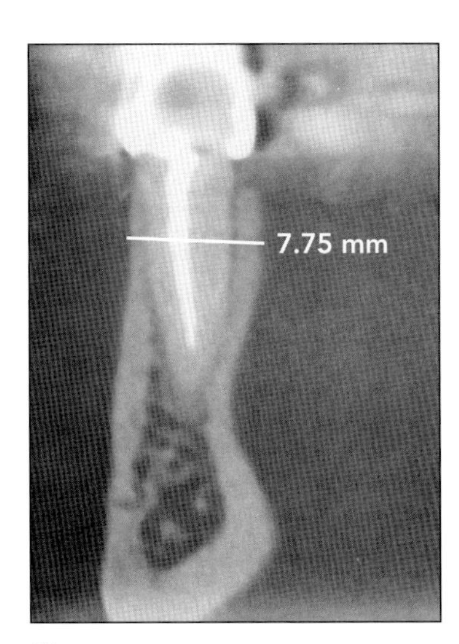

Fig 6-13c The orofacial slice confirms that there is sufficient crest width in the area of the remaining first premolar.

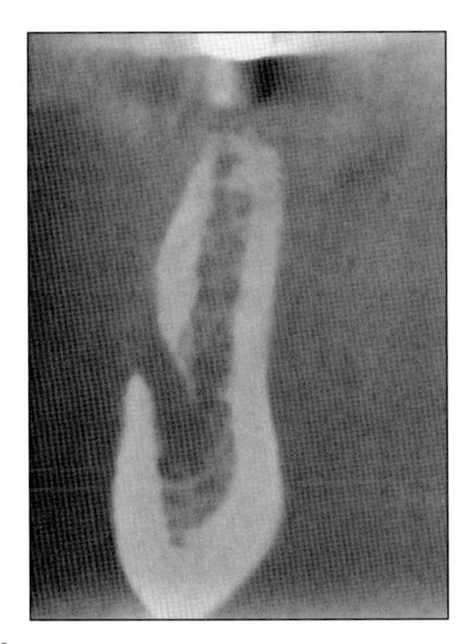

Fig 6-13d The crest is slightly reduced in width in the area of the mandibular right second premolar.

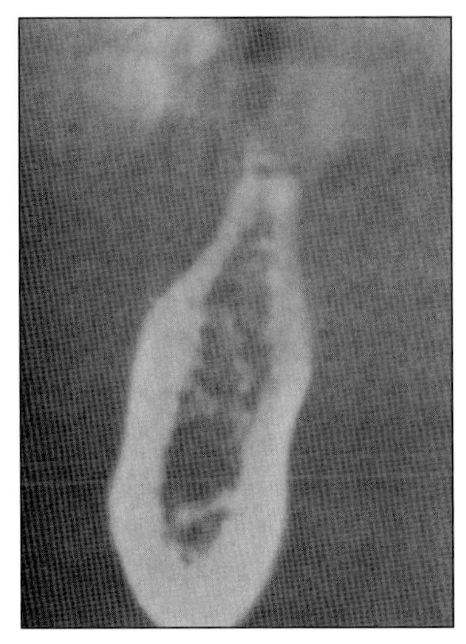

Fig 6-13e The crest is clearly reduced in the area of the mandibular right first molar.

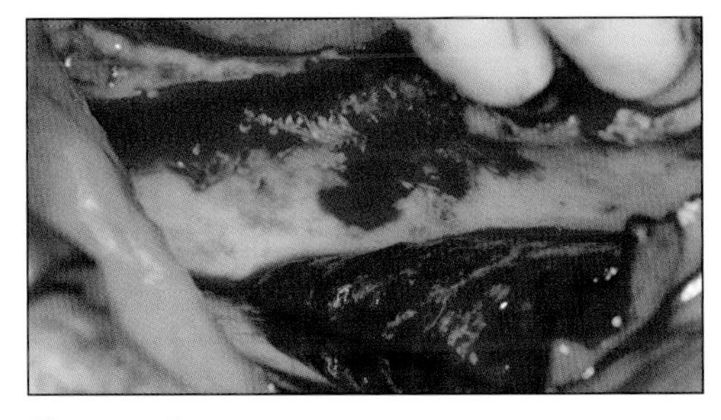

Fig 6-13f A mucoperiosteal flap that is vertically released at the canine is elevated.

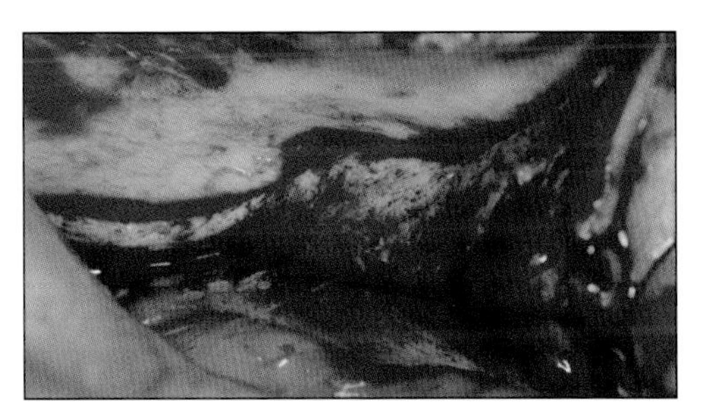

Fig 6-13g The mental nerve is clearly visible and has to be protected during surgery.

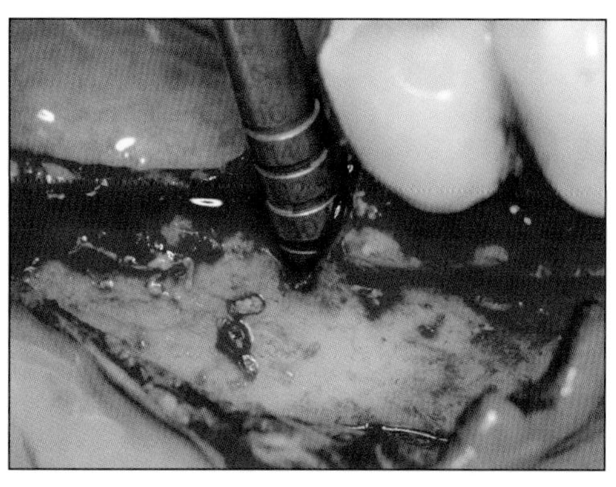

Fig 6-13h The implant bed is prepared for a standard 4.1-mm implant. A depth gauge is inserted. The small buccal defect is apparent.

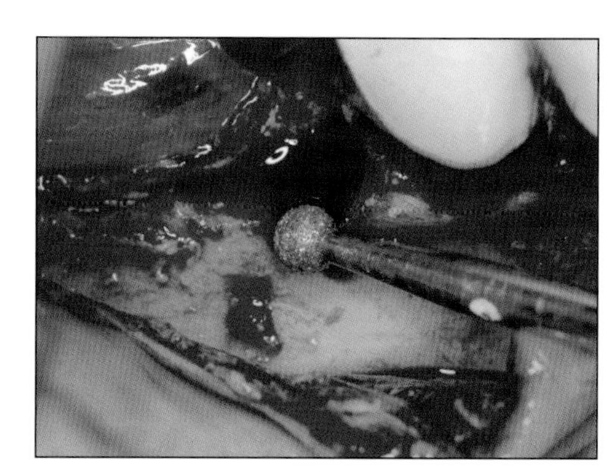

Fig 6-13i The thin buccal bone wall is reduced in height with a round diamond bur.

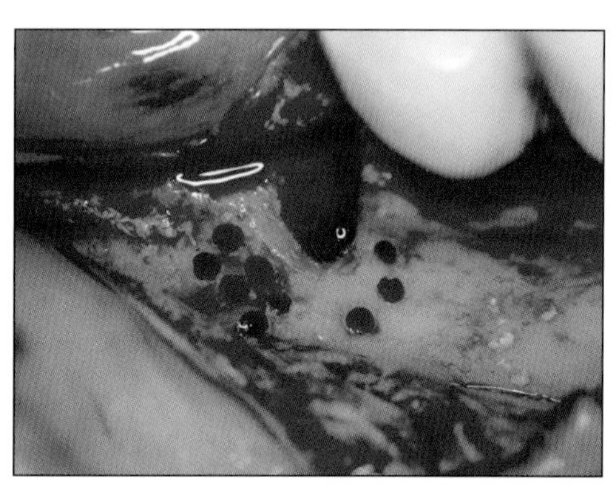

Fig 6-13j The buccal defect now has a flat bottom. In addition, the cortical bone has been perforated in the vicinity with a small round bur.

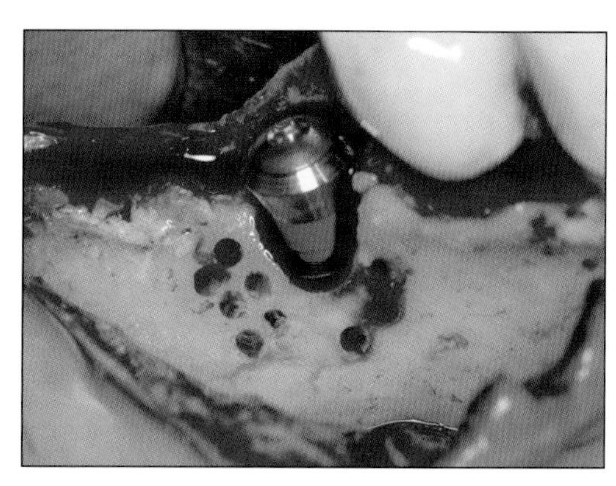

Fig 6-13k Following insertion of the standard-diameter implant, the extent of the buccal defect is apparent. A medium-sized defect remains.

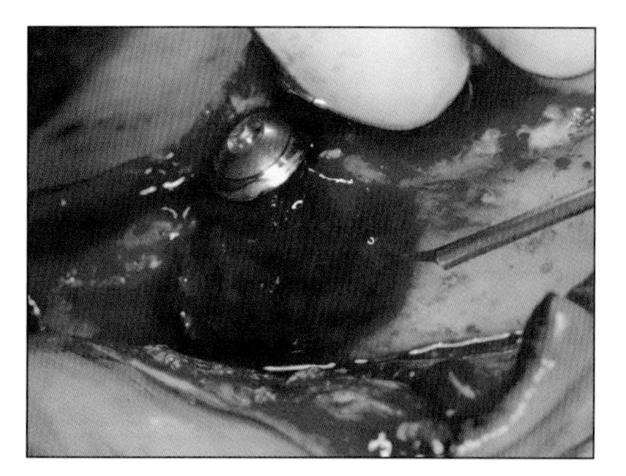

Fig 6-13l Autogenous bone chips are applied and stabilized with fibrin sealant.

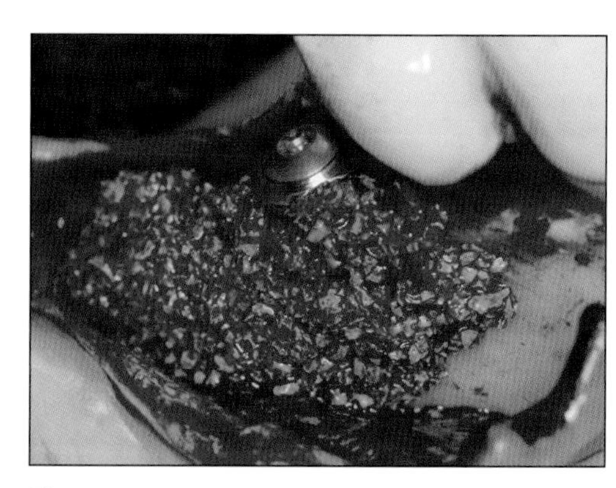

Fig 6-13m The autograft is covered with a layer of DBBM particles.

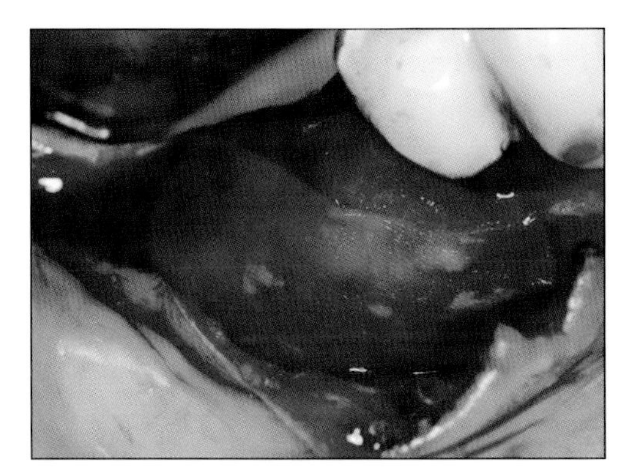

Fig 6-13n A collagen membrane is applied using a double-layer technique.

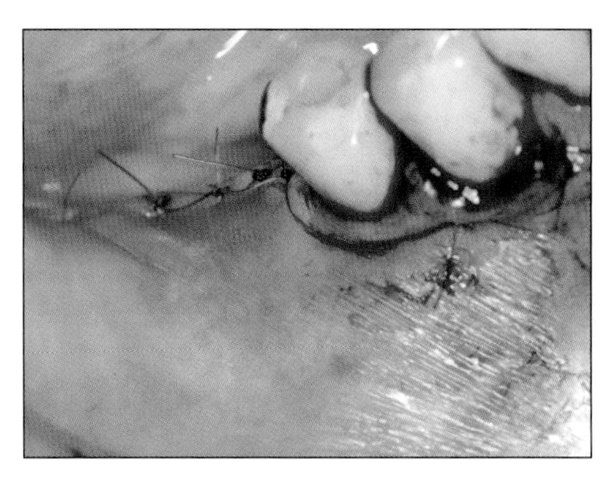

Fig 6-13o The surgery is completed with tension-free primary wound closure. Prior to suturing, the buccal flap was mobilized with a careful incision of the periosteum.

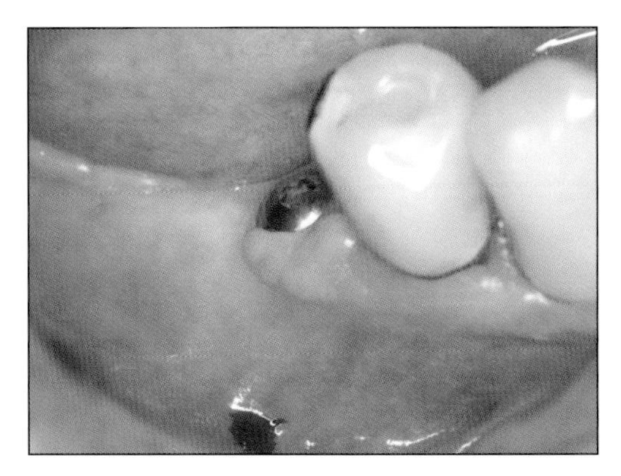

Fig 6-13p Clinical status a few days following a reopening procedure.

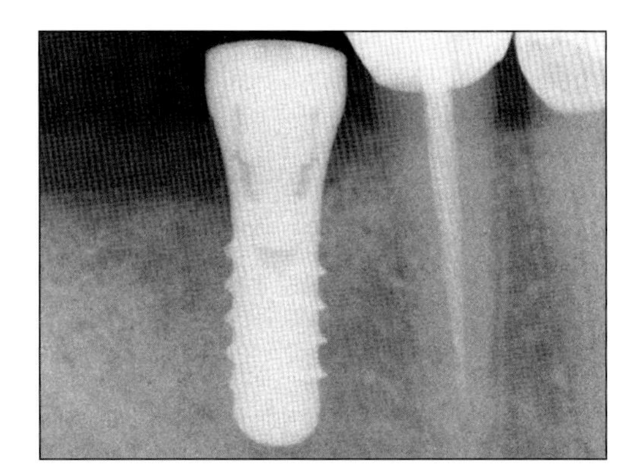

Fig 6-13q The periapical radiograph confirms that the standard-diameter 4.1-mm implant is well integrated.

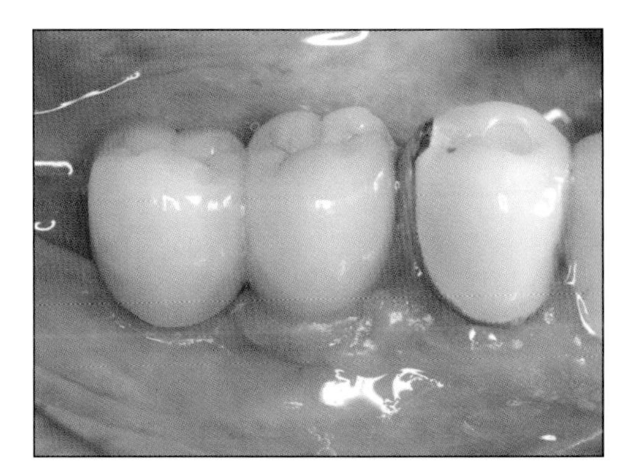

Fig 6-13r Clinical status 18 months following implant placement. The implant was restored by the referring dentist with a cemented metal-ceramic crown and a distal cantilever unit.

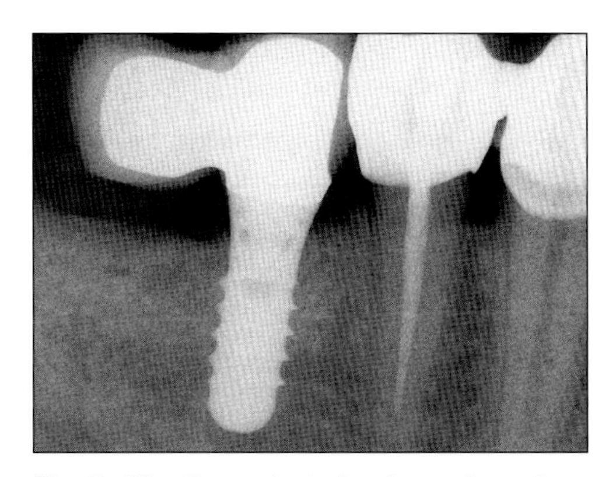

Fig 6-13s The periapical radiograph confirms the implant to be well integrated at the 18-month follow-up examination.

Postoperative Treatment and Healing Periods

Appropriate postoperative instructions and care are important aspects for successful outcomes as well. During the soft tissue healing period, chemical plaque control with chlorhexidine digluconate (0.1%) is routinely used for roughly 2 weeks. Mechanical toothbrushing is discontinued in the surgical site. Follow-up visits are scheduled at days 7, 14, and 21 to check the progress of wound healing. In sites with a large augmentation volume and a potential risk for the development of a postsurgical hematoma, an additional examination is often performed at day 3. The perioperative antibiotic prophylaxis is maintained for 3 days. Sutures are removed after 7 to 14 days.

The healing period until reopening depends on the extent of the peri-implant defect to be regenerated. In apical fenestration-type defects, a healing period of 8 weeks is routinely used. In crestal dehiscence and extraction socket defects, healing periods are based on the extent of the vertical defect dimension on the facial aspect.

For many years, a 6- to 12-week healing period following implant placement was used successfully with simultaneous GBR. Six weeks of healing were allowed for defect sites with a fully intact facial bone wall providing a 3-wall defect, whereas 8 weeks of healing were allowed for vertical bone defects of up to 2 mm in the facial bone wall. A 10-week healing period was used when 3- to 5-mm vertical defects were present in the facial bone wall. The longest healing period was 12 weeks, which was used for vertical bone defects of 6 mm or more on the facial aspect. Recently, these healing periods have been reduced with the introduction of implants with a chemically modified SLA surface into routine practice (see chapter 7).

Conclusion

Implant placement with a simultaneous GBR procedure in apical fenestration and crestal dehiscence defects is a common clinical procedure in implant dentistry. The presented surgical approach offers successful clinical outcomes with high predictability and is attractive not only for clinicians but also for patients. For the patient, it is important that successful treatment outcomes can be achieved with only one open flap procedure and with a rather short healing period of 8 to 12 weeks. Compared to implant placement in standard sites without bone deficiency, the surgical time is only extended by about 15 minutes.

For the clinician, the proposed surgical technique has been simplified compared with the original GBR procedures of 15 to 20 years ago that used ePTFE membranes. Significant progress was made with the introduction of resorbable non–cross-linked collagen membranes because these membranes are easy to handle during surgery, do not need a second surgical procedure for their removal, and are not susceptible to infection in case of a soft tissue dehiscence. These collagen membranes are combined with appropriate bone fillers. A synergistic combination of autogenous bone chips and a low-substitution, hydroxyapatite-based filler is preferred because it offers not only rapid healing but also stable volume of the augmented ridge over time.

References

1. Garber DA, Belser UC. Restoration-driven implant placement with restoration-generated site development. Compend Contin Educ Dent 1995;16:796, 798–802,804.
2. Belser UC, Bernard JP, Buser D. Implant-supported restorations in the anterior region: Prosthetic considerations. Pract Periodontics Aesthet Dent 1996;8: 875–883.
3. Brånemark PI, Breine U, Adell R, Hansson BO, Lindström J, Ohlsson A. Intra-osseous anchorage of dental prostheses. 1. Experimental studies. Scand J Plast Reconstr Surg 1969;3:81–100.
4. Schroeder A, Pohler O, Sutter F. Gewebsreaktion auf ein Titan-Hohlzylinderimplantat mit Titan-Spritzschichtoberfläche. Schweiz Monatsschr Zahnmed 1976;86: 713–727.
5. Albrektsson T, Brånemark PI, Hansson HA, Lindstrom J. Osseointegrated titanium implants. Requirements for ensuring a long-lasting, direct bone-to-implant anchorage in man. Acta Orthop Scand 1981;52: 155–170.
6. Schenk RK, Buser D. Osseointegration: A reality. Periodontol 2000 1998;17:22–35.
7. Schenk RK, Buser D, Hardwick WR, Dahlin C. Healing pattern of bone regeneration in membrane-protected defects: A histologic study in the canine mandible. Int J Oral Maxillofac Implants 1994;9: 13–29.
8. Sculean A, Nikolidakis D, Schwarz F. Regeneration of periodontal tissues: Combinations of barrier membranes and grafting materials—Biological foundation and preclinical evidence: A systematic review. J Clin Periodontol 2008;35:106–116.
9. Slotte C, Lundgren D, Sennerby L, Lundgren AK. Surgical intervention in enchondral and membranous bone: Intraindividual comparisons in the rabbit. Clin Implant Dent Relat Res 2003;5:263–268.
10. Nishimura I, Shimizu Y, Ooya K. Effects of cortical bone perforation on experimental guided bone regeneration. Clin Oral Implants Res 2004;15:293–300.
11. Buser D, Dula K, Belser U, Hirt HP, Berthold H. Localized ridge augmentation using guided bone regeneration. 1. Surgical procedure in the maxilla. Int J Periodontics Restorative Dent 1993;13:29–45.
12. Nevins M, Mellonig JT. The advantages of localized ridge augmentation prior to implant placement. A staged event. Int J Periodontics Restorative Dent 1994;14:97–111.
13. Buser D, Hoffmann B, Bernard JP, Lussi A, Mettler D, Schenk RK. Evaluation of filling materials in membrane-protected bone defects. A comparative histomorphometric study in the mandible of miniature pigs. Clin Oral Implants Res 1998;9:137–150.
14. Buser D, Schenk RK, Steinemann S, Fiorellini JP, Fox CH, Stich H. Influence of surface characteristics on bone integration of titanium implants. A histomorphometric study in miniature pigs. J Biomed Mater Res 1991;25:889–902.
15. Wennerberg A, Albrektsson T, Johansson C, Andersson B. Experimental study of turned and grit-blasted screw-shaped implants with special emphasis on effects of blasting material and surface topography. Biomaterials 1996;17:15–22.
16. Cochran DL, Schenk RK, Lussi A, Higginbottom FL, Buser D. Bone response to unloaded and loaded titanium implants with a sandblasted and acid-etched surface: A histometric study in the canine mandible. J Biomed Mater Res 1998;40:1–11.
17. Klokkevold PR, Nishimura RD, Adachi M, Caputo A. Osseointegration enhanced by chemical etching of the titanium surface. A torque removal study in the rabbit. Clin Oral Implants Res 1997;8:442–447.
18. Cochran DL, Buser D, ten Bruggenkate CM, et al. The use of reduced healing times on ITI implants with a sandblasted and acid-etched (SLA) surface: Early results from clinical trials on ITI SLA implants. Clin Oral Implants Res 2002;13:144–153.
19. Lazzara RJ, Porter SS, Testori T, Galante J, Zetterqvist L. A prospective multicenter study evaluating loading of Osseotite implants two months after placement: One-year results. J Esthet Dent 1998;10: 280–289.
20. Testori T, Del Fabbro M, Feldman S, et al. A multicenter prospective evaluation of 2-months loaded Osseotite implants placed in the posterior jaws: 3-year follow-up results. Clin Oral Implants Res 2002; 13:154–161.
21. Bornstein MM, Schmid B, Belser UC, Lussi A, Buser D. Early loading of non-submerged titanium implants with a sandblasted and acid-etched surface. 5-year results of a prospective study in partially edentulous patients. Clin Oral Implants Res 2005; 16:631–638.
22. Buser D, Broggini N, Wieland M, et al. Enhanced bone apposition to a chemically modified SLA titanium surface. J Dent Res 2004;83:529–533.
23. Ferguson SJ, Broggini N, Wieland M, et al. Biomechanical evaluation of the interfacial strength of a chemically modified sandblasted and acid-etched titanium surface. J Biomed Mater Res A 2006;78: 291–297.
24. Schwarz F, Herten M, Sager M, Wieland M, Dard M, Becker J. Bone regeneration in dehiscence-type defects at chemically modified (SLActive) and conventional SLA titanium implants: A pilot study in dogs. J Clin Periodontol 2007;34:78–86.
25. Schwarz F, Sager M, Ferrari D, Herten M, Wieland M, Becker J. Bone regeneration in dehiscence-type defects at non-submerged and submerged chemically modified (SLActive) and conventional SLA titanium implants: An immunohistochemical study in dogs. J Clin Periodontol 2008;35:64–75.
26. Hurzeler MB, Strub JR. Guided bone regeneration around exposed implants: A new bioresorbable device and bioresorbable membrane pins. Pract Periodontics Aesthet Dent 1995;7:37–47.

27. Hurzeler MB, Kohal RJ, Naghshbandi J, et al. Evaluation of a new bioresorbable barrier to facilitate guided bone regeneration around exposed implant threads. An experimental study in the monkey. Int J Oral Maxillofac Surg 1998;27:315–320.
28. Zitzmann NU, Naef R, Schärer P. Resorbable versus nonresorbable membranes in combination with Bio-Oss for guided bone regeneration. Int J Oral Maxillofac Implants 1997;12:844–852.
29. Zitzmann NU, Schärer P, Marinello CP. Long-term results of implants treated with guided bone regeneration: A 5-year prospective study. Int J Oral Maxillofac Implants 2001;16:355–366.
30. von Arx T, Broggini N, Jensen SS, Bornstein MM, Schenk RK, Buser D. Membrane durability and tissue response of different bioresorbable barrier membranes: A histologic study in the rabbit calvarium. Int J Oral Maxillofac Implants 2005;20:843–853.
31. Bornstein MM, Bosshardt D, Buser D. Effect of two different bioabsorbable collagen membranes on guided bone regeneration: A comparative histomorphometric study in the dog mandible. J Periodontol 2007;78:1943–1953.
32. Buser D, Bornstein MM, Weber HP, Grutter L, Schmid B, Belser UC. Early implant placement with simultaneous guided bone regeneration following single-tooth extraction in the esthetic zone: A cross-sectional, retrospective study in 45 subjects with a 2- to 4-year follow-up. J Periodontol 2008;79:1773–1781.
33. Buser D, Chen ST, Weber HP, Belser UC. The concept of early implant placement following single tooth extraction in the esthetic zone: Biologic rationale and surgical procedures. Int J Periodontics Restorative Dent 2008;28:440–451.
34. von Arx T, Buser D. Horizontal ridge augmentation using autogenous block grafts and the guided bone regeneration technique with collagen membranes: A clinical study with 42 patients. Clin Oral Implants Res 2006;17:359–366.
35. Simion M, Baldoni M, Rossi P, Zaffe D. A comparative study of the effectiveness of e-PTFE membranes with and without early exposure during the healing period. Int J Periodontics Restorative Dent 1994; 14:166–180.
36. Augthun M, Yildirim M, Spiekermann H, Biesterfeld S. Healing of bone defects in combination with immediate implants using the membrane technique. Int J Oral Maxillofac Implants 1995;10:421–428.
37. Machtei EE. The effect of membrane exposure on the outcome of regenerative procedures in humans: A meta-analysis. J Periodontol 2001;72:512–516.
38. Artzi Z, Nemcovsky CE. The application of deproteinized bovine bone mineral for ridge preservation prior to implantation. Clinical and histological observations in a case report. J Periodontol 1998;69: 1062–1067.
39. Schlegel KA, Fichtner G, Schultze-Mosgau S, Wiltfang J. Histologic findings in sinus augmentation with autogenous bone chips versus a bovine bone substitute. Int J Oral Maxillofac Implants 2003;18: 53–58.
40. Jensen SS, Broggini N, Hjørting-Hansen E, Schenk R, Buser D. Bone healing and graft resorption of autograft, anorganic bovine bone and beta-tricalcium phosphate. A histologic and histomorphometric study in the mandibles of minipigs. Clin Oral Implants Res 2006;17:237–243.
41. Jensen SS, Yeo A, Dard M, Hunziker E, Schenk R, Buser D. Evaluation of a novel biphasic calcium phosphate in standardized bone defects. A histologic and histomorphometric study in the mandibles of minipigs. Clin Oral Implants Res 2007;18: 752–760.
42. Jensen SS, Bornstein MM, Dard M, Bosshardt D, Buser D. Comparative study of biphasic calcium phosphates with different HA/TCP ratios in mandibular bone defects. A long-term histomorphometric study in minipigs. J Biomed Mater Res B Appl Biomater 2009;90B:171–181.
43. Scharf DR, Tarnow DP. Success rates of osseointegration for implants placed under sterile versus clean conditions. J Periodontol 1993;64:954–956.
44. Buser D, von Arx T, ten Bruggenkate C, Weingart D. Basic surgical principles with ITI implants. Clin Oral Implants Res 2000;11(suppl 1):59–68.
45. Buser D, Dula K, Belser UC, Hirt HP, Berthold H. Localized ridge augmentation using guided bone regeneration. 2. Surgical procedure in the mandible. Int J Periodontics Restorative Dent 1995;15:10–29.
46. Gomez-Roman G. Influence of flap design on periimplant interproximal crestal bone loss around single-tooth implants. Int J Oral Maxillofac Implants 2001;16:61–67.
47. Buser D, von Arx T. Surgical procedures in partially edentulous patients with ITI implants. Clin Oral Implants Res 2000;11(suppl 1):83–100.

CHAPTER 7

Implant Placement in Postextraction Sites

Daniel Buser
Stephen T. Chen

Implant placement in postextraction sites is a common situation in implant dentistry today. For the clinician, the timing of when to place an implant is critical for the achievement of the proposed primary and secondary objectives of implant therapy (see chapter 1). In postextraction sites, peri-implant bone defects are commonly encountered, requiring bone augmentation to ensure that the implant is completely surrounded by vital bone and to improve the contour of the ridge for esthetic reasons. Guided bone regeneration (GBR) procedures offer the ability to successfully achieve these goals with high predictability and a low risk of complications, thereby ensuring the long-lasting function and esthetics of the implant-supported restoration. These aspects are considered the primary objectives of implant therapy and are an absolute priority for the clinician to achieve.

Secondary objectives are to provide treatment with the least number of surgical interventions, low morbidity to the patient, and relatively short healing periods, thus increasing the attractiveness of implant therapy for patients. However, the pursuit of these secondary objectives should not compromise the primary objectives of treatment. In other words, techniques for reducing the number and duration of surgical interventions and decreasing healing periods should neither increase the risk of complications nor adversely affect the predictability for successful outcomes, long-term function, and esthetics. The clinician must carefully balance these aspects when selecting the most appropriate treatment approach in a given situation.

Implant placement after 6 to 12 months of healing following tooth extraction was considered the standard of care for postextraction sites in the late 1980s. This conservative concept offered good long-term results with osseointegrated titanium implants but was not very attractive to patients because of the long treatment time from extraction to implant restoration. Thus, many efforts have been made to improve the attractiveness of implant therapy for this particular indication. A first attempt was initiated by a German group under the leadership of Professor Willy Schulte, who recommended the so-called Tübinger Sofortimplantat (immediate implant).[1] They proposed the concept of immediate implant placement using aluminum oxide implants. This attempt was unsuccessful not because of the treatment approach but rather the failure of the biomaterial itself. These aluminum oxide implants showed a high rate of complications and failures, mainly arising from implant fractures.[2]

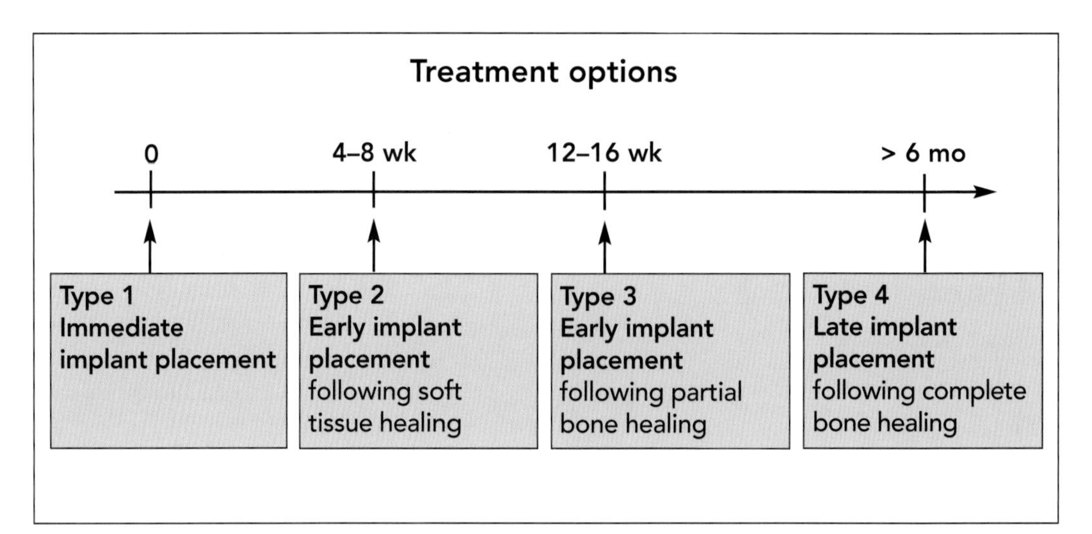

Fig 7-1 Four treatment options for implant placement in postextraction sites.

With the introduction of the GBR technique in the late 1980s, new surgical techniques with barrier membranes have been proposed in postextraction sites, involving either immediate implant placement at the day of extraction[3,4] or delayed or early implant placement after a few weeks of soft tissue healing.[5] These recommendations have received much attention because their aim was to improve the aforementioned secondary objectives of implant therapy in postextraction sites. For many years, case reports and clinical studies reporting on implant survival rates have dominated the literature.[6–9]

In recent years, the International Team for Implantology (ITI) has reviewed the current literature concerning existing scientific evidence about implants placed in postextraction sites twice in ITI consensus conferences. The first review took place in August 2003 in Gstaad, Switzerland, and resulted in the publication of the proceedings with clinical recommendations and a literature review.[10,11] The authors presented a classification concerning the timing of implant placement, comprising type 1 through type 4 placement. They also concluded that implants placed in extraction sockets demonstrated survival rates comparable to those of implants placed in healed sites. However, they also noted that there were only a few studies examining esthetic outcomes up to 2003.

The classification concerning the timing of postextraction implants was adopted for the third *ITI Treatment Guide*[12] and for the proceedings of the recent ITI consensus conference that took place in Stuttgart, Germany, in August 2008.[13] For both publications, the classification was expanded with descriptive terms to allow the clinician an easier understanding of the various treatment options (Fig 7-1).

Decision Criteria for Treatment Approach

Implant placement in postextraction sites in most cases involves a localized bone augmentation procedure to regenerate bone in the peri-implant bone defect that remains following implant insertion. The goal is the reestablishment of sufficient bone volume at the implant site to ensure that the implant will provide long-lasting function and esthetics. Whenever possible, implant placement is combined with a simultaneous GBR procedure to avoid a staged approach, which involves two open flap procedures. The simultaneous approach fulfills the secondary objectives of treating patients with the least possible number of surgical procedures and reducing morbidity. This approach also requires the use of a resorbable collagen membrane to eliminate the need for an additional surgery for membrane removal.

Implant placement with simultaneous GBR has three prerequisites: *(1)* the ability to achieve implant insertion in a correct three-dimensional position, *(2)* the ability to achieve implant insertion with good primary stability, and *(3)* the existence of a favorable defect morphology with at least two bone walls to allow predictable bone regeneration of the defect. The last aspect is most critical when the timing of implant placement is decided because an extended healing period of 6 months or longer following extraction can lead to a significant reduction of the crest width and thus compromise the predictability of GBR procedures.[14]

In esthetic sites, the bone tissue primarily determines the esthetic outcome because the peri-implant soft tissues have a constant dimension, often referred to as the *biologic width*.[15–17] In postextraction sites, the facial bone and soft tissues are most critical for the clinician to consider because significant dimensional alterations take place following extraction in this area. In the past 5 years, researchers and clinicians have developed a much better understanding of ridge alterations that occur following extraction.[14,18–21] Preclinical and clinical studies showed that significant resorption of the facial bone wall occurred in a horizontal and/or vertical direction during the first 8 to 12 weeks of healing, irrespective of whether an implant was inserted into the extraction socket. Today it is believed that this bone resorption process is a physiologic healing response to the interruption of blood supply to the bundle bone lining the extraction socket from the periodontal ligament of the extracted tooth.[19]

The clinician must have an understanding of these ridge alterations to decide on the best time point for implant placement following extraction and, hence, to select the appropriate treatment approach to achieve the treatment objectives. The clinician has the choice of one of four treatment options. Each has its advantages and disadvantages, and each can be used in specific clinical situations. The decision should be based on objective criteria but may also be influenced by personal preferences and by the clinical skills and experience of the involved clinician.

In the following paragraphs, the advantages of, disadvantages of, and indications for various treatment options will be discussed. These clinical recommendations may seem conservative but are based on more than 20 years of clinical experience with implants placed in postextraction sites.

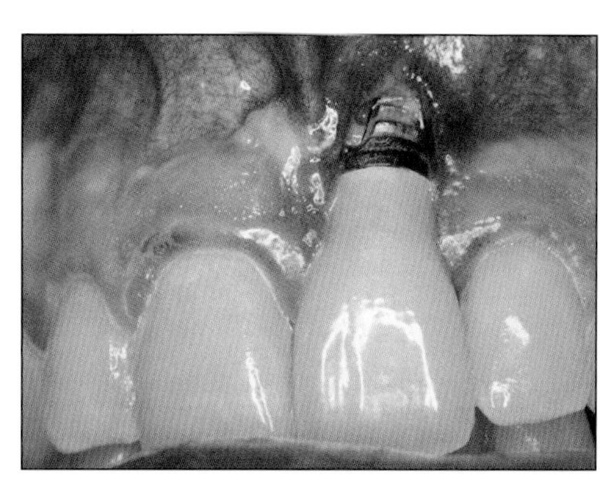

Fig 7-2a A severe esthetic complication has followed immediate implant placement. The oversized implant, malpositioned apically and facially, has caused a severe mucosal recession with an exposed implant surface.

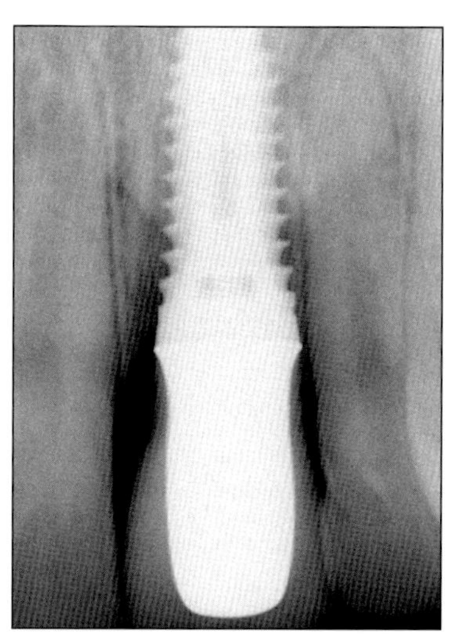

Fig 7-2b The periapical radiograph reveals the oversized, wide-platform implant in an apical malposition.

Immediate Implant Placement (Type 1)

Advantages and disadvantages

Initiated by the first two case reports on immediate implant placement with GBR,[3,4] this new treatment option received much attention at implant conferences in the 1990s. Immediate implants had the obvious advantages of reducing the overall treatment time and having a maximum amount of local bone volume available at the time of implant placement. Within a few years, several retrospective and prospective clinical studies reported acceptable implant survival rates for immediate implants.[6–9,11]

The most recent literature review,[13] however, clearly demonstrated that immediate implants are associated with a significant risk for esthetic complications, in particular the development of mucosal recession on the facial aspect. Several clinical studies, some of them randomized clinical trials with high levels of evidence, reported a high frequency of mucosal recession with immediate implants.[22–26] This complication was also observed for immediate implants placed with a flapless surgery[27] or with an immediate restoration.[28] The frequency of recession of 1 mm or more ranged from 8% to 40.5% in the cited studies. These clinical studies confirmed what had already been seen clinically by the late 1990s and early 2000s. Several severe esthetic complications had been observed within this period, when immediate implant placement was often used in daily practice by dentists (Figs 7-2 and 7-3).

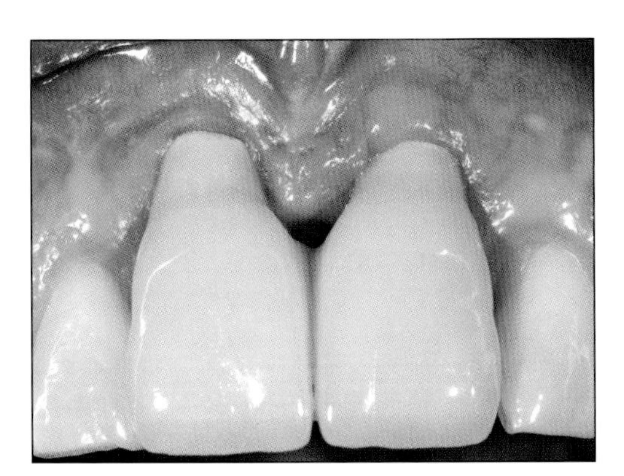

Fig 7-3a Mucosal recession at two immediate implants placed in central incisor sites has resulted in a nonharmonious gingival margin, extralong clinical crowns, and a short interimplant papilla.

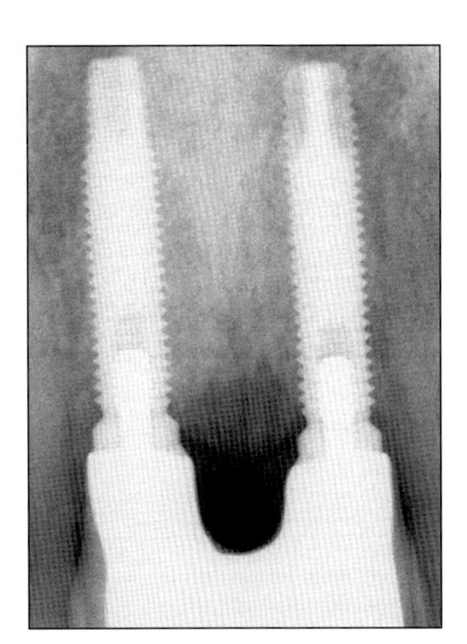

Fig 7-3b The radiograph reveals that the two implants are in an apical malposition.

In the cited clinical studies, it was noted that the risk of mucosal recession increased in patients with thin tissue biotypes, in extraction sites with damage of the facial socket wall, and with facial malpositioning of the implant within the extraction socket. Facial malpositioning of the implant is a common complication with immediate implants. At the time of implant insertion, the dense cortical bone of the palatal wall can often cause the implant to deflect toward the facial aspect. This deflection may go undetected by the clinician during surgery. An additional problem is the relative lack of soft tissue to achieve submerged or semisubmerged healing. The facial flap must be well mobilized and coronally advanced, often changing the position of the mucogingival junction in relation to the adjacent teeth.[26]

Another risk factor is a clinician with insufficient skills and clinical experience to perform such a delicate surgical procedure. Immediate implant placement is considered a complex procedure in most clinical situations according to the SAC classification (S = straightforward, A = advanced, C = complex).[29]

Indications

Immediate implant placement should only be used by skilled and very experienced clinicians in well-selected cases because aspects of case selection and precise surgical execution of the procedure are of utmost importance for a successful esthetic outcome. For appropriate case selection, each patient must be analyzed with an esthetic risk assessment to establish an individual risk profile.[30] Immediate implant placement can only be

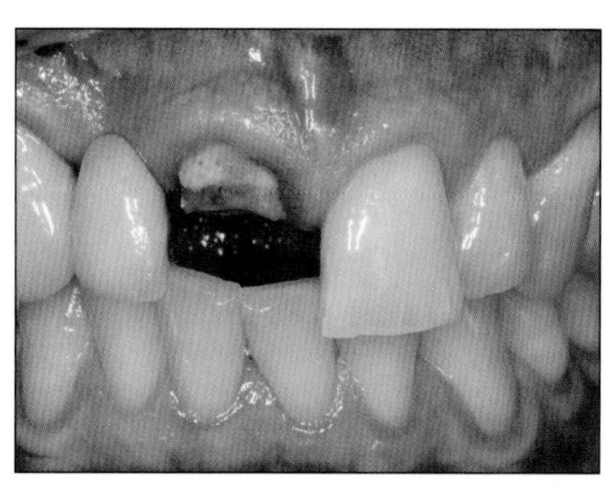

Fig 7-4a A 40-year-old man has a subgingival fracture of the maxillary right central incisor, which served as an abutment for a three-unit fixed partial denture replacing the maxillary right lateral incisor. The partial denture has been sectioned, leaving the pontic in place. The tissue biotype is medium-thick, and the patient has a low lip line.

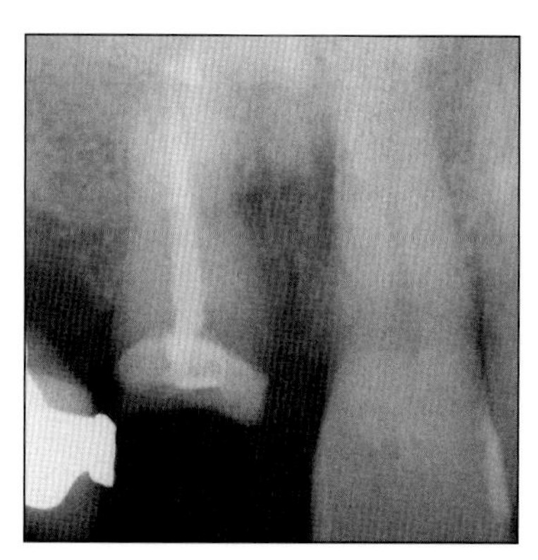

Fig 7-4b The preoperative radiograph shows the root of the maxillary right central incisor.

recommended for patients with a single-rooted tooth extraction and a low-risk profile in ideal clinical conditions. Such conditions include a healthy, nonsmoking patient with a low lip line, a thick gingival biotype, an intact and thick facial bone wall, absence of acute infection in the extraction site, and good vertical bone levels at adjacent teeth. Review of these conditions indicates that such clinical situations are rarely found in patients with extraction sites in the anterior maxilla.

Conversely, immediate implants are not recommended in extraction sites of multi-rooted teeth, in smoking patients, in patients with a medium or high lip line and/or a thin gingival biotype, and in extraction sites with either an acute infection or a bone deficiency on the facial aspect or at adjacent teeth.

In ideal cases, where the site exhibits an intact and thick facial bone wall, a flapless surgical approach is often used today, although such a procedure further complicates the surgical treatment.

Case reports

Case 1: Flapless approach

The patient had a low lip line and medium-thick tissue biotype, and the facial bone of the maxillary right central incisor socket was thick and undamaged. The esthetic demands were relatively low. For these reasons, flapless implant placement immediately after tooth extraction was recommended (Fig 7-4).

The placement technique included a graft of deproteinized bovine bone mineral (DBBM) in the peri-implant defect and a small connective tissue graft to support the facial mucosa. The connective tissue graft served to compensate for the anticipated dimensional change following physiologic modeling of the facial bone by increasing the thickness of the facial mucosa.

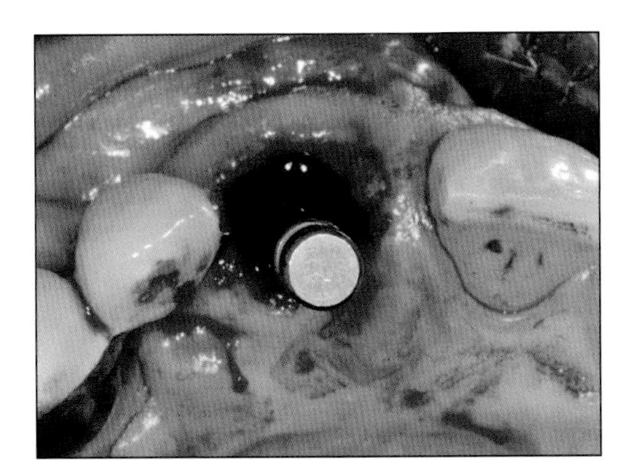

Fig 7-4c The root is carefully extracted without elevation of a flap. The facial bone is checked to confirm that it is intact. The osteotomy is prepared, with a correct axial inclination, in the palatal aspect of the socket.

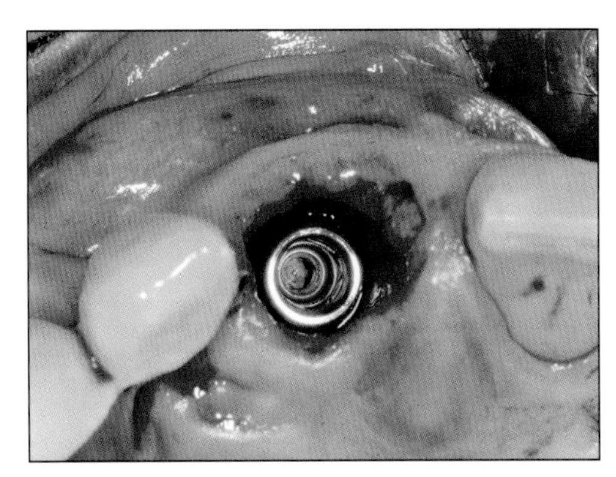

Fig 7-4d On insertion of the implant, a 2-mm distance is maintained between the implant and the facial socket wall.

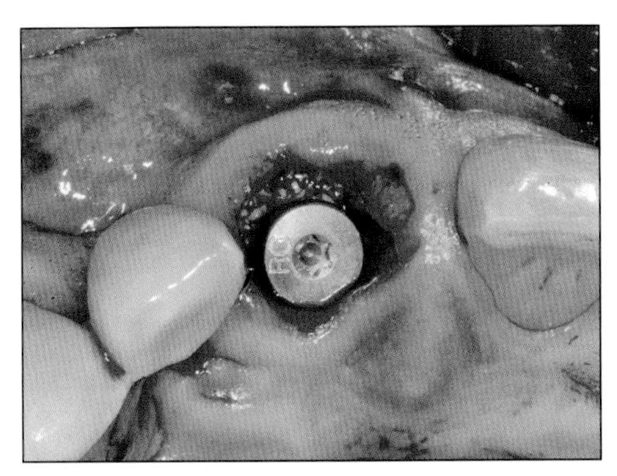

Fig 7-4e A healing abutment is connected to the implant. Deproteinized bovine bone mineral is lightly packed in the defect on the facial aspect of the implant. Care has been taken not to overfill the defect and to place the graft only to the level of the facial crestal bone.

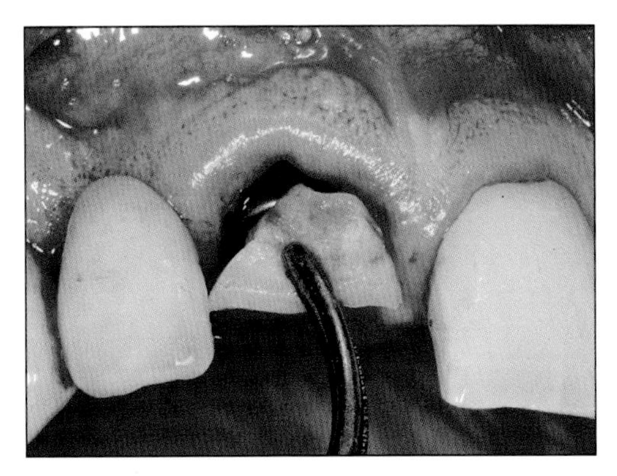

Fig 7-4f A small connective tissue graft harvested from the palate is inserted in the soft tissue pouch between the healing abutment and the facial mucosa.

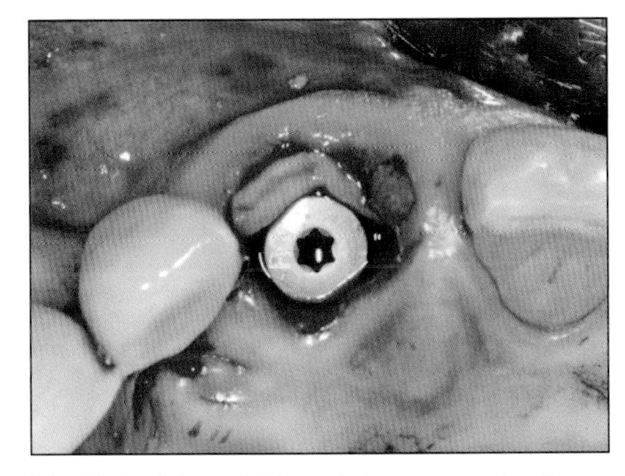

Fig 7-4g The addition of the connective tissue graft helps to support the facial mucosa and to contain the particulate graft in the peri-implant defect.

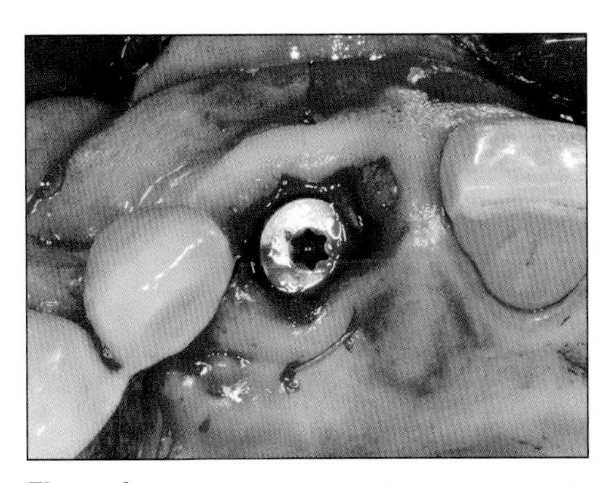

Fig 7-4h An internal horizontal mattress suture is used to loosely adapt the palatal and facial mucosa to the healing abutment.

(Fig 7-4 continues on next page.)

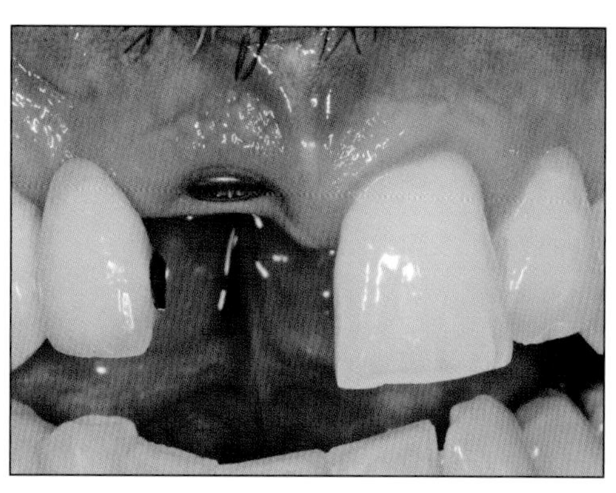

Fig 7-4i The implant in the maxillary right central incisor site is shown after 6 weeks of healing.

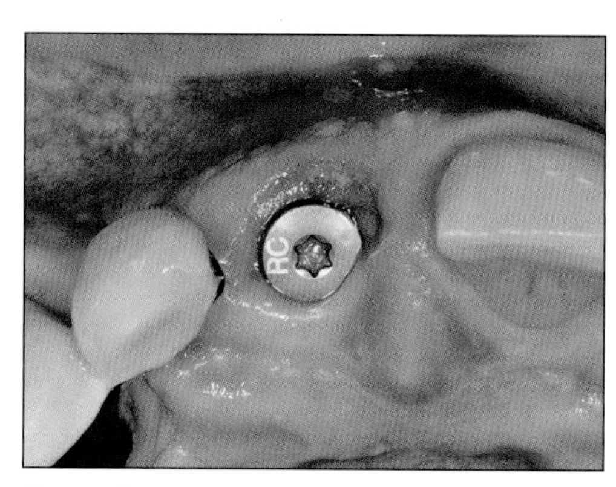

Fig 7-4j After 6 weeks of healing, the connective tissue graft has incorporated into the site and has maintained the thickness of the facial mucosa.

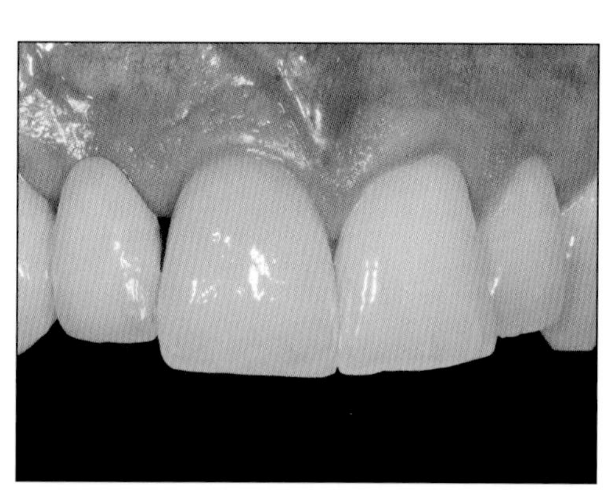

Fig 7-4k The completed restoration replacing the maxillary right central incisor is shown 1 year after surgery.

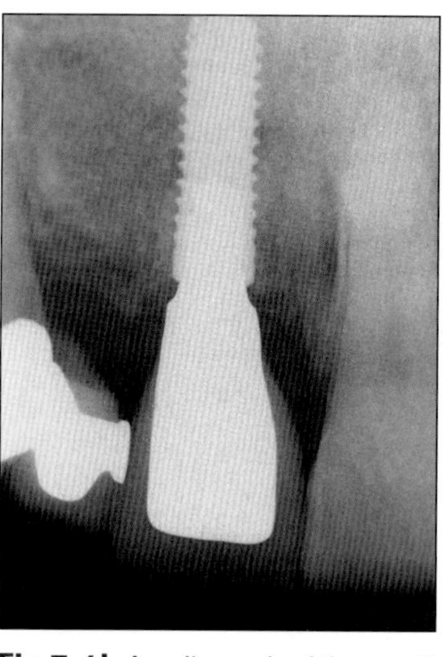

Fig 7-4l A radiograph of the maxillary right central incisor site 1 year after surgery reveals the stability of the implant.

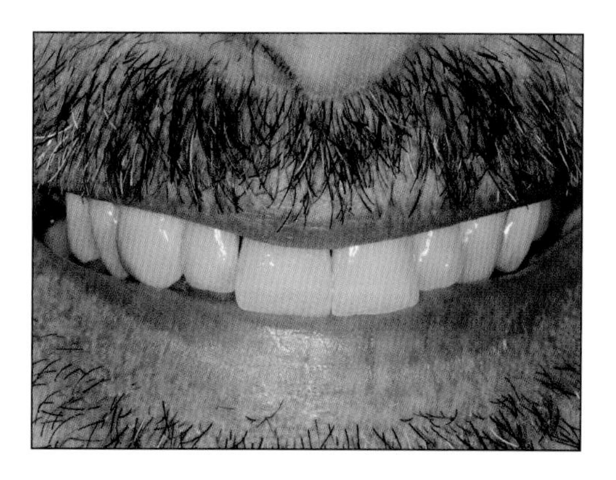

Fig 7-4m The patient's smile at the 1-year follow-up examination reveals that function and esthetics have been restored.

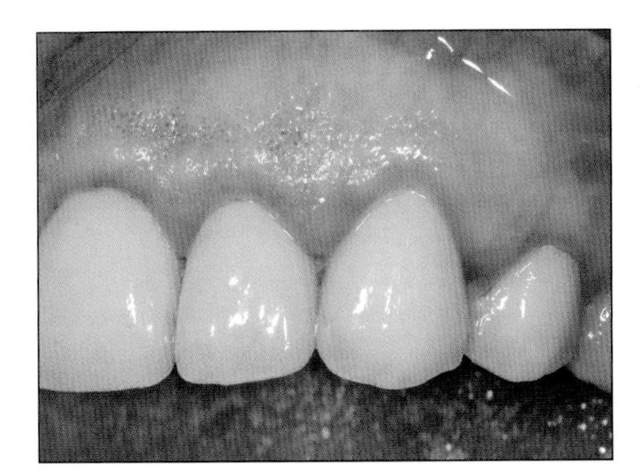

Fig 7-5a Caries has undermined the crown of the maxillary left canine, and there is insufficient tooth structure remaining to replace the crown.

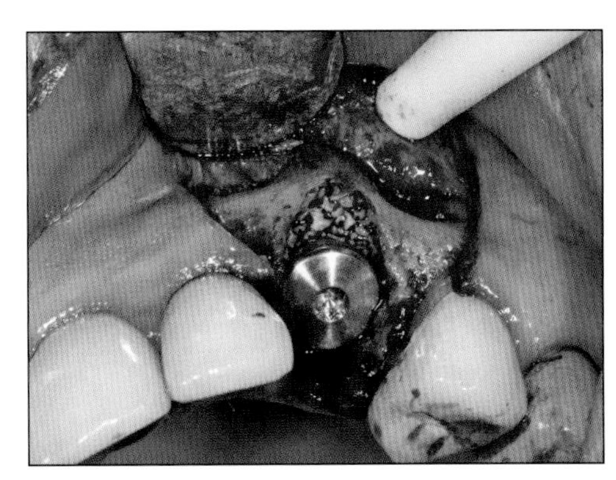

Fig 7-5b Following reflection of a full-thickness mucoperiosteal flap, the root has been carefully removed with a combination of luxators and root forceps. The facial bone wall is intact. An implant is placed in an ideal three-dimensional position. The marginal defect on the facial aspect is 3 mm in horizontal depth. This defect is filled with loosely packed DBBM particles. A short (2-mm) healing cap is attached.

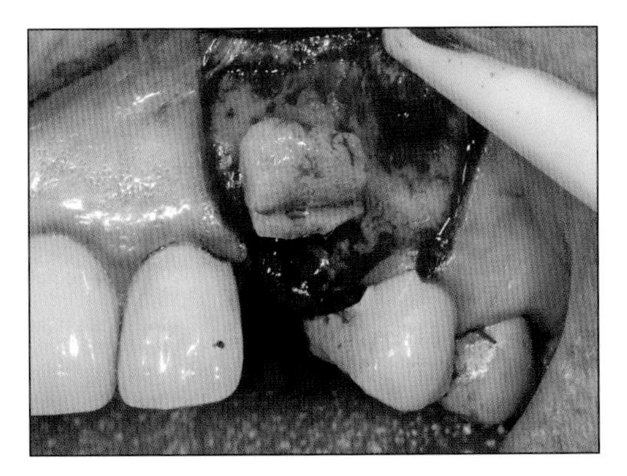

Fig 7-5c A connective tissue graft is harvested from the palate and placed over the facial aspect of the implant shoulder.

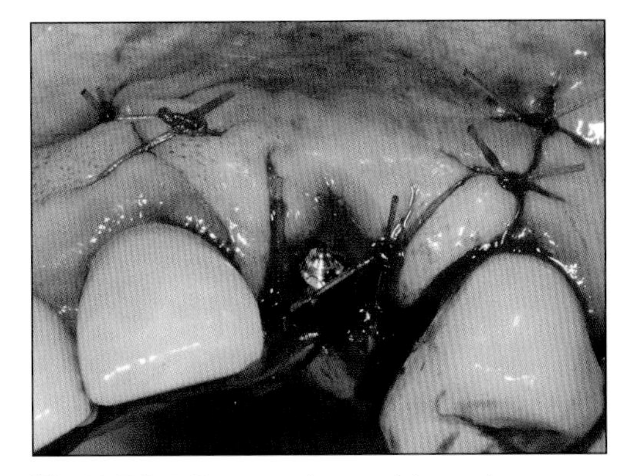

Fig 7-5d Following release of the periosteum at its base, the facial flap is advanced to partially submerge the healing cap.

(Fig 7-5 continues on next page.)

Case 2: Elevation of a flap

A 64-year-old woman required replacement of the maxillary left canine with an implant. The tooth was restored with a post-retained metal-ceramic crown, which had loosened because of recurrent caries. The dentition was extensively restored with crowns. The clinical conditions included a low lip line, thick tissue biotype, and an intact and thick facial bone wall. This was favorable for immediate implant placement (Fig 7-5).

Because it was anticipated that the extraction might be difficult as a result of the recurrent caries, the treatment plan included elevation of a surgical flap to facilitate access for tooth removal and subsequent implant placement. The procedure included the application of DBBM particles in the peri-implant defect and a connective tissue graft to maintain mucosal thickness and to compensate for anticipated dimensional change following physiologic modeling of the facial bone.

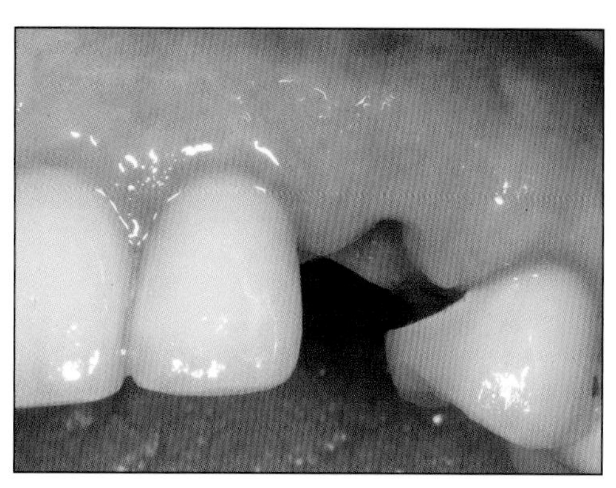

Fig 7-5e Six weeks after surgery, healing has progressed well. A longer healing cap is attached to the implant to expand the soft tissue cuff in preparation for restorative procedures.

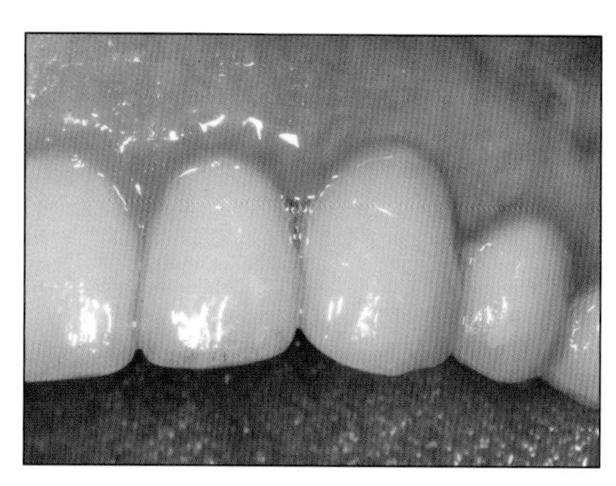

Fig 7-5f The completed implant crown replacing the maxillary left canine is shown 6 months after implant placement.

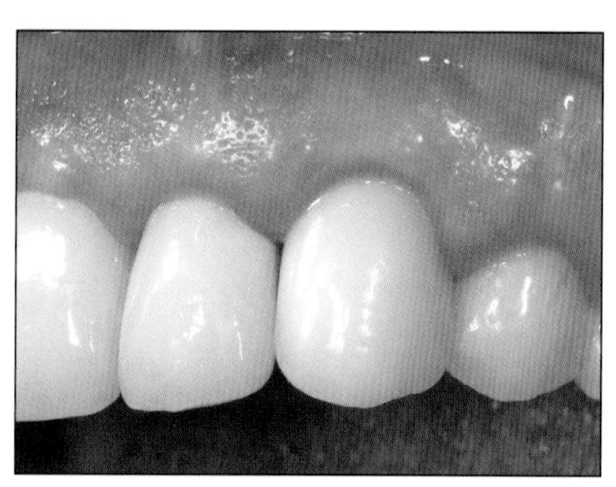

Fig 7-5g The 3-year follow-up of the implant reveals a pleasing esthetic outcome and no mucosal recession.

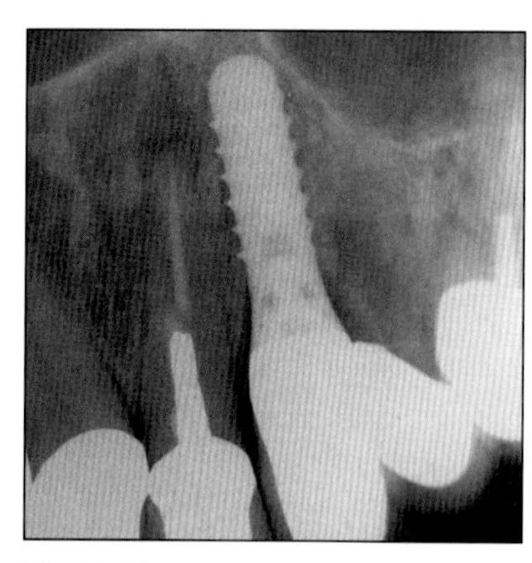

Fig 7-5h A radiograph of the implant at the 3-year follow-up reveals stable bone conditions. The adjacent lateral incisor has developed a periapical lesion but is not causing clinical symptoms.

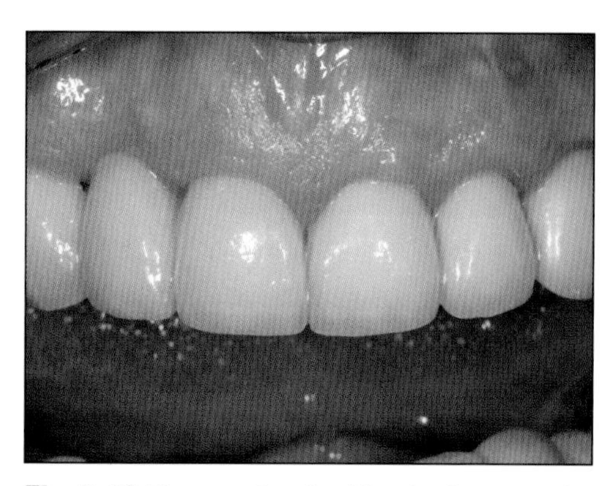

Fig 7-5i The anterior dentition is shown at the 3-year follow-up examination.

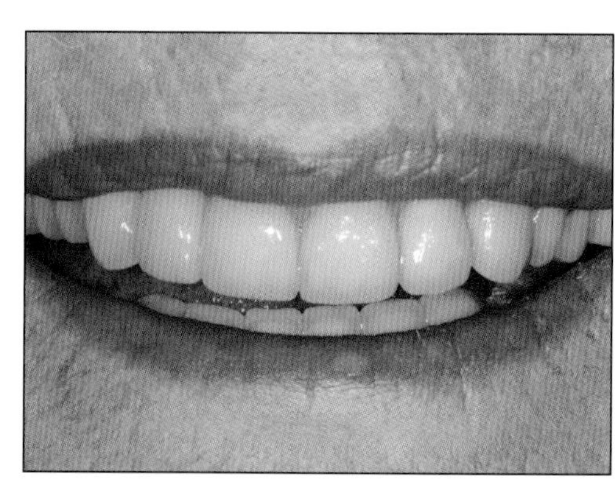

Fig 7-5j The patient's smile at the 3-year follow-up examination reveals the successful outcome of treatment.

Early Implant Placement Following Soft Tissue Healing (Type 2)

Advantages and disadvantages

The main advantage of this approach is the increased amount of keratinized mucosa available in the implant site. The soft tissue spontaneously heals following extraction and creates 3 to 5 mm of additional keratinized mucosa. The same effect can be accomplished without extraction simply by reducing the root in height to the bone level, as described by Langer.[31] The increased amount of keratinized mucosa simplifies attainment of tension-free primary wound closure of the released mucoperiosteal flap without displacing the mucogingival line too far coronally.

The time for soft tissue healing varies from 4 to 8 weeks, depending on the orofacial dimension of the extracted tooth. Lateral incisors in the maxilla and premolars in both jaws normally require only 4 weeks of soft tissue healing, whereas a healing of 6 to 8 weeks is frequently used for central incisors and canines in the maxilla.

During this soft tissue healing period of 4 to 8 weeks, a certain degree of ridge alteration takes place. However, this bone resorption is mainly limited to the bundle bone, which, from a clinical point of view, only affects the facial aspect in the anterior maxilla because this area of the bone structure is typically thin. To avoid additional bone resorption on the facial aspect at interproximal areas of adjacent teeth, extraction must be carried out without flap elevation whenever possible. Elevation of a mucoperiosteal flap not only increases morbidity and necessitates an additional follow-up examination for suture removal but also causes additional superficial bone resorption, as shown in clinical and experimental studies.[32,33] Extraction without flap elevation is an essential point of this surgical concept.

The healing period of 4 to 8 weeks is sufficient to gain the advantage of healed soft tissues but avoids the disadvantage of resorption that reduces crest width. Clinical experience of more than 10 years with a large number of patients has confirmed that the crest width is not reduced in the interproximal area of an extraction socket after 4 to 8 weeks of healing. Although flattening of the facial bone is routinely observed, this is confined to the middle of the extraction site (Fig 7-6).

Therefore, this timing protocol provides the conditions for a favorable two- or three-wall defect on the facial aspect, with the exposed implant surface contained within the alveolar crest. The defect conditions at this time point are comparable to those of sites treated with immediate implants. It makes no difference to the regenerative outcome if the facial bone wall in the middle of the extraction socket is intact or deficient at the time of implant placement because the facial contour is always augmented with autogenous bone chips and a low-substitution bone filler. A further advantage of this concept is the fact that a tension-free primary wound closure can be attained relatively easily following the release of the periosteum and without altering the position of the mucogingival line too far coronally. Details of the surgical procedure for single-tooth replacement in the anterior maxilla with this early implant placement protocol have been described recently.[34]

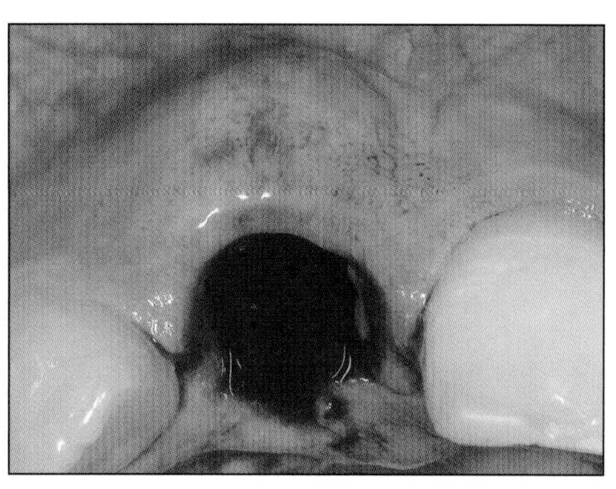

Fig 7-6a A central incisor with an acute infection, which has caused local swelling in the alveolar process, has been extracted.

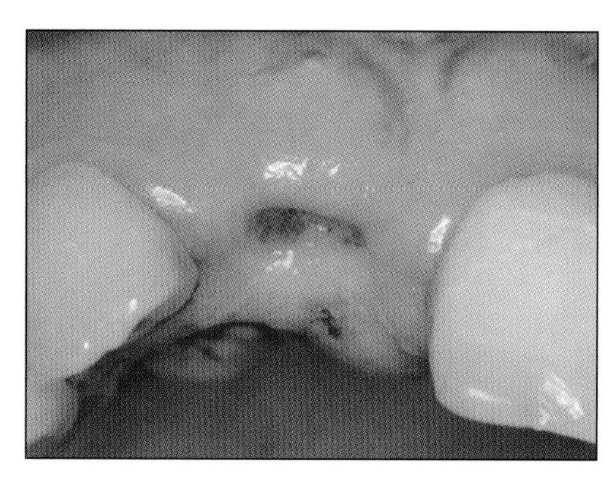

Fig 7-6b After 8 weeks of healing, flattening of the ridge in the middle of the healing socket is visible, but the interproximal crest width at adjacent teeth is well maintained.

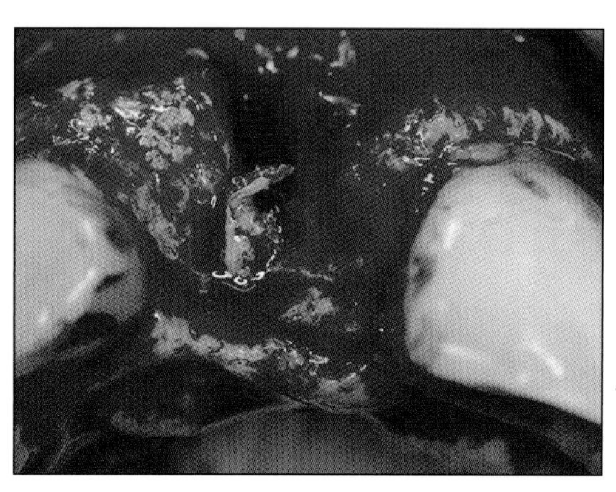

Fig 7-6c These findings are confirmed after elevation of a mucoperiosteal flap. In the middle of the socket, the facial bone wall has been resorbed, whereas the interproximal crest width at adjacent teeth is maintained, measuring more than 6 mm.

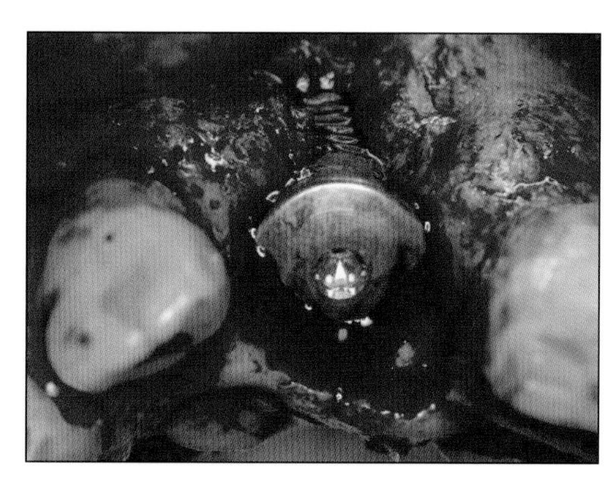

Fig 7-6d The optimal crest volume results in a two-wall defect morphology on the facial aspect following implant placement in a correct three-dimensional position. This defect morphology, when combined with applied autogenous bone chips, is favorable for predictable bone regeneration.

Another advantage of type 2 placement is the elimination of acute or chronic infections in the extraction socket during the healing period prior to implant placement. Once the etiologic factor, ie, the tooth, is removed, the immune system of the patient efficiently clears infection from the site and rapidly restores health to the local environment. This is considered very important for acute infection or for teeth with fistulae.

It may be argued that a potential disadvantage of early implant placement is an increased number of surgical procedures, which include extraction, implant placement with simultaneous GBR, and the reopening procedure. However, only the implant placement requires a flap procedure, whereas the extraction and reopening procedures are routinely carried out without flap elevation. The additional surgical procedures with type 2 placement are therefore only minor, with minimal postoperative morbidity to the patient.

A further option for early implant placement is a flapless surgical approach. Flapless implant placement should only be used in ideal clinical situations. Flapless placement has two main disadvantages: The surgery is more difficult for the clinician, and it does not allow simultaneous contour augmentation to be carried out. Therefore, this approach is only used in sites with a crest width of at least 8 mm and a thick facial bone wall of 1 to 2 mm. Such clinical situations are rare but can be found, primarily in maxillary premolar sites. Preoperative analysis with cone-beam computed tomography (CBCT) is essential to enable the clinician to identify such ideal clinical situations.

Indications

Early implant placement (type 2) is the most commonly used approach today in postextraction sites. In particular, this approach is widely favored in esthetic sites because it offers the most advantages and the fewest disadvantages, as outlined earlier. In contrast to immediate implants, this approach is characterized by a low risk for mucosal recession, as demonstrated by recent clinical studies.[35,36] The concept is also applied in premolar sites but much less frequently in molar sites of both jaws. In molar sites, early implant placement with partial bone healing (type 3 placement) is preferred in most patients.

Type 2 placement is not recommended if the implant cannot be placed with sufficient primary stability. A lack of primary stability is most often the result of medium-sized periapical lesions or radicular cysts.

Healing period

The overall treatment period between tooth extraction and implant restoration is defined by the healing of the soft tissues following extraction and the bone and soft tissue healing following implant placement. The duration of the anticipated healing period depends on the tissue volume to be regenerated. Postextraction, the healing varies between 4 and 8 weeks.

For many years, 6 to 12 weeks of healing following implant placement with simultaneous GBR has been successfully used in postextraction sites. A healing period of 6 weeks was used for defect sites with a fully intact facial bone wall that provided a three-wall defect, whereas 8 weeks was used for sites with vertical bone defects of up to 2 mm in the facial bone wall. A healing period of 10 weeks was selected when vertical defects of 3 to 5 mm were present in the facial bone wall. The longest healing period, 12 weeks of healing, was recommended for sites with vertical bone defects of 6 mm or more on the facial aspect.

The current healing period protocols are much shorter than those suggested in the early 1990s because 4 to 6 months of healing was recommended at the beginning of the development of GBR.[4,37] A shortening of the healing period was made feasible by the use of autogenous bone chips at the exposed implant surface because autogenous bone chips clearly expedite new bone formation in membrane-protected defects.[38–41]

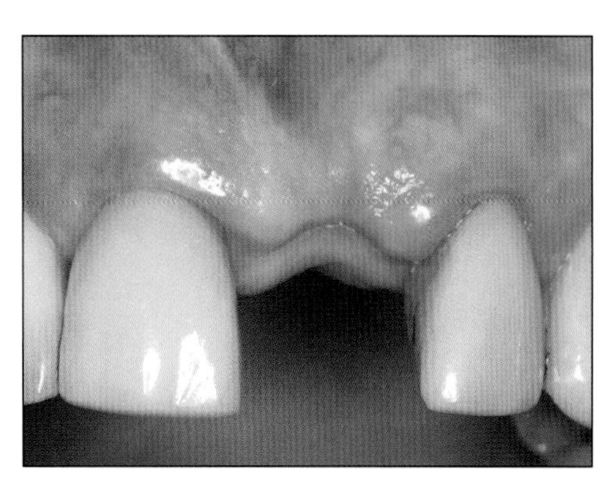

Fig 7-7a A single-tooth gap is present 8 weeks after extraction of a maxillary left central incisor.

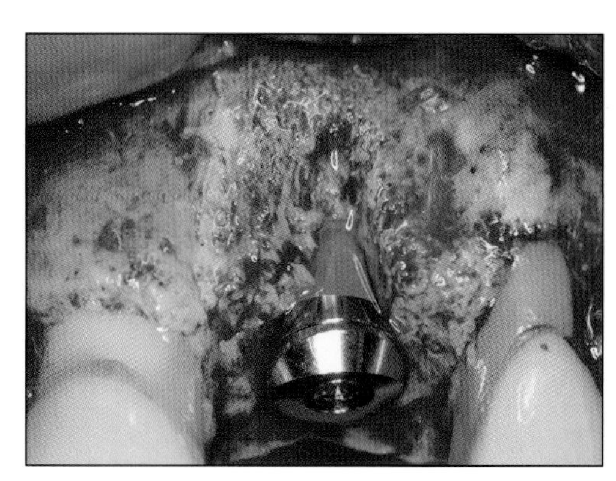

Fig 7-7b Following flap elevation and implant placement in a correct three-dimensional position, a craterlike bone defect is apparent. The exposed implant surface is located inside the alveolar crest, resulting in a favorable two-wall defect.

Recently, healing periods have been shortened further for patients with implant placement and simultaneous GBR. This reduction was made possible by the introduction of the chemically modified SLA surface (SLActive, Straumann) to routine clinical practice. This hydrophilic implant surface showed promising results and enhanced bone apposition at the bone-implant interface during initial healing in preclinical studies.[42–45] This success allowed a further reduction of healing periods to 3 weeks in standard sites without bone defects.[46,47] In addition, this new implant surface also demonstrated better bone fill in dehiscence-type defects in preclinical studies.[48,49] Consequently, healing periods were modified to 6 weeks of healing for vertical defects of up to 2 mm in the facial bone walls and to 8 weeks for vertical defects of 3 mm and more in the facial bone wall. These healing periods of 6 and 8 weeks further help to reduce the overall treatment time between tooth extraction and implant restoration.

Case reports

Case 3: Single-tooth replacement, trapezoidal flap design

A 61-year-old woman had a history of generalized periodontal disease, which had been successfully treated by the referring dentist. The maxillary left central incisor had to be extracted and replaced with an implant-borne single crown. She exhibited an extremely high smile line and a thin gingival tissue biotype.

A conventional trapezoidal flap design was chosen 8 weeks following extraction. Two divergent releasing incisions were made at adjacent teeth to allow contour augmentation with GBR following implant placement (Fig 7-7).

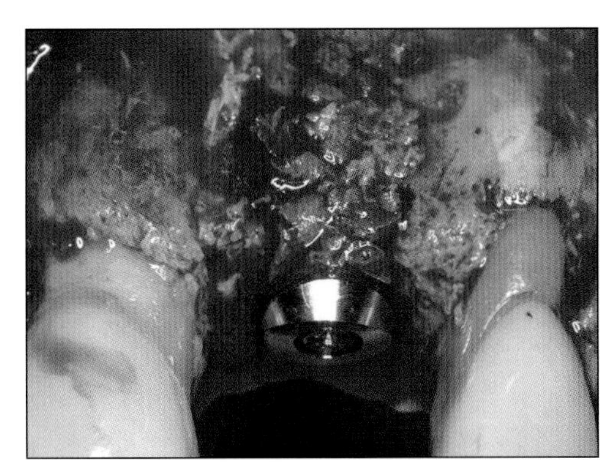

Fig 7-7c The bone defect has been filled with locally harvested autogenous bone chips to expedite new bone formation in the defect area during initial wound healing.

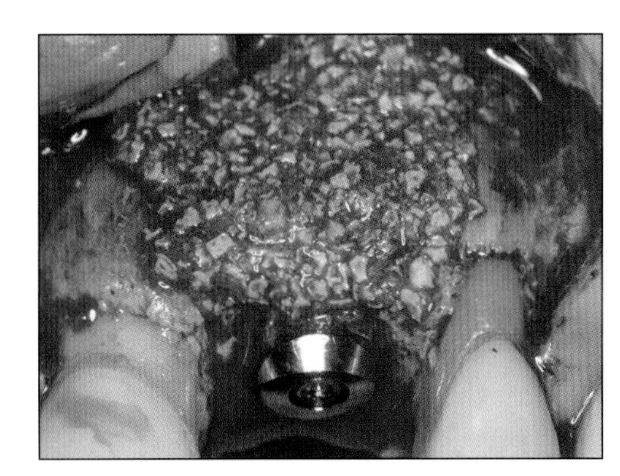

Fig 7-7d Contour augmentation is achieved with the application of DBBM particles to overcontour the alveolar process on the facial aspect of the implant site.

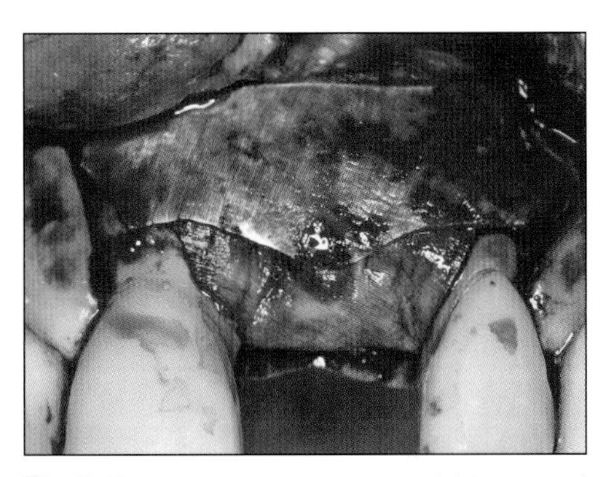

Fig 7-7e The augmentation material is covered with a collagen membrane applied with a double-layer technique. The membrane is soaked with blood to achieve good stability.

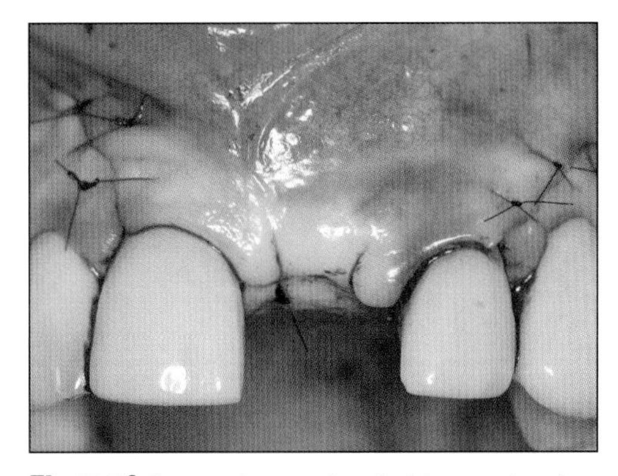

Fig 7-7f Surgery is completed with a tension-free primary wound closure following the release of the periosteum.

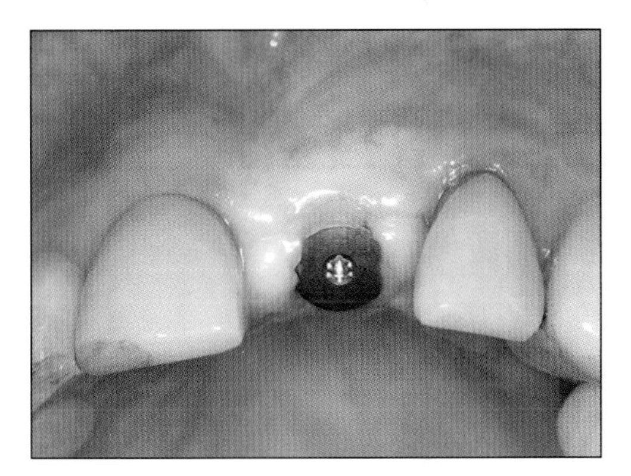

Fig 7-7g The site is reopened with a punch to gain access to the integrated implant 10 weeks following placement. A longer healing cap is inserted, causing blanching of the mucosa on the facial aspect.

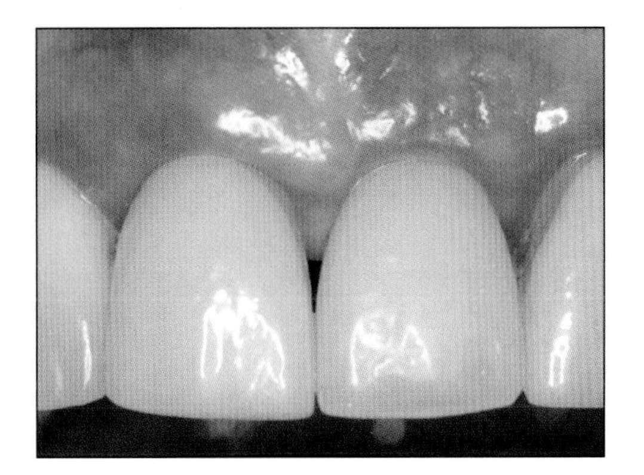

Fig 7-7h An acrylic resin provisional crown is used for soft tissue conditioning.

(Fig 7-7 continues on next page.)

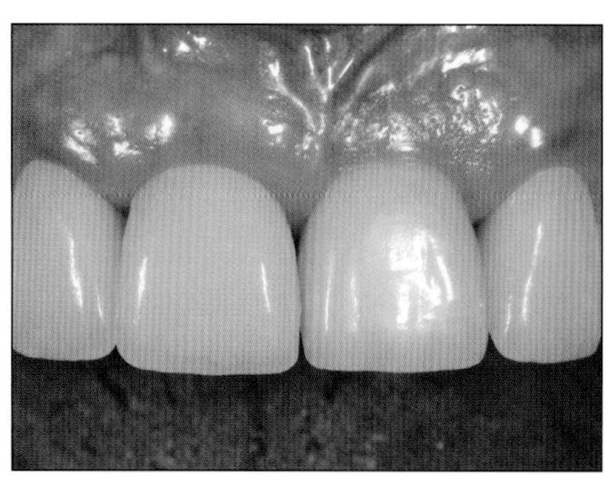

Fig 7-7i The 5-year examination reveals that over time the dentition has been extensively restored with ceramic crowns, not only for the implant but also for adjacent teeth. The esthetic outcome is pleasing; there is a harmonious gingival margin, and there are no abrupt changes in tissue height.

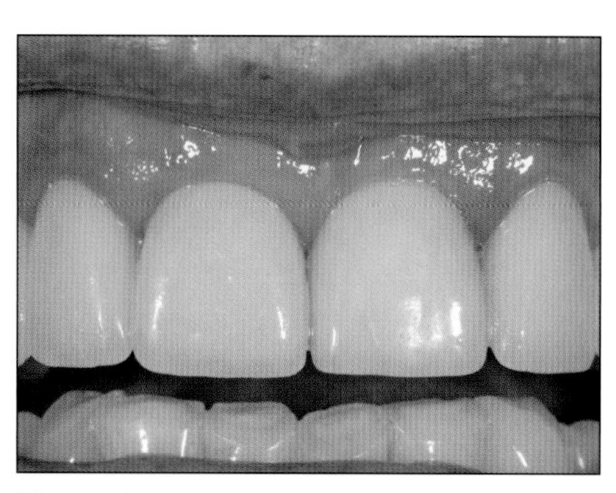

Fig 7-7j The patient's smile is shown at the 5-year follow-up examination.

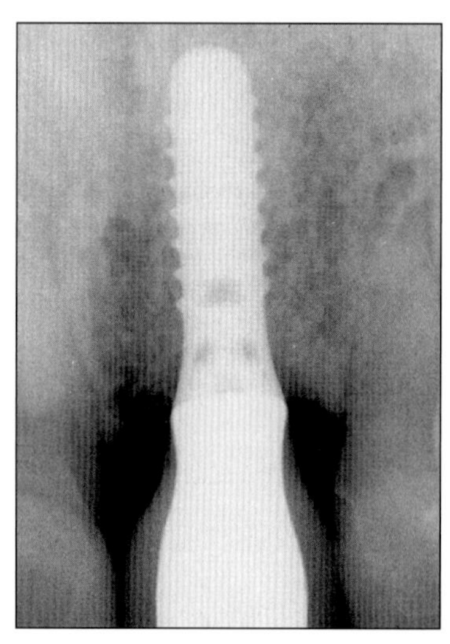

Fig 7-7k A periapical radiograph at the 5-year examination shows stable bone crest levels around the well-integrated implant.

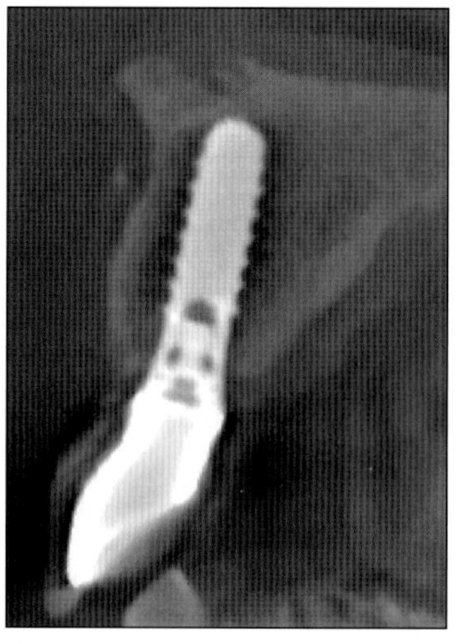

Fig 7-7l A CBCT at the 5-year examination confirms excellent stability of the contour augmentation on the facial aspect of the implant. The facial bone wall shows a thickness of roughly 3 mm.

Case 4: Single-tooth replacement, triangular flap design

A 28-year-old woman had a posttraumatic complication involving the maxillary left central incisor. The detailed esthetic risk assessment showed several high risk factors, such as a patient with high esthetic expectations, an extremely "gummy" smile because of her high lip line, an extended periradicular infection with a fistula in the apical area, an extensive horizontal and vertical bone defect on the facial aspect, and a restored adjacent tooth. Thus, immediate implant placement was contraindicated.

Early implant placement with soft tissue healing (type 2) was chosen. The treatment included bone-level implant placement, a triangular flap design, and a vertical releasing incision outside the esthetic zone (Fig 7-8).

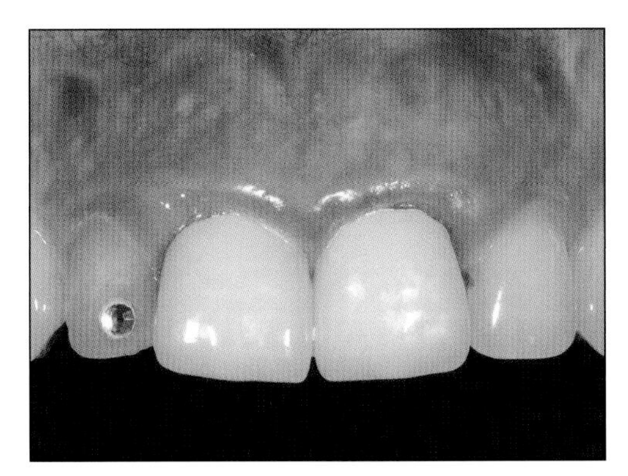

Fig 7-8a A long-term complication of trauma has resulted in a fistula at the maxillary left central incisor. Both incisors had been restored, and the right lateral incisor was discolored.

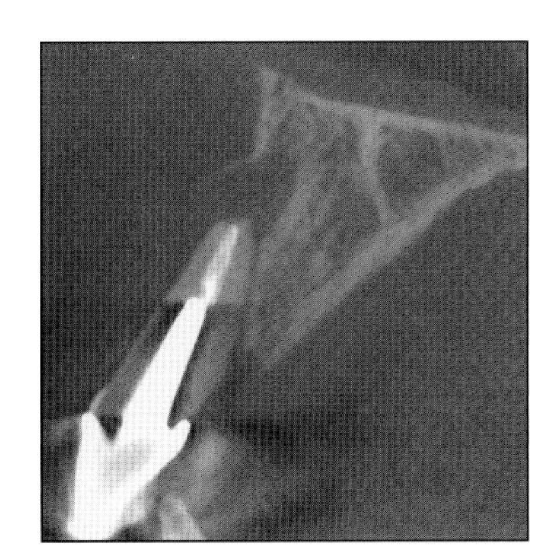

Fig 7-8b The CBCT clearly reveals a complete loss of the facial bone wall because of the chronic periradicular infection. The tooth has to be removed.

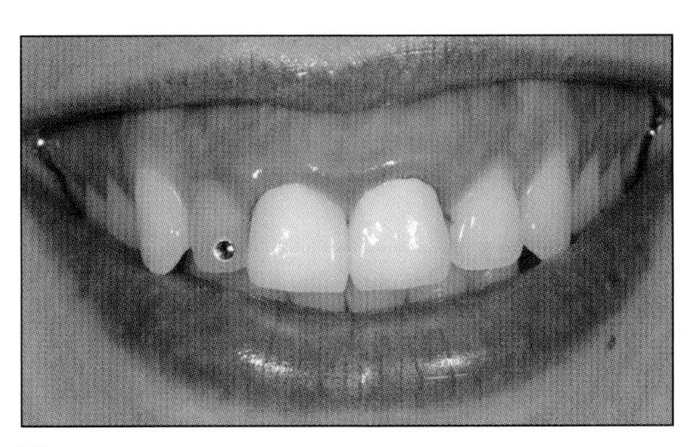

Fig 7-8c The patient exhibits an extremely gummy smile because of her high lip line. A medium-thick gingival biotype represented a less critical risk factor.

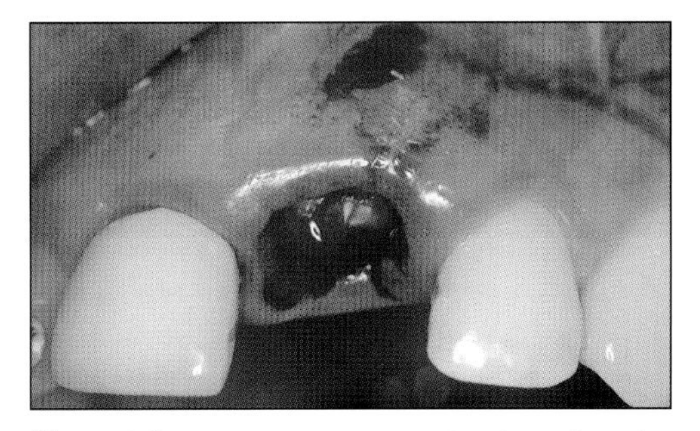

Fig 7-8d The tooth is extracted without flap elevation. Careful debridement is performed to remove granulation tissue.

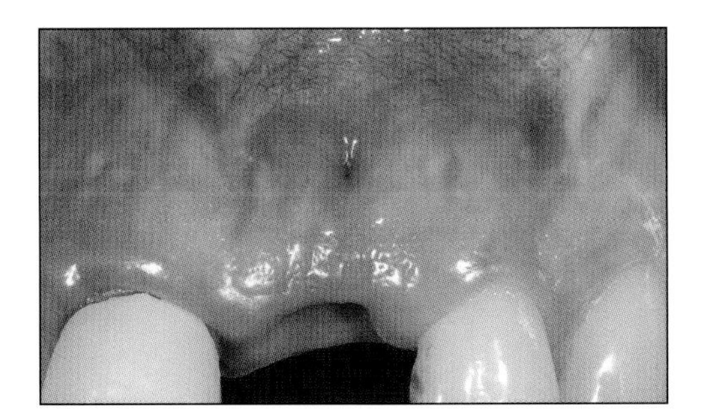

Fig 7-8e Eight weeks postextraction, the fistula is still visible but is closed.

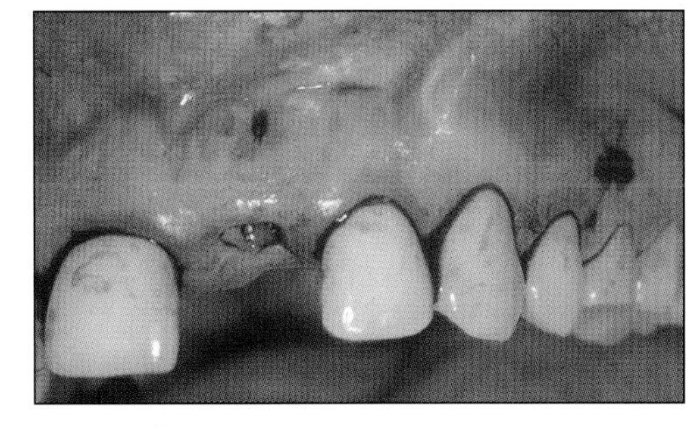

Fig 7-8f A triangular flap design with only one vertical releasing incision outside the esthetic zone at the left first premolar is chosen.

Fig 7-8g Following flap elevation, the extent of the large bone defect in the extraction site is apparent.

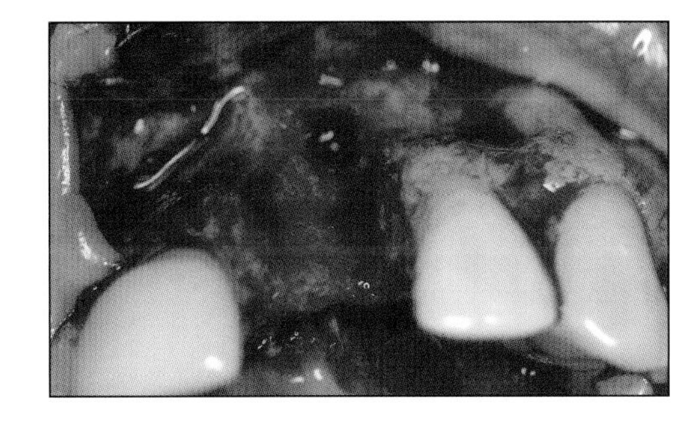

(Fig 7-8 continues on next page.)

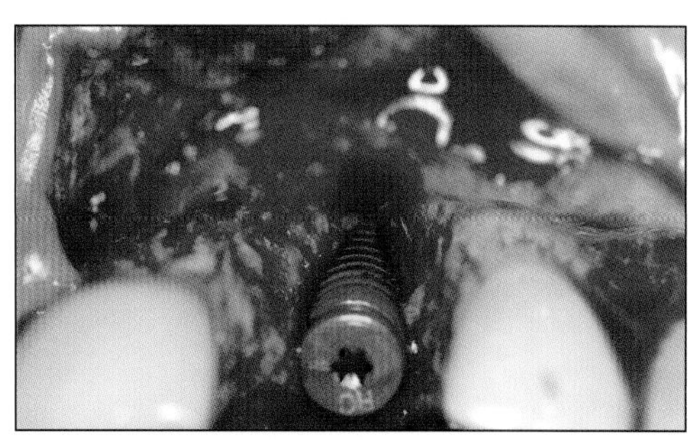

Fig 7-8h The crest width of more than 6 mm at adjacent teeth has resulted in a two-wall defect on the facial aspect following placement of a bone-level implant. The exposed, chemically modified SLA surface is clearly located inside the alveolar crest, favoring predictable bone regeneration in the defect area.

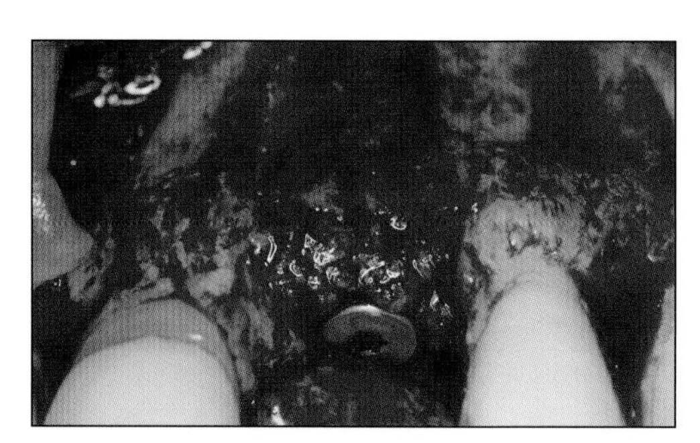

Fig 7-8i To expedite new bone formation in the defect area, locally harvested autogenous bone chips soaked in blood are applied to fill the defect up to the applied healing cap.

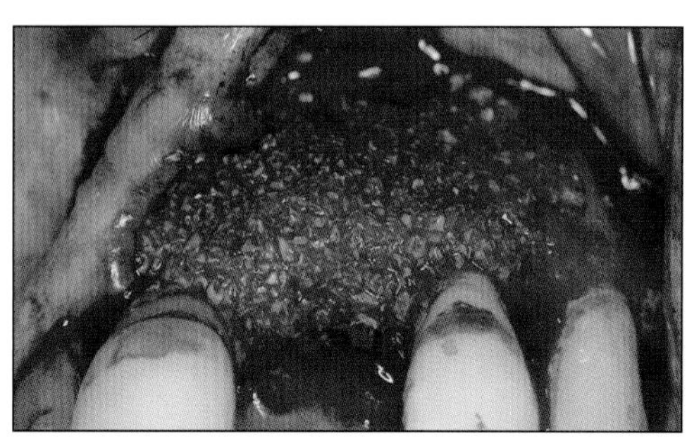

Fig 7-8j DBBM particles are applied to overcontour the local anatomy. This well-documented bone filler has a low substitution rate and is an important part of successful contour augmentation.

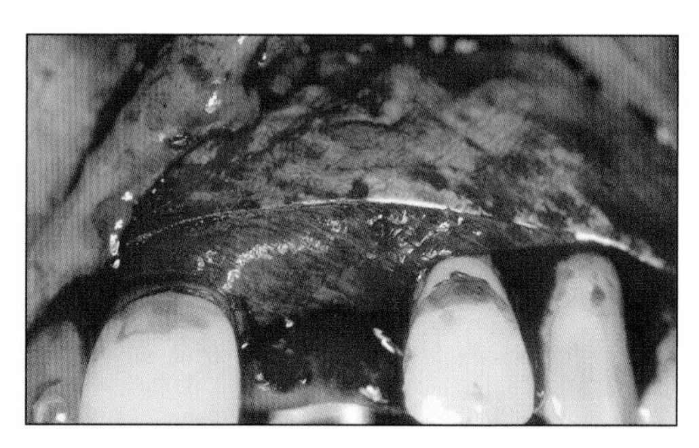

Fig 7-8k The bone fillers are covered with a non-cross-linked collagen membrane applied in a double-layer technique to improve membrane stability. The resorbable membrane is used as a temporary barrier and does not require a reopening procedure for membrane removal.

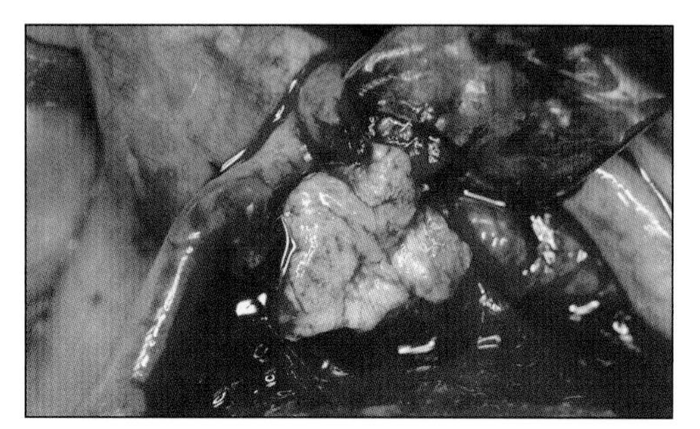

Fig 7-8l A small connective tissue graft, harvested from the palatal aspect, is used underneath the flap to support the soft tissues in the area of the previous fistula.

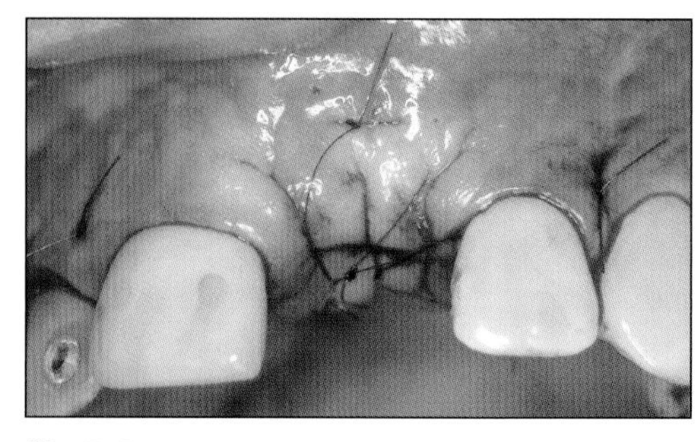

Fig 7-8m Following the release of the periosteum, tension-free primary wound closure is achieved using 5-0 and 6-0 nonresorbable sutures.

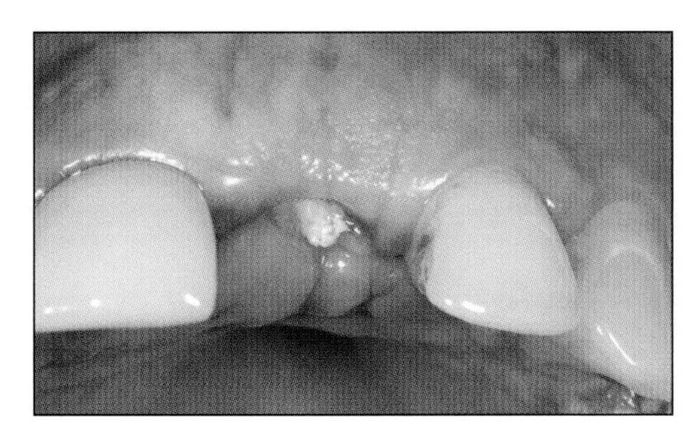

Fig 7-8n Although soft tissue healing progressed well, a small soft tissue dehiscence is apparent in the crestal area at 3 weeks, leaving the collagen membrane slightly exposed. The exposed membrane is kept clean by local application of chlorhexidine gel (0.2%) applied with an extrasoft toothbrush.

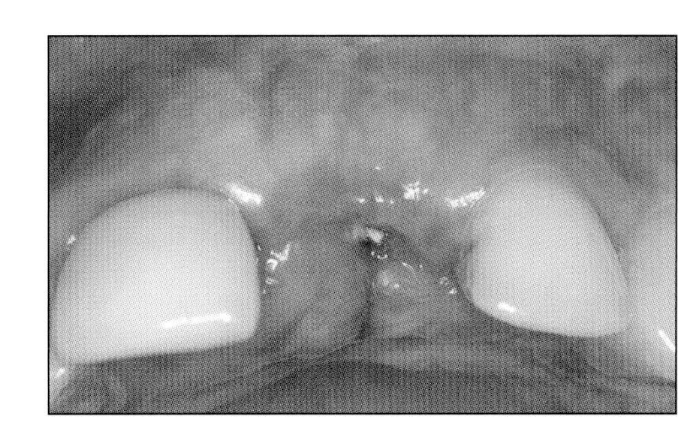

Fig 7-8o By 8 weeks of healing, the soft tissue dehiscence has spontaneously reduced in size by secondary granulation and has not caused any further complication.

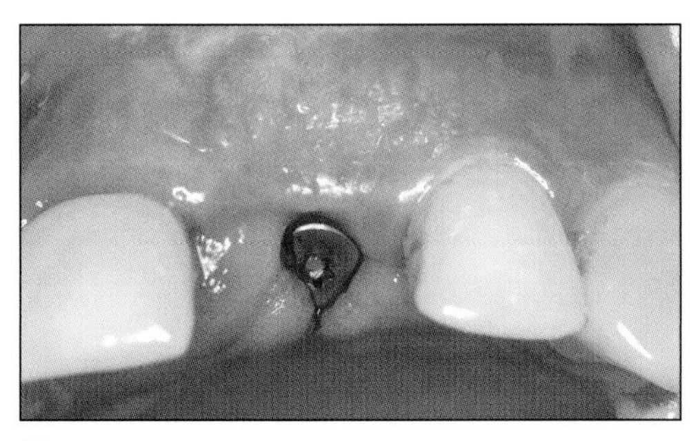

Fig 7-8p A reopening procedure was performed with a punch technique. A longer healing abutment with a 4-mm diameter at the top is inserted

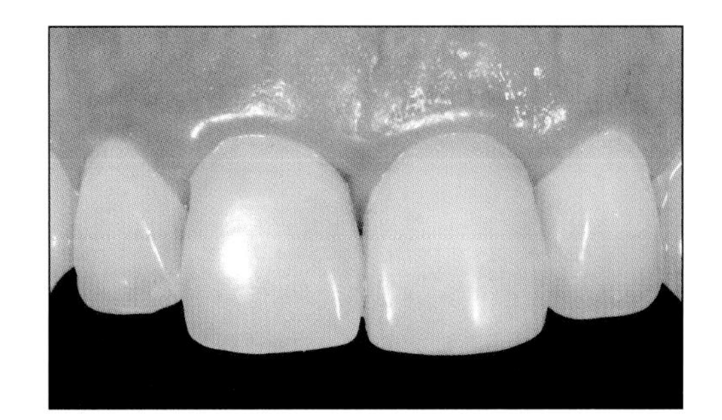

Fig 7-8q After impression taking with a transfer coping, a screw-retained provisional crown is inserted to initiate the soft tissue conditioning. A new provisional crown is also placed onto the contralateral incisor. Soft tissue maturation will take at least 3 months, at which time final all-ceramic crowns will be fabricated.

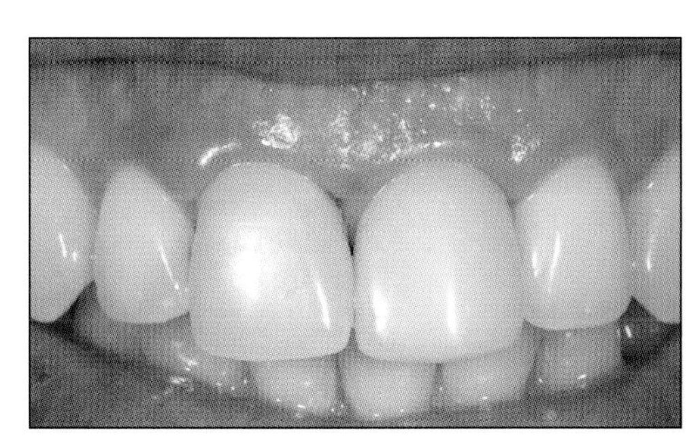

Fig 7-8r The extraoral view of the extremely gummy smile shows that the esthetic situation has clearly improved, even with provisional crowns.

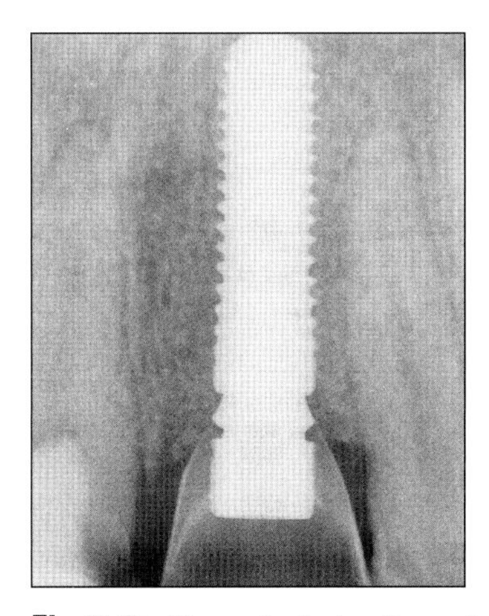

Fig 7-8s The periapical radiograph reveals that the peri-implant bone crest level is stable.

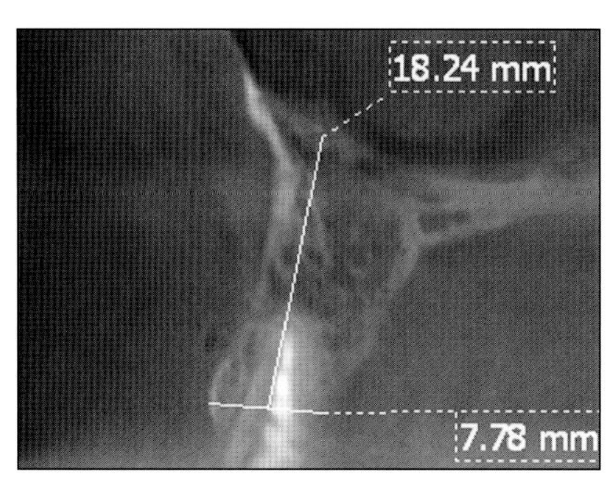

Fig 7-9a The CBCT of the maxillary right second premolar reveals a thick facial bone wall and excellent bone volume of the alveolar crest, both in width and in height.

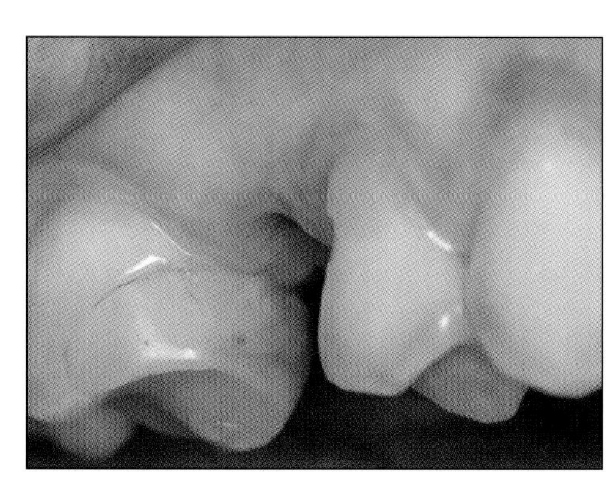

Fig 7-9b Examination 6 weeks following extraction of the second premolar indicates that the alveolar crest has excellent contour and the gingival biotype is thick.

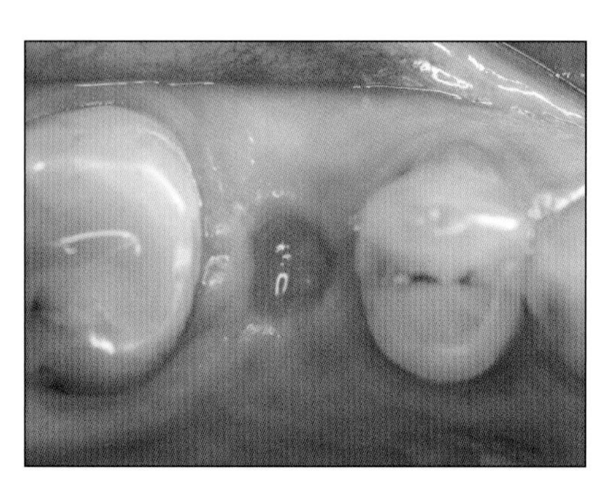

Fig 7-9c No facial flattening is apparent because of the extremely thick facial bone wall at the extraction site. Flapless implant placement can be used in such an ideal clinical situation.

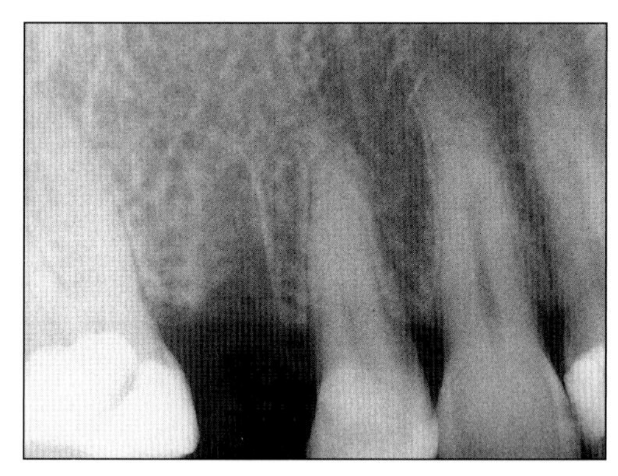

Fig 7-9d The extraction socket is still visible in the periapical radiograph taken prior to implant placement.

Case 5: Single-tooth replacement, flapless approach

A 44-year-old woman had a maxillary second premolar that had to be removed because of a crack in the root. The CBCT (Fig 7-9a) revealed an unusually thick facial bone wall of more than 2 mm and a crest width of almost 8 mm without any undercuts. In addition, the bone height measured 18 mm, allowing the placement of a 12-mm implant without interference with the maxillary sinus.

The treatment plan was to extract the tooth and to place an implant 6 weeks later (Figs 7-9b to 7-9d). The excellent bone volume allowed a flapless approach to implant placement without the need for surgical guides (Figs 7-9e to 7-9n).

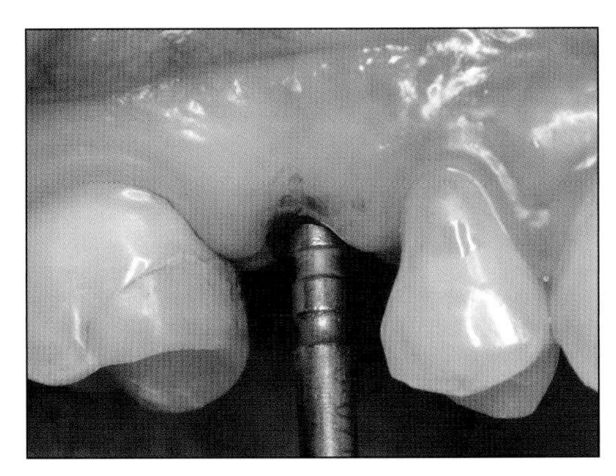

Fig 7-9e Initial implant bed preparation is performed with the smallest spiral drill (2.2-mm diameter), and a depth gauge is inserted to obtain an intraoperative radiograph.

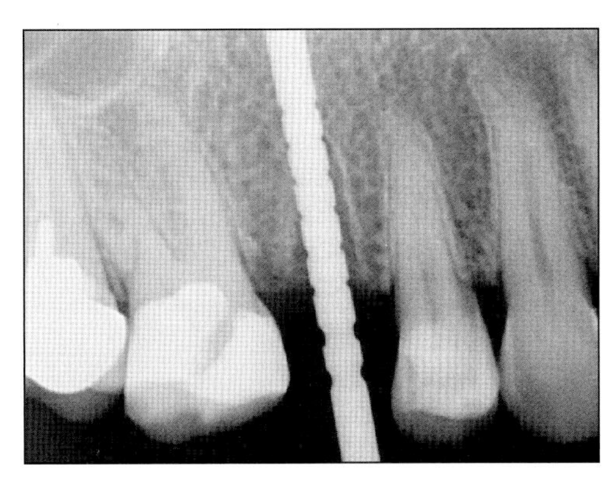

Fig 7-9f The intraoperative radiograph confirms the correct mesiodistal positioning of the implant preparation.

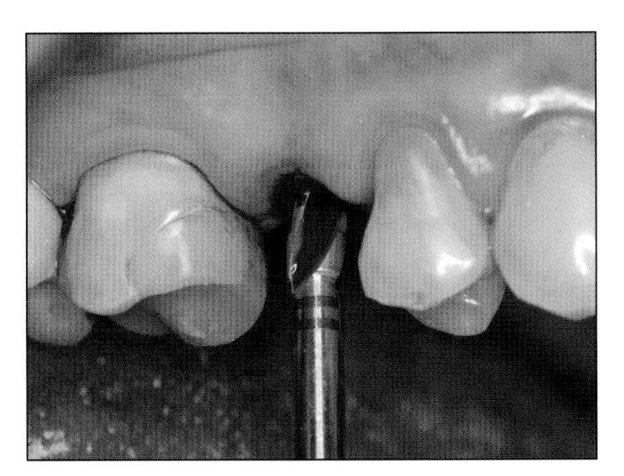

Fig 7-9g Further implant bed preparation is performed with spiral and profile drills of increasing diameters.

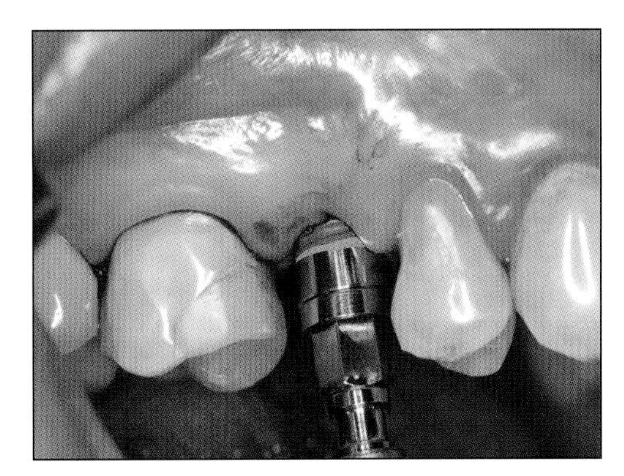

Fig 7-9h A 12-mm, tissue-level implant is transmucosally inserted. The intention is to position the implant shoulder roughly 3 mm below the mucosal surface.

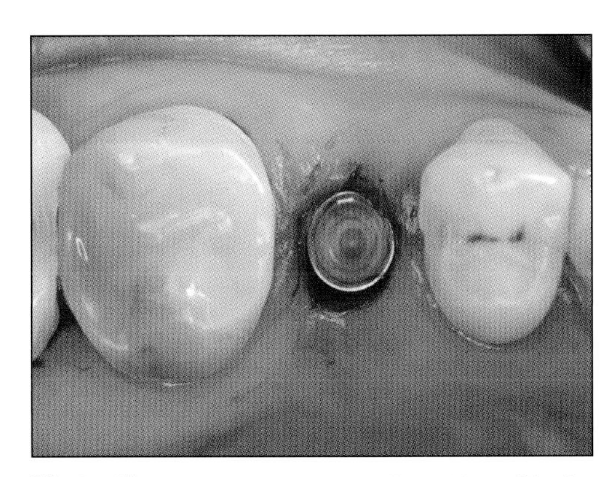

Fig 7-9i The implant is also well positioned in the orofacial direction. There is no need for any grafting procedure.

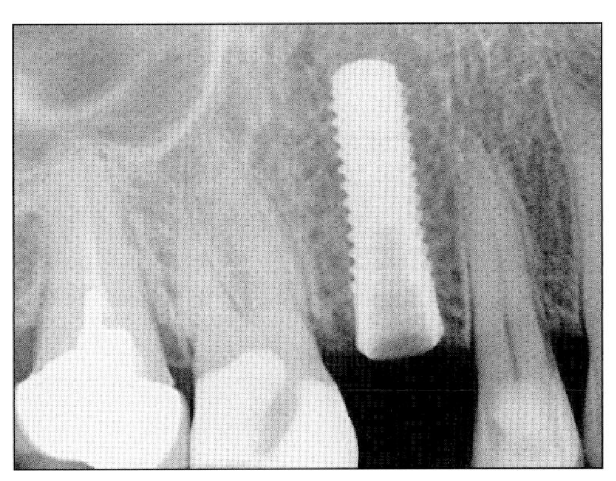

Fig 7-9j The postsurgical radiograph shows the well-positioned implant.

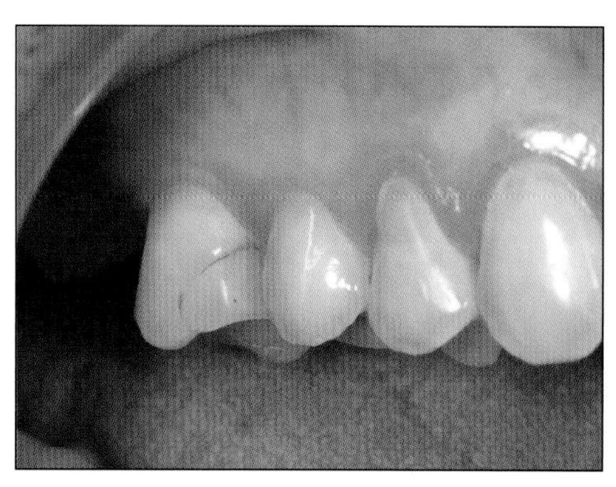

Fig 7-9k At 6 weeks, the implant is restored with a provisional acrylic resin crown seated on a titanium coping.

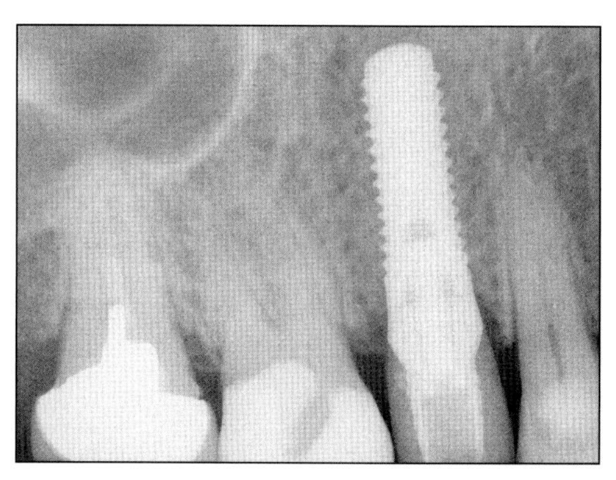

Fig 7-9l A periapical radiograph taken with the provisional crown still in place reveals signs of remodeling at the peri-implant bone crest and the development of a peri-implant bone saucer, which is typical for tissue-level implants.

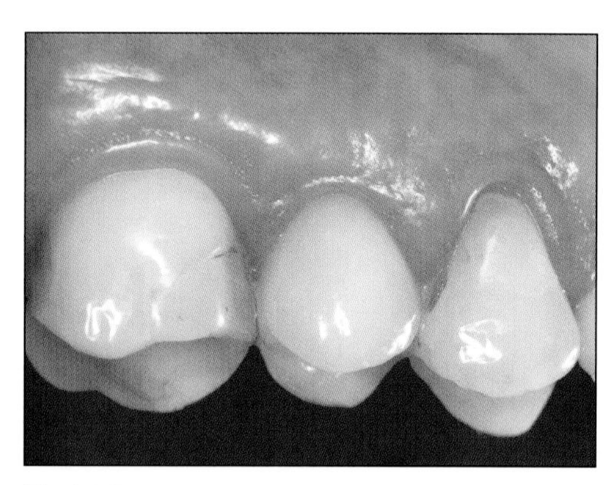

Fig 7-9m At the 3-year follow-up examination, the peri-implant soft tissues are stable.

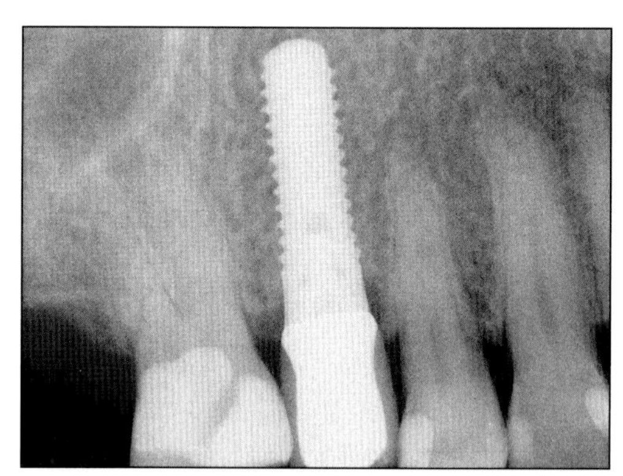

Fig 7-9n The 3-year follow-up radiograph confirms stable bone crest levels around the tissue-level implant.

Case 6: Two missing central incisors

A 27-year-old woman was referred to the clinic for extraction of her maxillary central incisors because of external root resorption resulting from dental trauma that had occurred a few years earlier. The patient had several high esthetic risk factors, including a high lip line and a thin gingival biotype. In addition, the extraction of both central incisors required the placement of two adjacent implants. In such a situation, the establishment of an interimplant papilla is challenging. Thus, implant placement 8 weeks following extraction was combined with a simultaneous contour augmentation, which was particularly important in the interimplant area. To improve the augmentation volume in this crucial area, applied DBBM particles were stabilized with fibrin sealant (Fig 7-10).

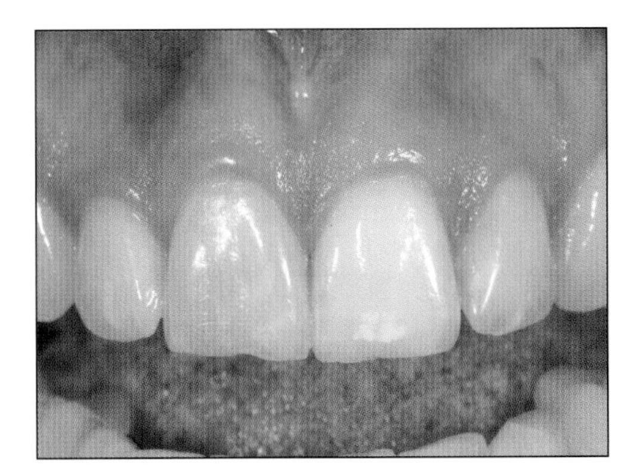

Fig 7-10a The slightly discolored right central incisor has increased probing depths. The patient has a thin gingival biotype, which is a high esthetic risk factor.

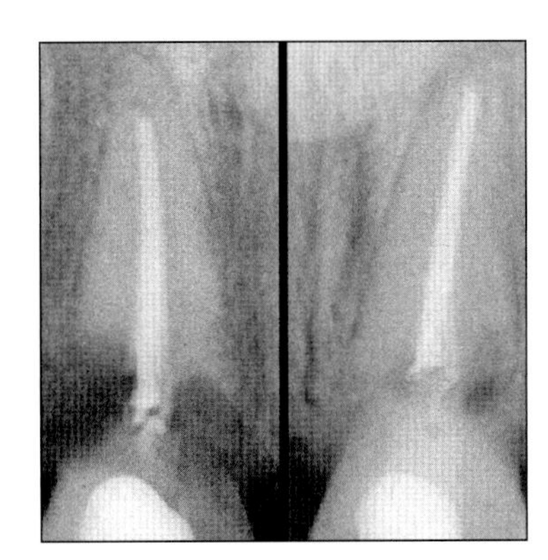

Fig 7-10b The periapical radiograph shows extensive external root resorption of the right central incisor caused by previous dental trauma. The contralateral root also shows initial signs of resorption. Both central incisors have to be removed, which represents another high esthetic risk factor.

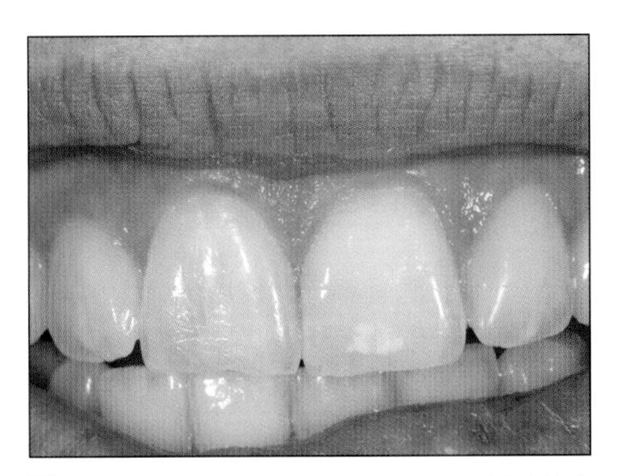

Fig 7-10c A view of the lips reveals a third high esthetic risk factor—a high lip line.

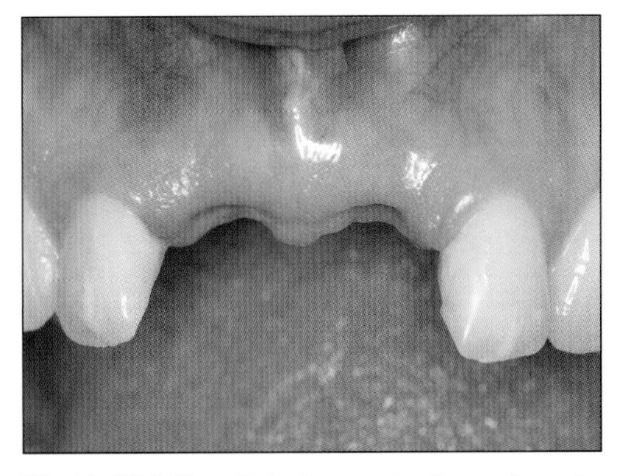

Fig 7-10d The clinical status is shown 8 weeks following extraction without flap elevation.

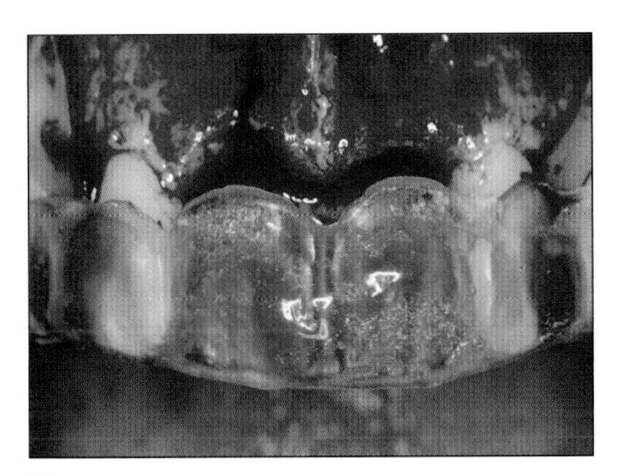

Fig 7-10e Following flap elevation, surgery is performed with a translucent surgical stent, which is standard in implant sites with multiple missing teeth. The stent defines the incisal edge and the facial margins of the two future crowns.

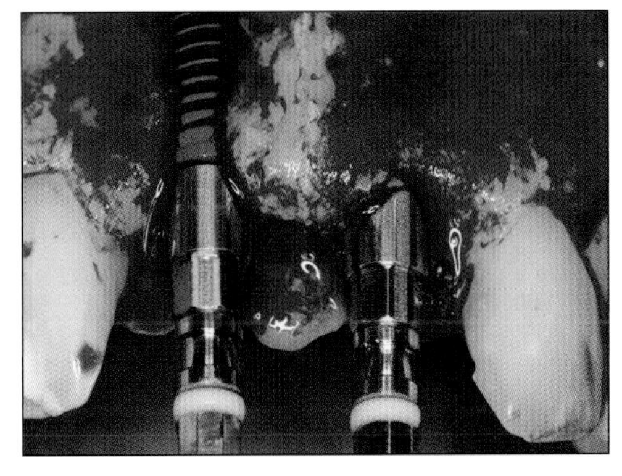

Fig 7-10f Two bone-level implants have been placed so that the implant platform is positioned approximately 3 mm apical to the future crown margins on the midfacial aspect. The right implant shows a dehiscence defect on the facial aspect.

(Fig 7-10 continues on next page.)

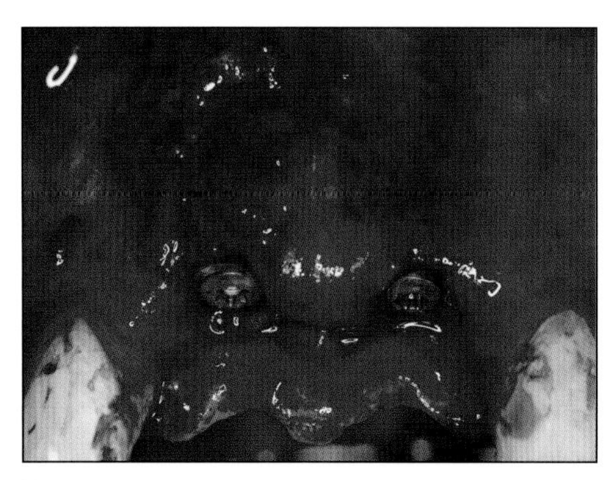

Fig 7-10g The peri-implant bone defects are augmented with autogenous bone grafts harvested at the nasal spine.

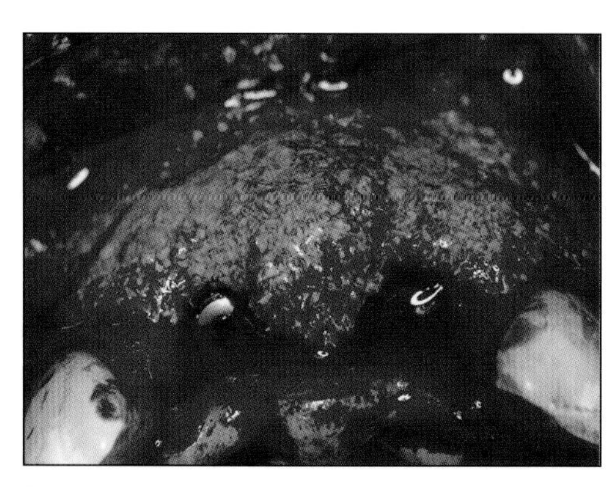

Fig 7-10h Contour augmentation is achieved with a layer of DBBM particles stabilized with fibrin sealant. The interimplant area is also vertically augmented to optimize the future shape of the interimplant papilla.

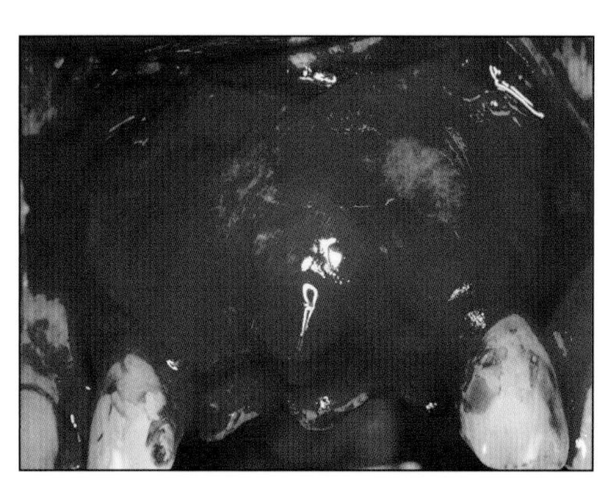

Fig 7-10i The augmentation material is covered with a collagen membrane applied with a double-layer technique.

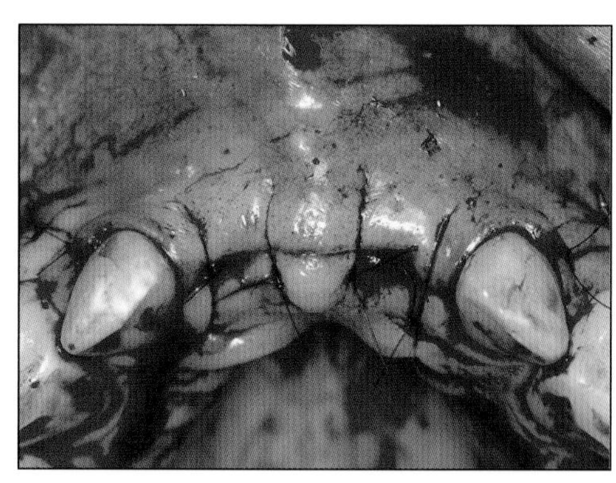

Fig 7-10j The surgery is completed with tension-free primary wound closure. To achieve that, an incision of the periosteum was necessary to release the flap.

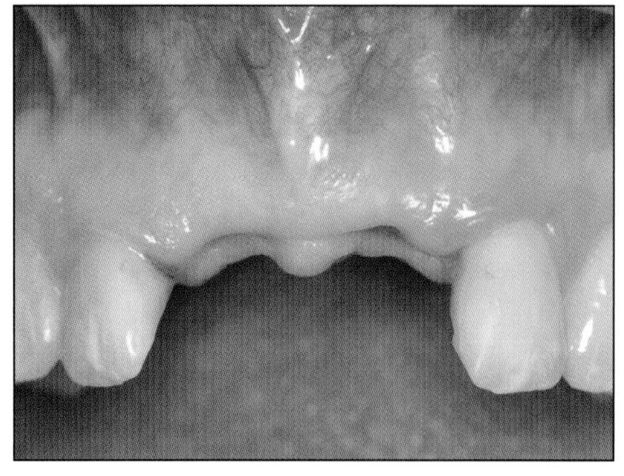

Fig 7-10k After 8 weeks of healing without complications, the implant sites are ready for a reopening procedure.

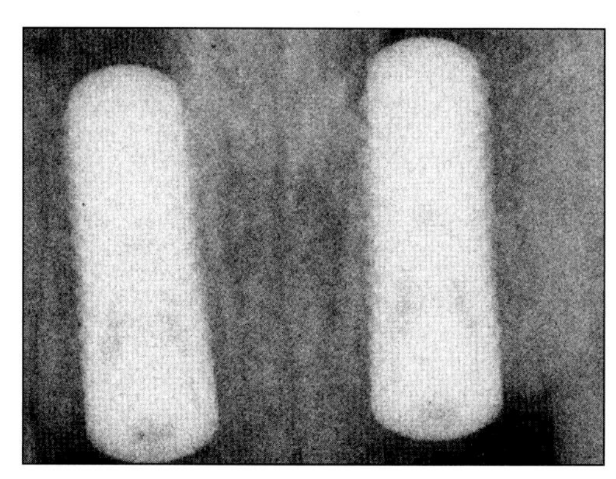

Fig 7-10l The periapical radiograph taken 2 months following implant placement indicates that both implants are well integrated.

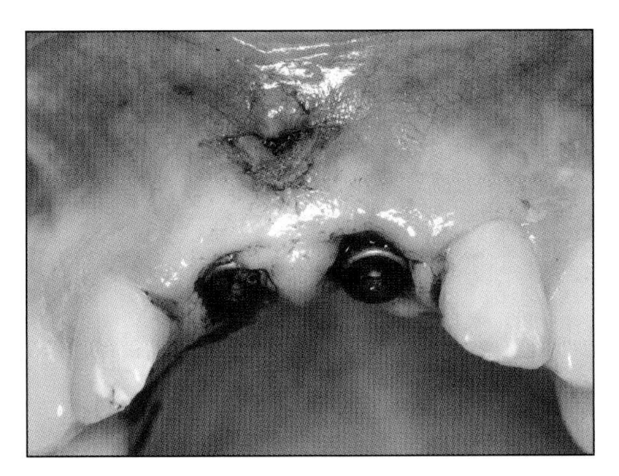

Fig 7-10m A punch technique is used to gain access to both implants. Longer 4-mm healing caps are inserted. In addition, the frenulum has been resected with a carbon dioxide laser.

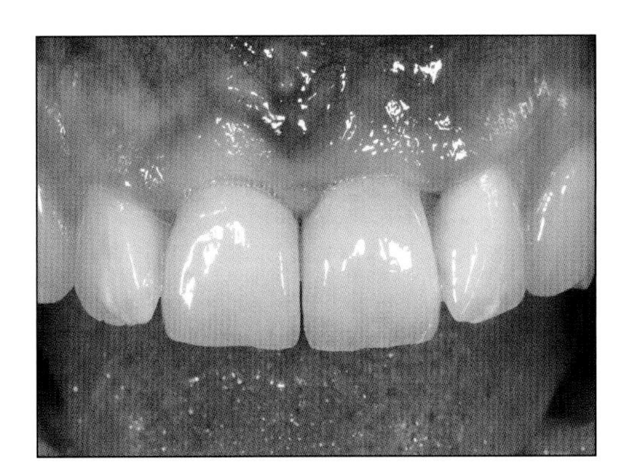

Fig 7-10n Two provisional crowns are placed to initiate the soft tissue conditioning phase.

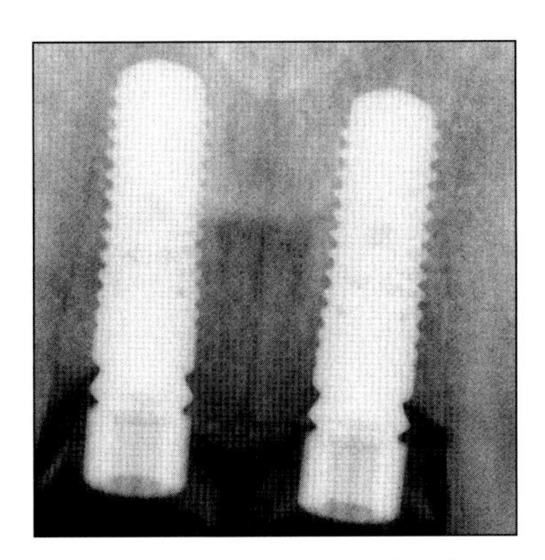

Fig 7-10o The periapical radiograph of both implants with their provisional crowns reveals that bone crest levels are well maintained around the implants as well as in the interimplant area.

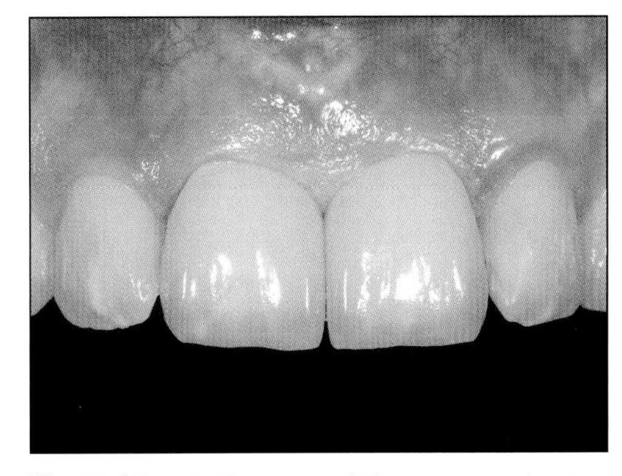

Fig 7-10p At the 2-year follow-up examination, the esthetic treatment outcome with definitive all-ceramic crowns is excellent. The interimplant papilla has a pleasing shape.

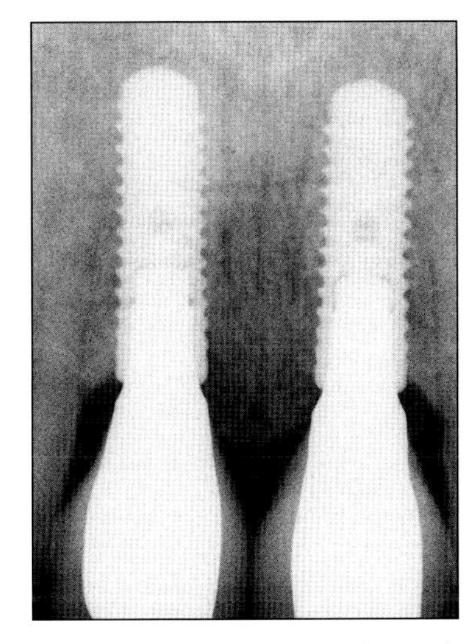

Fig 7-10q The 2-year follow-up radiograph shows stable peri-implant bone levels and excellent bone structure between the implants.

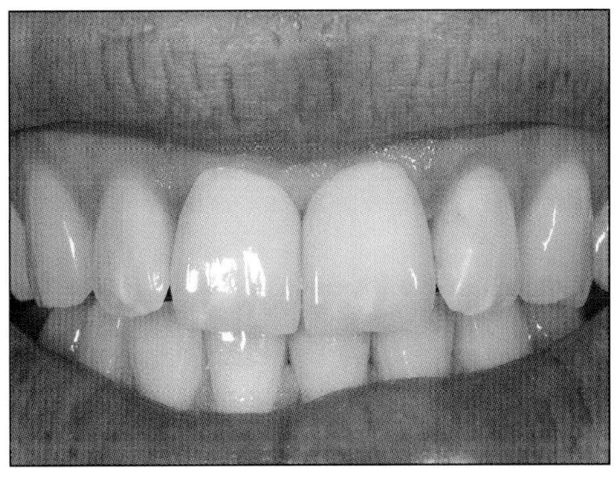

Fig 7-10r The two implant-borne single crowns display excellent esthetics. (Prosthodontics by Prof U. Belser, University of Geneva, Switzerland.)

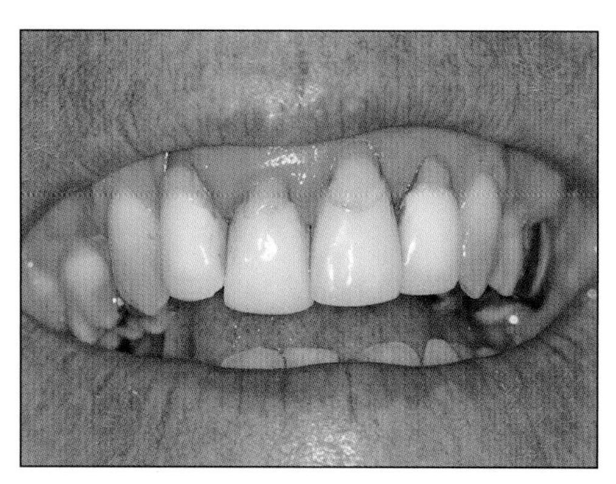

Fig 7-11a Female patient with a severe esthetic problem because of a high lip line, gingival recession, and discolored teeth.

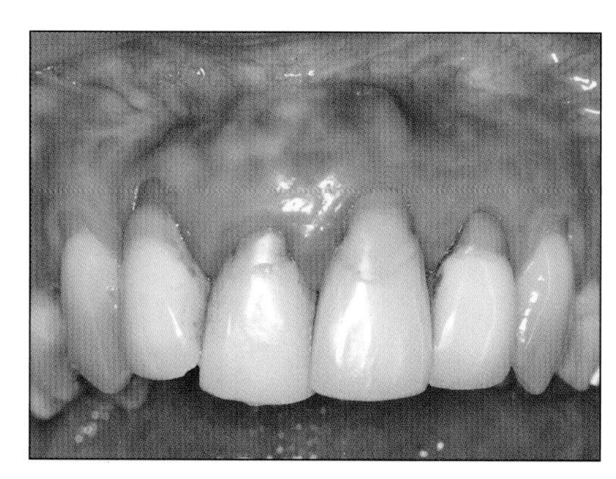

Fig 7-11b Generalized recession has caused a nonharmonious gingival margin. Three maxillary incisors have a chronic fistula and show extended probing depths on the facial aspect.

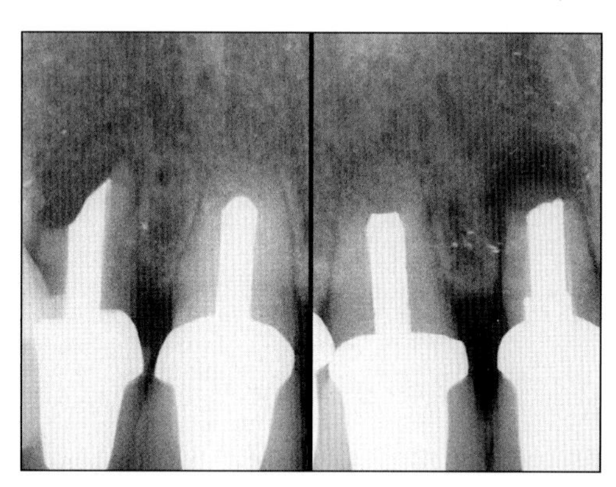

Fig 7-11c All four incisors have had endodontic surgery with apicoectomies. The two lateral incisors have osteolytic apical lesions. All four incisors have to be removed.

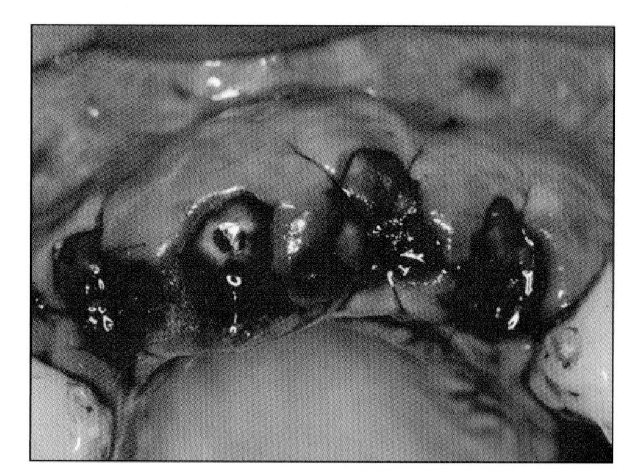

Fig 7-11d Only the three teeth with fistulas have been removed. The right central incisor has been cut back to the bone level and left in place to maintain the crest width in that area during the soft tissue healing period of 8 weeks.

Case 7: Four missing maxillary incisors

A 50-year-old woman was referred with a severe esthetic problem in the anterior maxilla. The four maxillary incisors had to be extracted, resulting in an extended edentulous space representing a category C situation (complex) according to the SAC classification (Figs 7-11a to 7-11c). Three roots with a fistula had to be removed, whereas one root was shortened and left temporarily in place, as proposed by Langer.[31] This technique is useful prior to implant placement to maintain the crest width (Figs 7-11d to 7-11f).

Implant placement was carried out 8 weeks following extraction and combined with a simultaneous GBR procedure (Figs 7-11g to 7-11m). The local bone anatomy dictated the placement of two implants in the two central incisor sites to avoid a staged approach in the lateral incisor sites. Following 3 months of healing, the two implant sites were reopened to initiate the restorative treatment, first with a provisional fixed prosthesis, followed by a metal-ceramic fixed partial denture (Figs 7-11n to 7-11s).

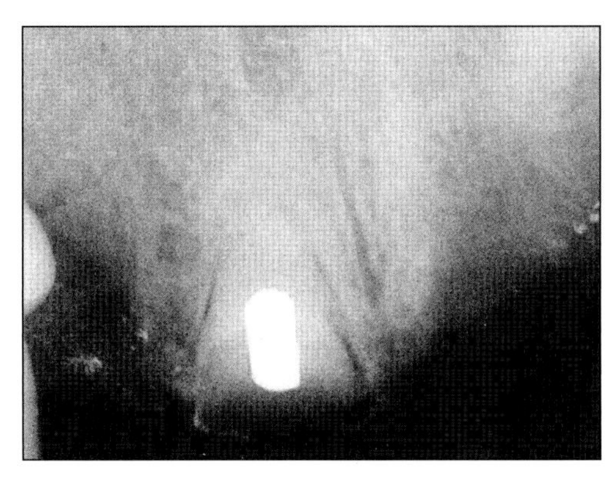

Fig 7-11e The small root has been left in place to prevent resorption of bundle bone in that area.

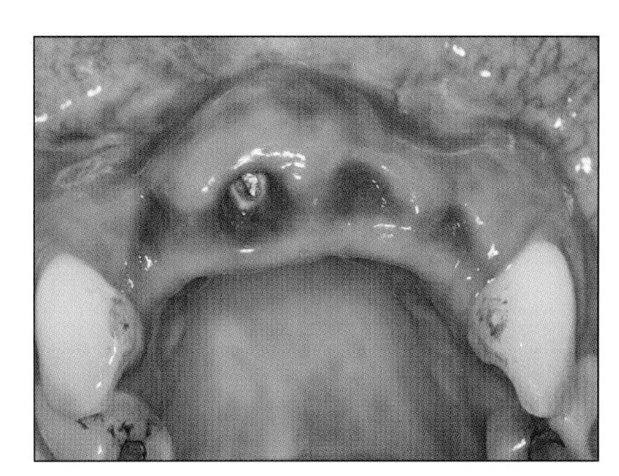

Fig 7-11f After 8 weeks, the crest width is well maintained in the area with the small root remnant, whereas the crest width clearly has collapsed, as expected, in both lateral incisor sites.

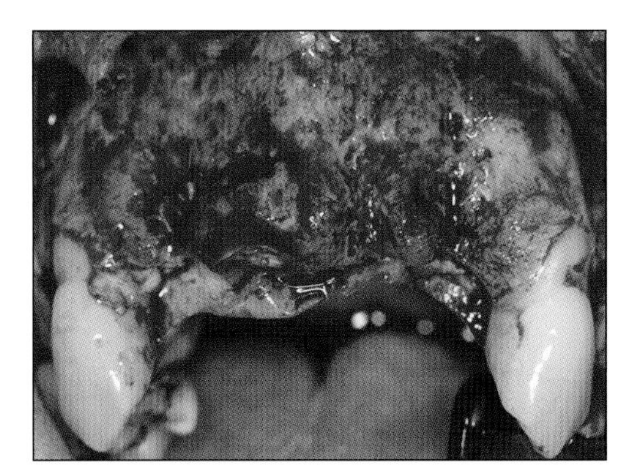

Fig 7-11g Elevation of a mucoperiosteal flap reveals that bone atrophy is pronounced in both lateral incisor sites, which does not allow implant placement with simultaneous GBR.

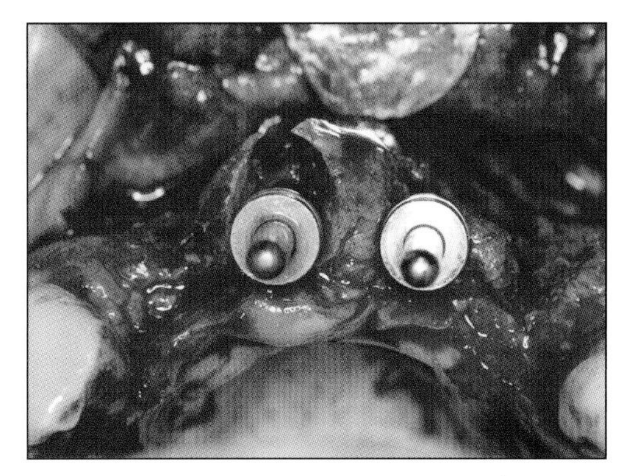

Fig 7-11h Two tissue-level implants are placed in the central incisor sites. The volume of bone is excellent where the root was left in place.

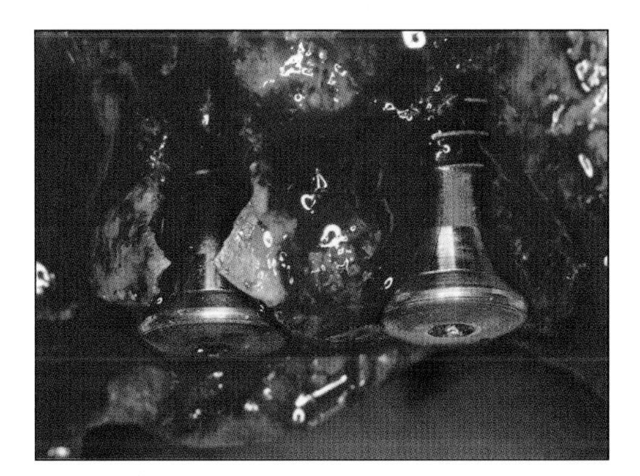

Fig 7-11i Two tissue-level implants and 1.5-mm healing caps are placed. The right implant has an excellent two-wall defect morphology, whereas the defect morphology at the left implant is much less favorable.

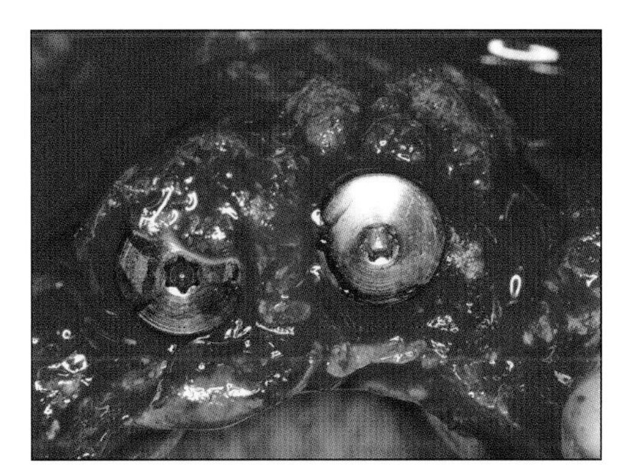

Fig 7-11j The facial bone defects are augmented with autogenous bone chips harvested locally with a chisel.

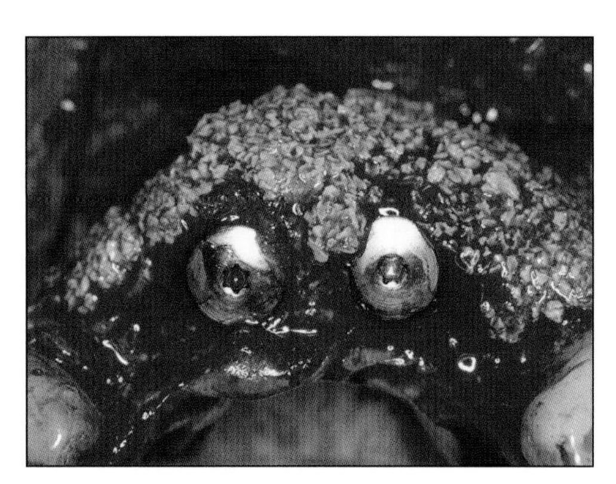

Fig 7-11k The local bone anatomy is overcontoured with DBBM particles to provide a facial bone wall with a sufficient thickness and a convex contour.

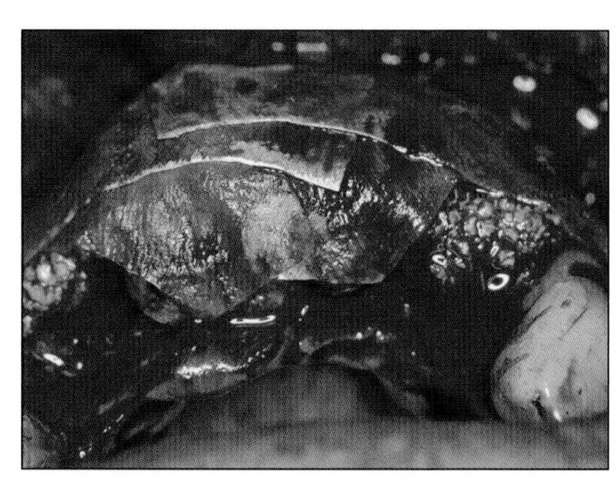

Fig 7-11l The bone fillers are covered with a non-cross-linked collagen membrane applied with various layers to improve membrane stability.

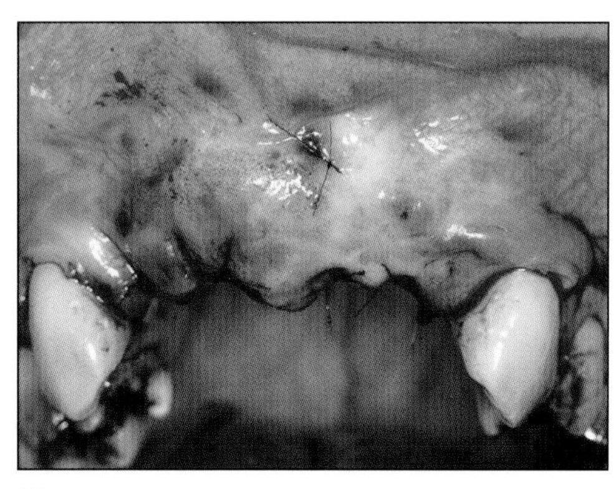

Fig 7-11m The surgery is completed with a tension-free primary wound closure following the release of the periosteum.

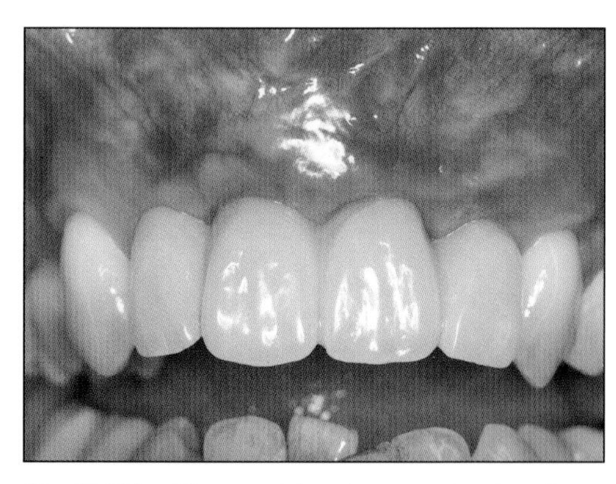

Fig 7-11n The provisional restoration is a four-unit fixed partial denture with a distal cantilever unit on both sides.

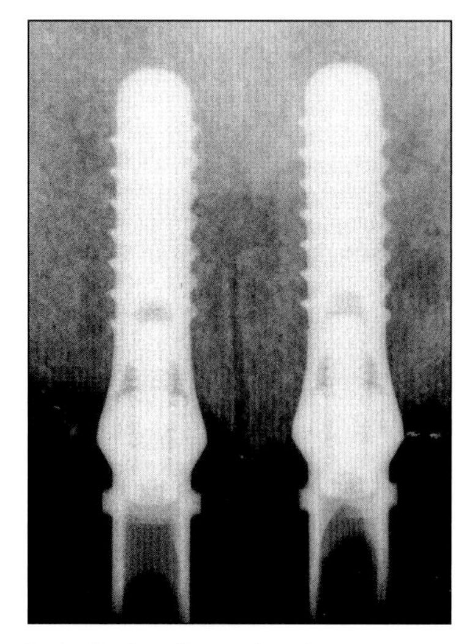

Fig 7-11o Periapical radiographs show the two well-integrated implants. The bone crest levels are stable around both implants.

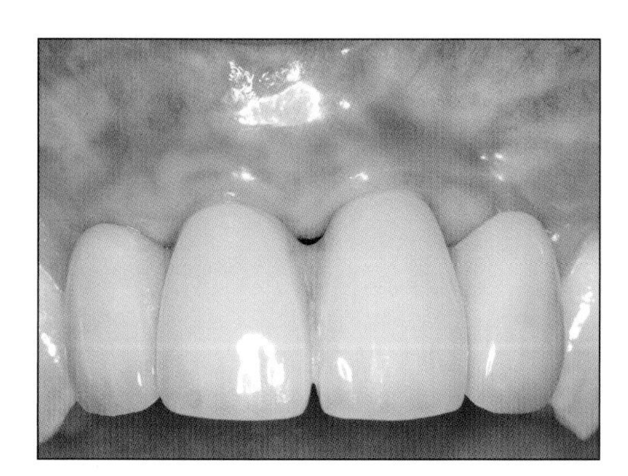

Fig 7-11p At the 5-year follow-up examination, the esthetic outcome is more than satisfactory considering the severely compromised esthetic situation at initiation of therapy.

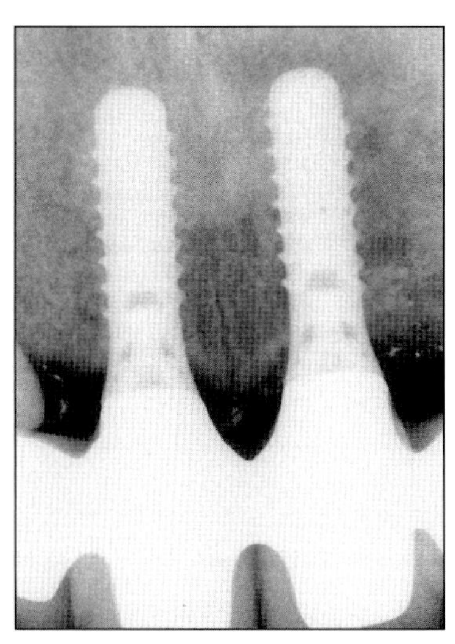

Fig 7-11q The 5-year follow-up radiograph confirms the stable bone crest levels around the two tissue-level implants.

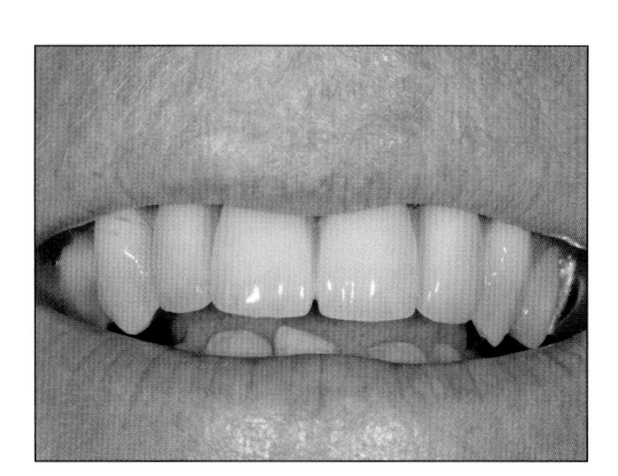

Fig 7-11r Extraoral view at the 5-year examination.

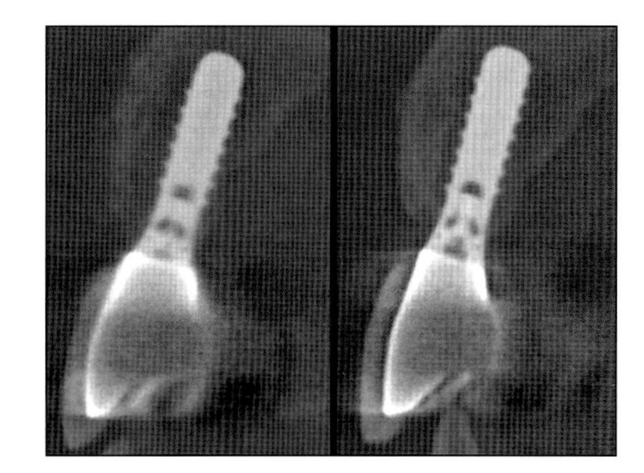

Fig 7-11s The CBCT at the 5-year examination confirms the excellent stability of the facial contour augmentation. The facial bone wall clearly exceeds 2 mm of thickness for both implants.

Early Implant Placement Following Partial Bone Healing (Type 3)

Advantages, disadvantages, and indications

Early implant placement with partial bone healing (type 3) provides for a healing period of 12 to 16 weeks prior to implant placement to allow more bone healing in the future implant site. As discussed previously, this approach is only used in the anterior maxilla if primary implant stability cannot be achieved or expected with type 2 placement. This situation may occur in patients with medium-to-large periapical or periodontal bone lesions but is not frequently encountered (Fig 7-12).

However, type 3 placement can be a valuable treatment option in mandibular molar sites following extraction. If molar sites show a crest width of more than 8 mm and in-

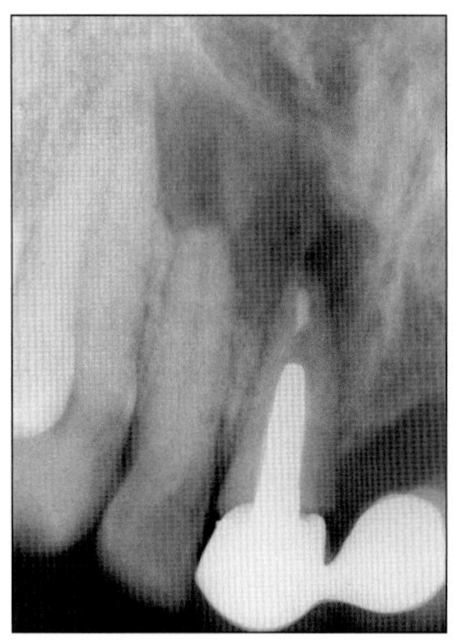

Fig 7-12a The maxillary right central incisor has a large periapical defect. The adjacent lateral incisor tests normally to pulpal vitality testing. The site is not suitable for early implant placement following soft tissue healing (type 2). A type 3 approach (early placement following partial bone healing) is the preferred option to ensure primary stability following implant insertion.

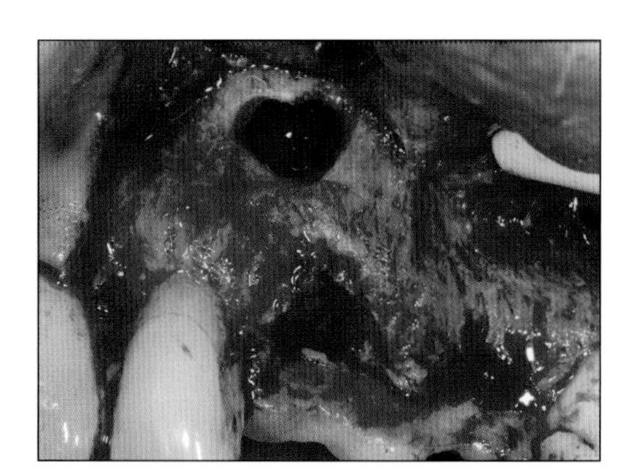

Fig 7-12b The extent of the bone defect is apparent following extraction of the tooth and removal of the periapical granuloma.

tact socket walls, 12 to 16 weeks of healing are sufficient in most patients to achieve an almost complete fill of the socket with newly formed bone but without significant reduction in crest width. At implant placement, remnants of granulation tissue might still be present in central portions of the previous socket. However, these remnants are mostly removed during the preparation of the implant bed. If a small peri-implant bone defect remains, this defect is filled with autogenous bone chips harvested from the vicinity, as long as the defect is contained within intact bone walls. In many cases, this approach allows implant placement without the use of bone substitutes and barrier membranes, hence offering a more cost-effective treatment than GBR procedures.

In addition, such a standard implant placement without bone augmentation usually allows short healing periods of 6 to 8 weeks. This early loading concept is well documented today; clinical studies with up to 5 years of follow-up have shown excellent success rates for SLA implants.[50–53] In ideal clinical situations, an even shorter healing period is used today with SLActive implants, when resonance frequency analysis shows an implant stability quotient of greater than 70.[46,47] Hence, shorter healing periods following implant placement compensate for the disadvantage of a longer healing period after extraction. In mandibular molar sites, this treatment is the preferred approach today.

In mandibular molar sites with significant loss of the facial bone wall because of infection, implant placement after 8 weeks of soft tissue healing (type 2) is recommended because a simultaneous GBR procedure has to be performed anyway. Thus, there is no benefit to waiting 12 to 16 weeks after extraction because this delay bears the risk of significant horizontal bone resorption.

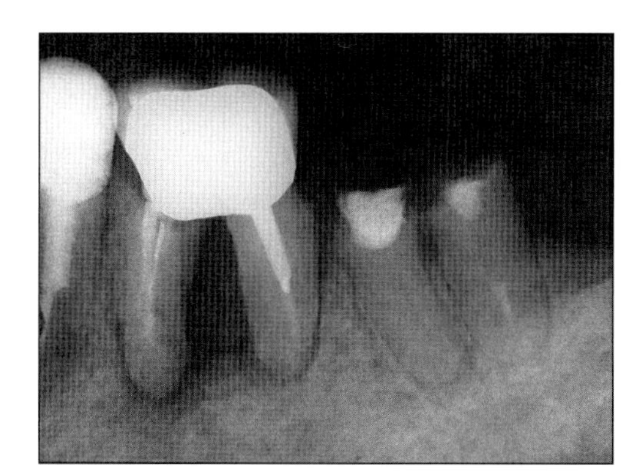

Fig 7-13a The mandibular left first molar shows a large bone lesion. Both molars were extracted by the referring dentist, who reported that the facial bone wall was missing in the first molar site.

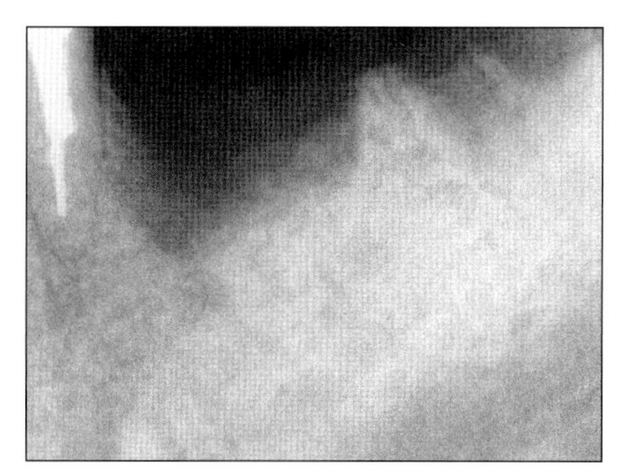

Fig 7-13b Four months later, partial bone healing is apparent, which will provide sufficient primary stability following implant insertion.

Case reports

Case 8: Distal-extension situation

A 59-year-old woman was referred following the extraction of two mandibular left molars. The first molar had a chronic infection, causing a large bone defect at the first molar site (Fig 7-13a). It was decided that an extended healing period of more than 3 months following extraction would achieve partial bone healing in the defect area. This extended healing period would ensure good primary implant stability following implant insertion.

Simultaneous GBR was performed according to the usual procedures; autogenous bone chips harvested from the retromolar area within the same flap were applied, a superficial layer of DBBM particles was added, a collagen membrane was applied, and primary wound closure was achieved.

A bone healing period of 5 months was required because the 3-month radiograph revealed unsatisfactory bone density in the defect area (Figs 7-13b to 7-13j). This was an unusual situation because in most cases restorative treatment can proceed 3 months after implant placement. A provisional acrylic resin crown was placed to initiate implant loading 5 months after implant placement in order to trigger bone remodeling in the peri-implant area. This approach was finally successful, and the bone density quickly improved (Figs 7-13k and 7-13l). At the 5-year follow-up examination, the clinical and radiographic images showed a successfully integrated implant supporting a metal-ceramic crown (Figs 7-13m and 7-13n).

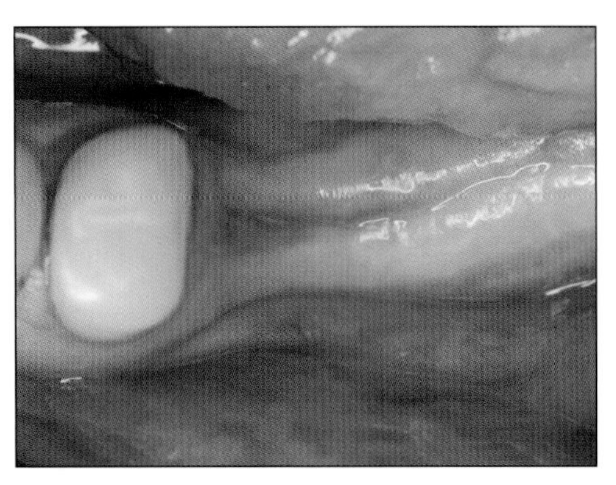

Fig 7-13c The day of implant surgery, a bone deficiency is visible on the facial aspect.

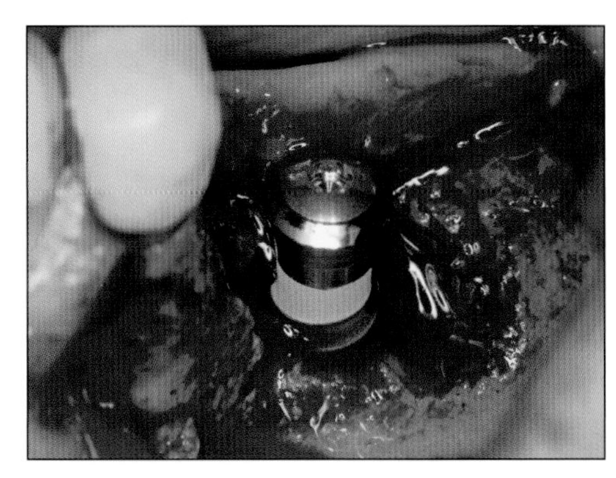

Fig 7-13d Following flap elevation, a tissue-level implant is inserted. On the facial aspect, a large bone defect with a two-wall defect morphology is present.

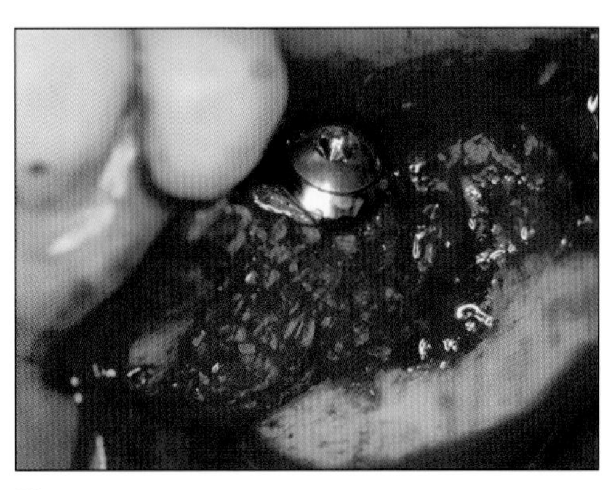

Fig 7-13e The bone defect is augmented with locally harvested autogenous bone chips. They are vertically stabilized by the horizontal bone wall of the defect.

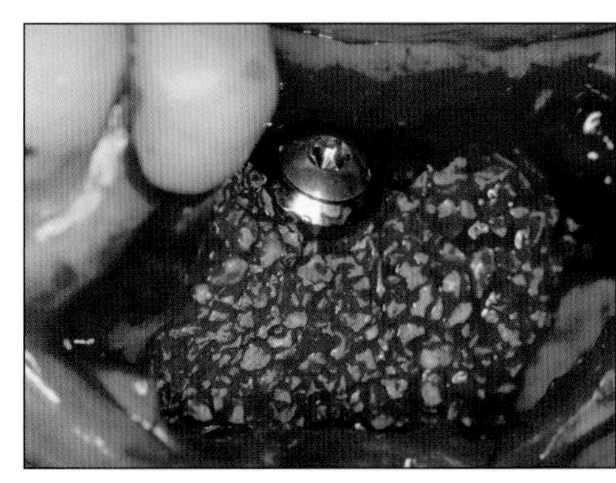

Fig 7-13f A second layer of DBBM particles is applied for contour augmentation.

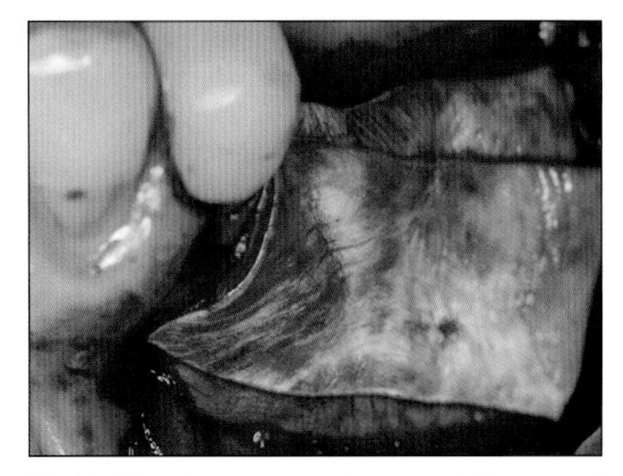

Fig 7-13g The augmentation material is covered by a collagen membrane applied in a double-layer technique.

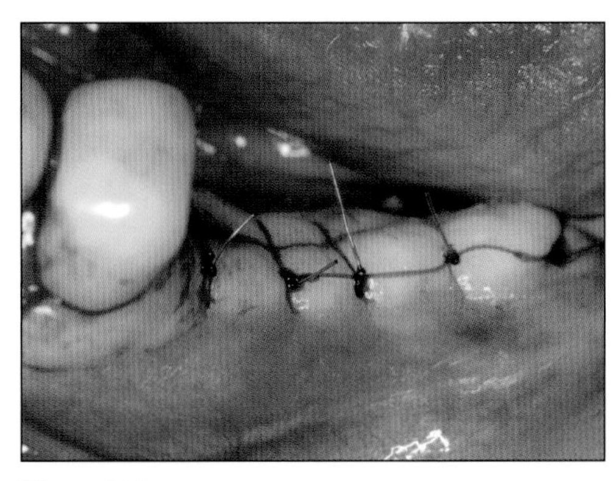

Fig 7-13h The surgery is completed with tension-free primary wound closure to protect the applied biomaterials from the bacteria in the oral cavity.

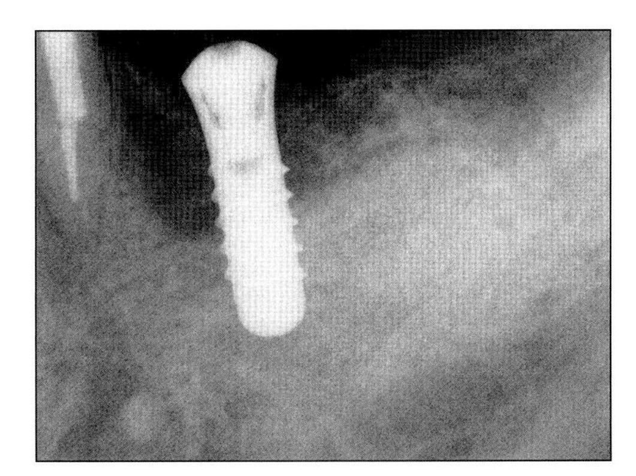

Fig 7-13i Three months following placement, a large area with a low bone density is still present mesial to the implant. It was decided to extend the healing period by 2 months.

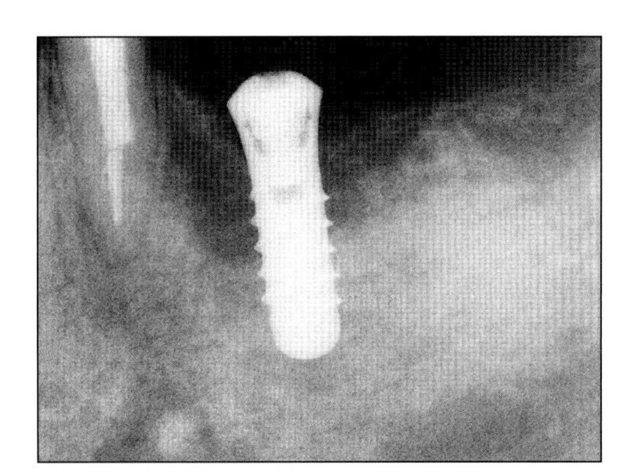

Fig 7-13j A radiograph taken at 5 months reveals the increased bone density mesial to the implant. It was decided to initiate implant function with the insertion of a provisional crown. Loading of the implant should enhance bone remodeling in the peri-implant bone structure.

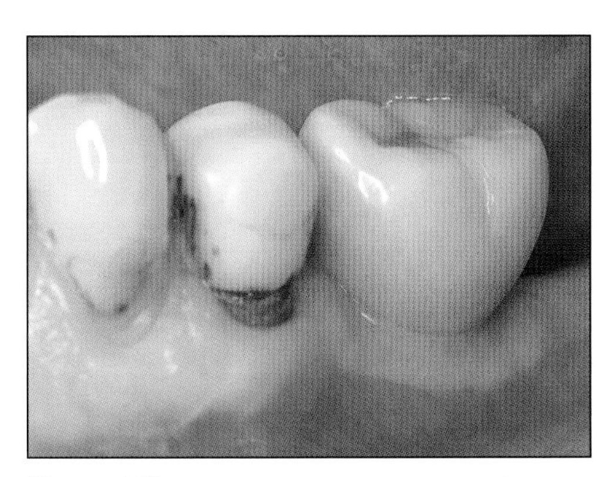

Fig 7-13k The provisional crown is shown 4 months following its placement.

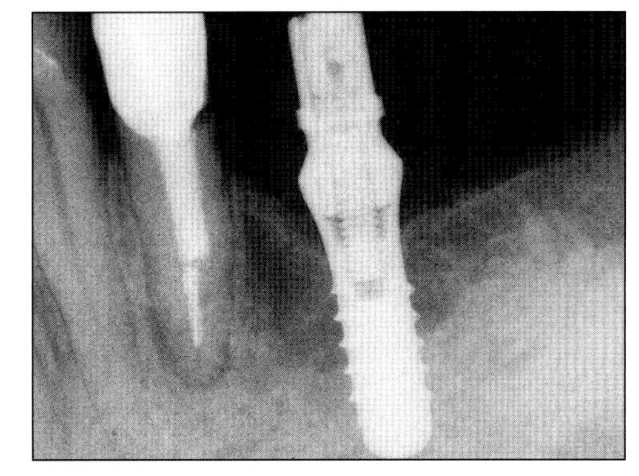

Fig 7-13l The radiograph taken after 4 months of implant loading reveals increased bone density in the defect area.

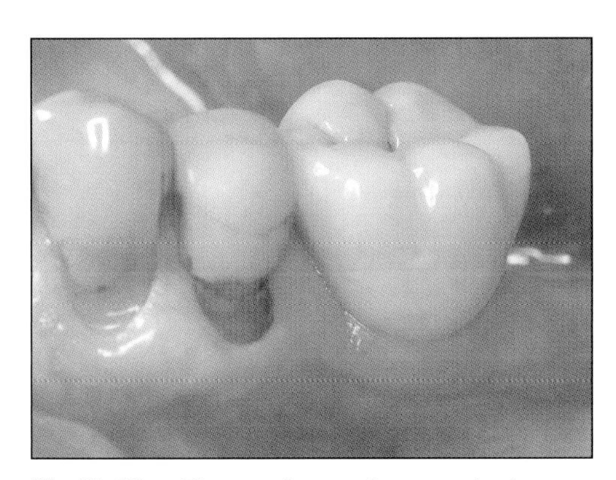

Fig 7-13m The metal-ceramic crown is shown 5 years following implant insertion. The peri-implant soft tissues are healthy and without signs of infection.

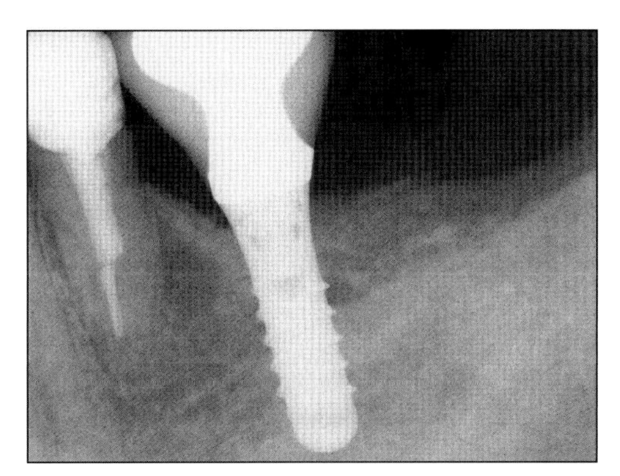

Fig 7-13n At the 5-year follow-up examination, the peri-implant bone structure and bone crest level appear completely normal following a remarkable remodeling process.

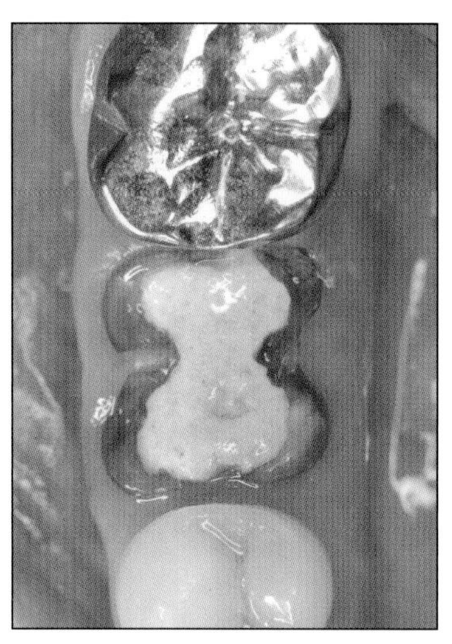

Fig 7-14a Only the roots of the mandibular right first molar are left following extensive secondary caries that undermined the crown.

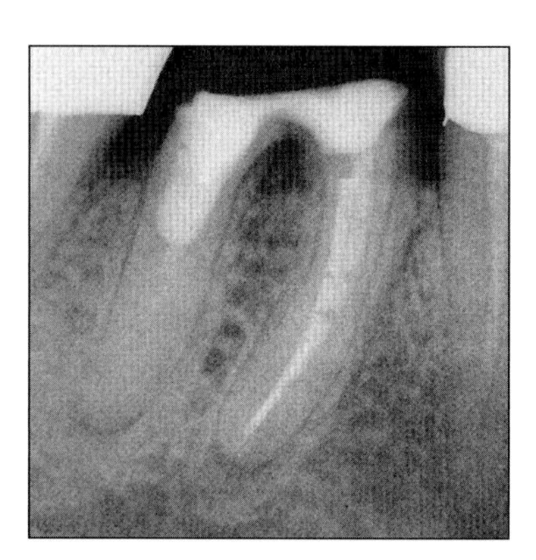

Fig 7-14b The corresponding radiograph reveals an inadequate root canal filling. The referring dentist decided to remove the root.

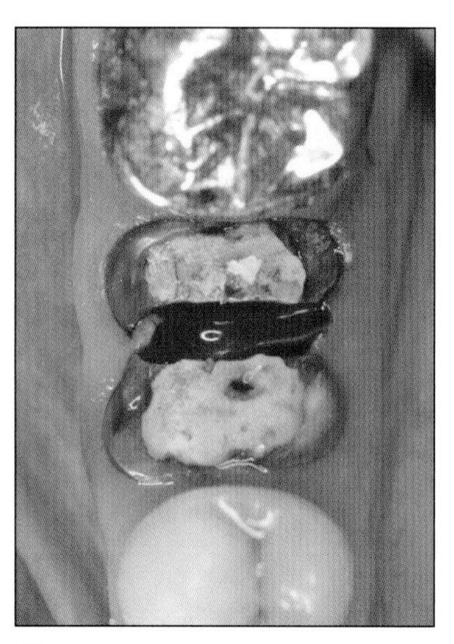

Fig 7-14c Mandibular molars are always removed after separation of the two roots to facilitate removal of each root.

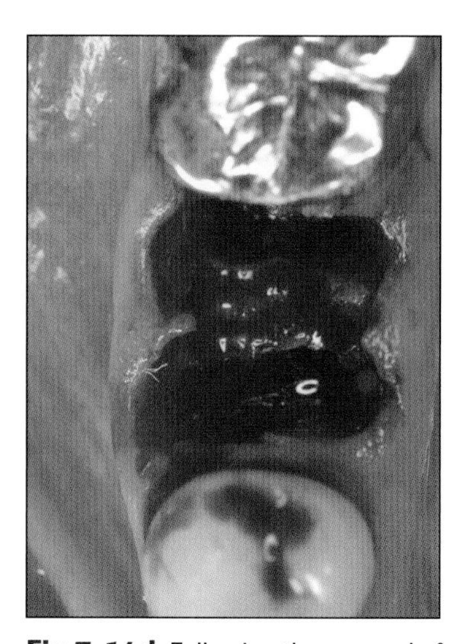

Fig 7-14d Following the removal of the two roots, it is important to carefully remove granulation tissue from the extraction socket, if present.

Case 9: Single-tooth replacement in a mandibular molar site

A 56-year-old woman presented with a mandibular right first molar that had to be removed. Mandibular molars should always be removed with the separation technique so that the mesial and distal roots are removed independently (Figs 7-14a to 7-14d).

At the time of extraction, the buccal socket wall was fully intact. Thus, it was decided to choose type 3 implant placement with 4 months of healing to allow implant placement without a bone grafting procedure. In mandibular molar sites, this is an often used and elegant clinical approach because it simplifies the implant surgery, reduces morbidity,

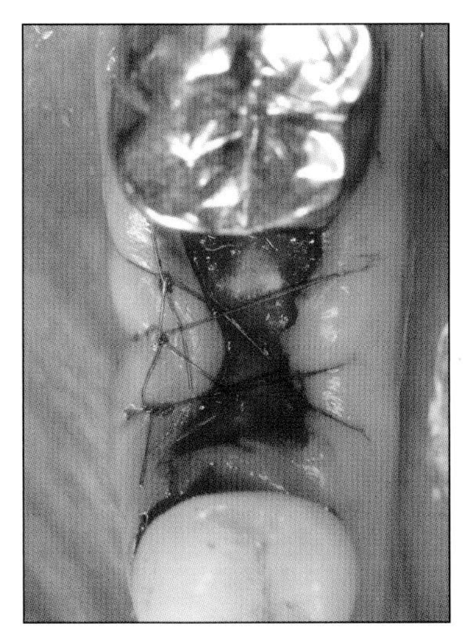

Fig 7-14e The extraction socket is filled with collagen fleece cut into pieces to stabilize the blood clot. Mattress sutures are applied.

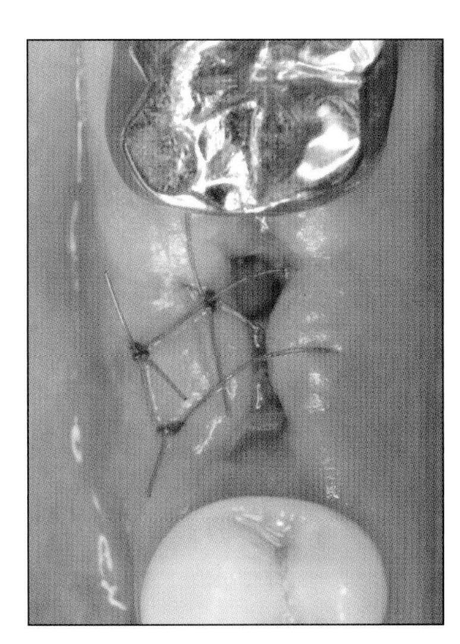

Fig 7-14f The 1-week follow-up examination demonstrates normal wound healing in the extraction site.

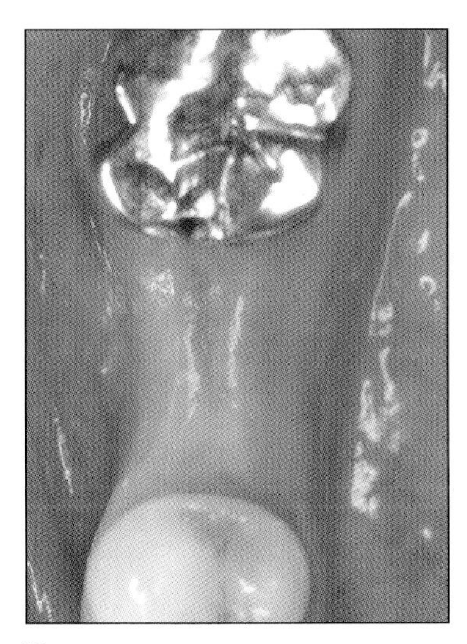

Fig 7-14g At 4 months, the site has healed without complications. The crest width is sufficient for the placement of a wide-platform implant.

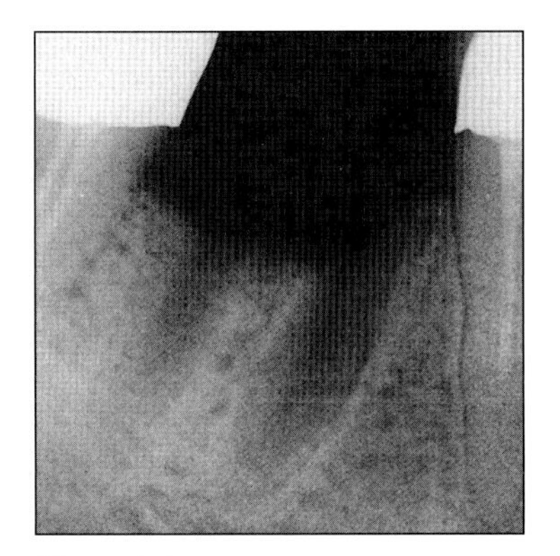

Fig 7-14h The corresponding radiograph still shows the outline of the extraction socket. Signs of partial bone healing are visible.

and decreases expenses for the patient because the GBR technique and biomaterials do not have to be used.

Implant surgery was performed 4 months following extraction in a well-healed implant site. Following preparation of the implant bed, no peri-implant defect was present, as was anticipated in the preoperative assessment (Figs 7-14e to 7-14l). Following a complication-free, nonsubmerged healing period of 6 weeks (Figs 7-14m and 7-14n), the implant was restored with a cemented metal-ceramic crown (Figs 7-14o and 7-14p).

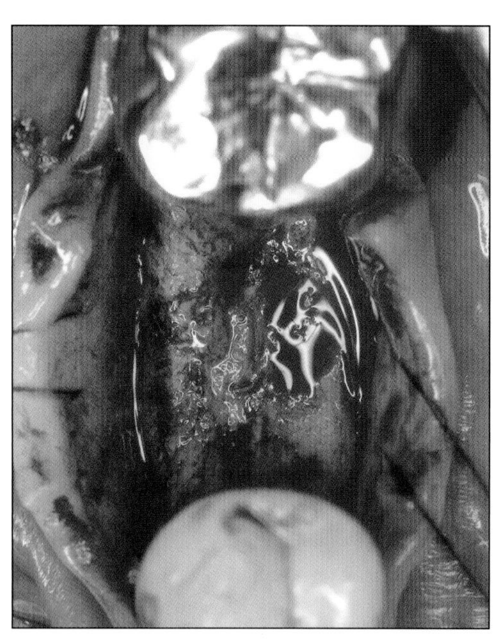

Fig 7-14i Following flap elevation without releasing incisions, the site shows well-progressed healing in the extraction site.

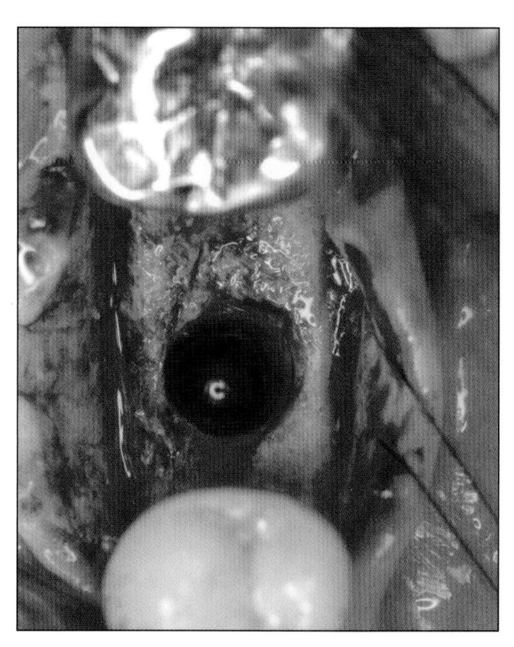

Fig 7-14j Following preparation of the implant bed, no bone defect is visible, allowing implant placement without the need for a bone grafting procedure.

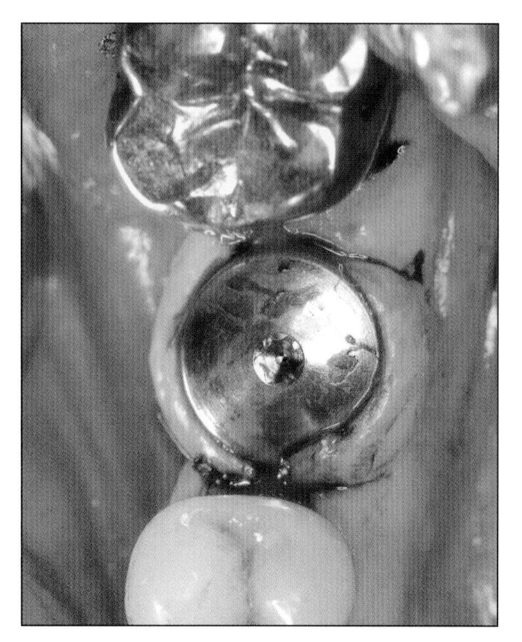

Fig 7-14k Following implant insertion and placement of a 3-mm titanium healing cap, the wound margins are adapted and secured in place with two interrupted sutures to allow nonsubmerged healing.

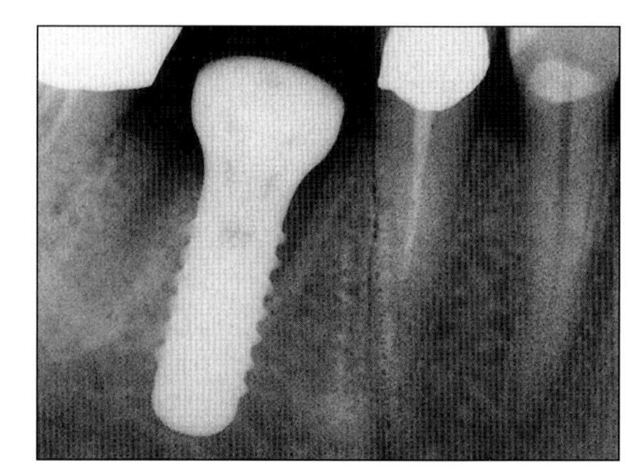

Fig 7-14l The postoperative radiograph shows the position and axis of the inserted implant in relation to the previous extraction socket.

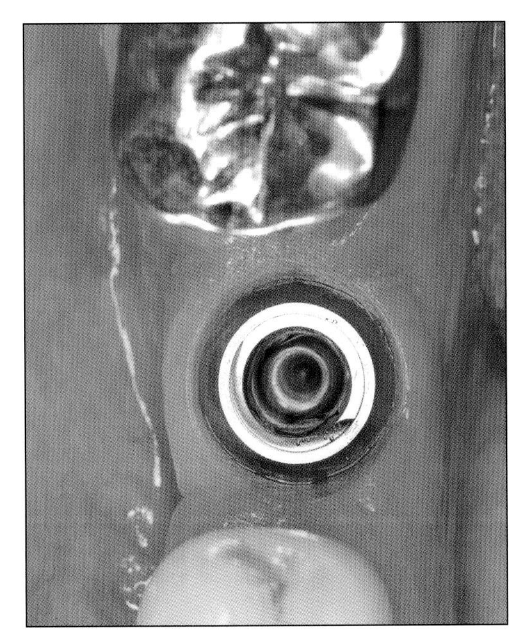

Fig 7-14m At 6 weeks postplacement, tissue integration is well advanced, allowing restoration of the implant with a metal-ceramic crown.

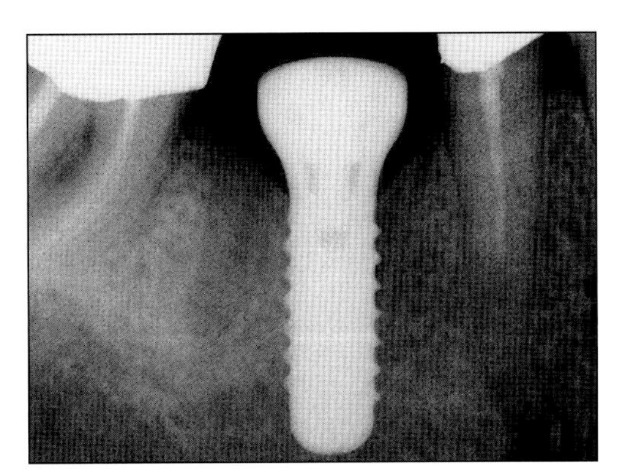

Fig 7-14n A periapical radiograph taken 6 weeks postplacement demonstrates excellent bone integration of the wide-neck implant with an SLA surface.

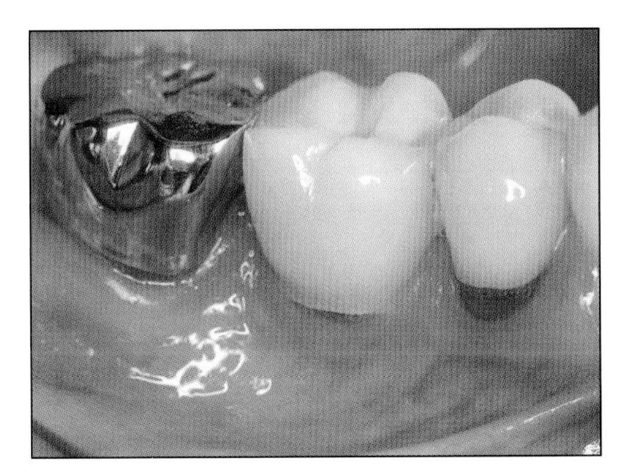

Fig 7-14o At the 4-year follow-up examination, the peri-implant soft tissues are healthy.

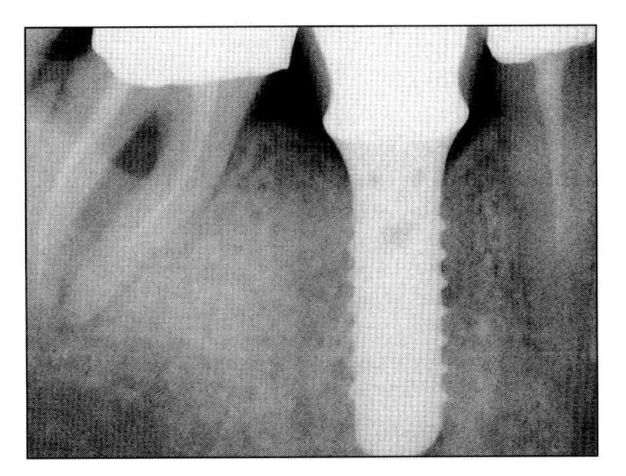

Fig 7-14p The corresponding 4-year radiograph reveals a well-integrated implant, but the interradicular bone lesion at the second molar shows some progression.

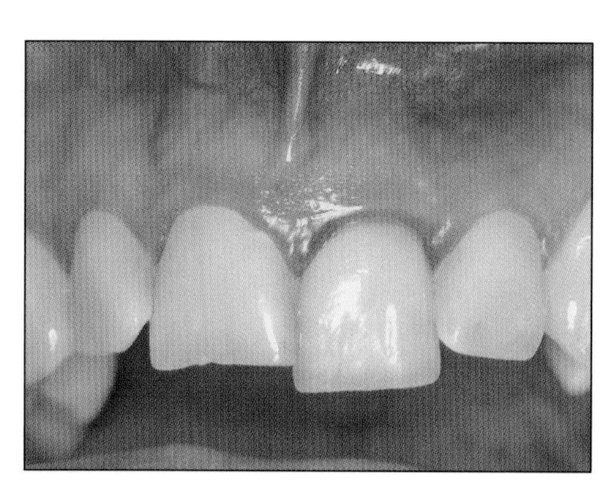

Fig 7-15a A soft swelling is present at the apical area of the elongated maxillary left central incisor.

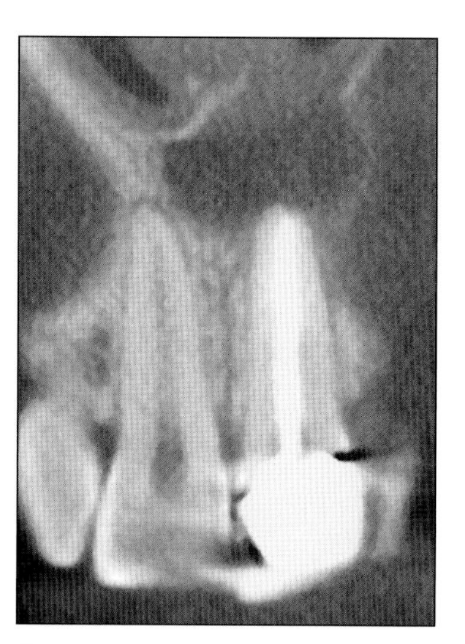

Fig 7-15b Digital volume tomography reveals the cause of the swelling and the elongation of the tooth: A large periapical bone lesion, indicating a large radicular cyst, is apparent.

Late Implant Placement Following Complete Bone Healing (Type 4)

Advantages, disadvantages, and indications

Late implant placement (type 4) with a postextraction healing period of at least 6 months is used by the authors only in exceptional clinical situations. Most frequently, it is used in adolescent patients who are too young for implant placement and when extraction of a tooth cannot be delayed. In esthetic sites, the age limit ranges between 18 and 20 years; in nonesthetic sites, younger patients may be considered. Another potential indication for late implant placement is the presence of an extensive bone lesion in the periapical area (eg, a large radicular cyst). This situation requires at least 6 months of bone healing before an implant can be inserted with sufficient primary stability (Fig 7-15). Late implant placement may also be used for patients who are not available or ready for implant therapy following extraction for personal reasons, which can include temporary financial restrictions.

The major disadvantage of waiting 6 months or longer is the potential collapse of the facial ridge anatomy, leading to a reduced crest width of less than 6 mm. This risk is significantly higher in the anterior maxilla and in premolar sites than in molar sites. In addition, such an extended healing period is not attractive to most patients.

A reduced crest width must be avoided whenever possible because it might require a staged GBR procedure with initial ridge augmentation prior to implant placement

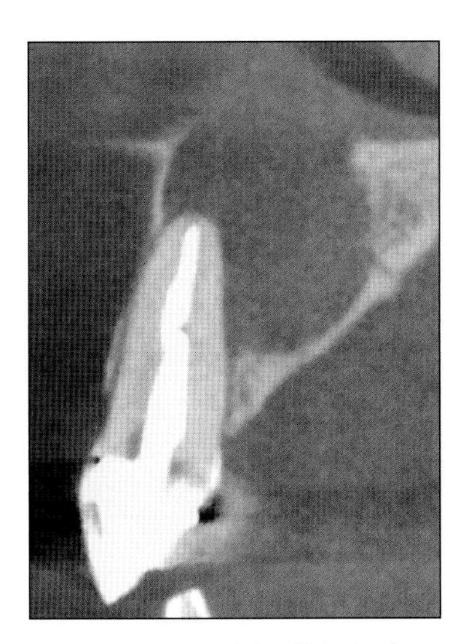

Fig 7-15c An orofacial slice of the digital volume tomogram reveals the extent of the cyst and resorption of the nasal floor. The large bone defect necessitates late implant placement (type 4) with at least 6 months of bone healing following cystectomy and a ridge preservation technique in the future implant site.

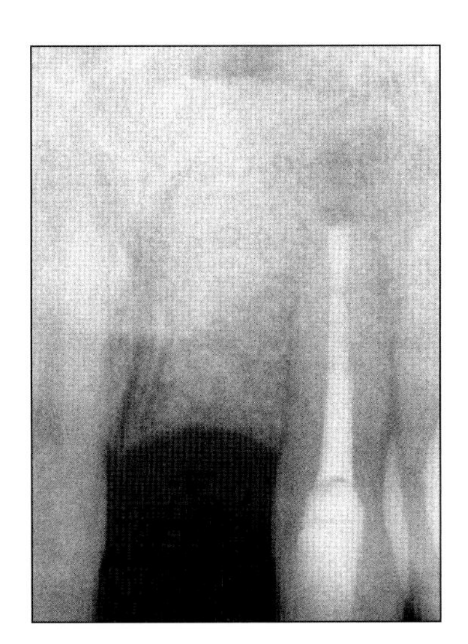

Fig 7-15d The periapical radiograph reveals the condition following cystectomy, an apicoectomy of the lateral incisor with a root-end filling, and a ridge preservation technique in the edentulous area. Implant placement will be possible when bone healing is completed, which requires at least 6 months.

(see chapter 8). Therefore, if late implant placement has to be selected, the use of a ridge preservation technique is highly recommended.[54] This ridge preservation procedure can be performed at the time of tooth extraction or a few weeks later. In the past 5 to 10 years, several techniques have been described in the literature, most of them using a bone filler with a low substitution rate.[55]

Conclusion

The four treatment options for postextraction implant placement are all used in daily practice but with different preference and frequency. Each has advantages, disadvantages, and typical clinical indications. Overall, selection of the appropriate treatment approach is driven by the primary objectives of therapy: successful regenerative outcomes with a high predictability and a low risk of complications. Early implant placement (types 2 and 3) dominates daily practice today; together, these protocols are used in about 90% of patients with postextraction implant placement.

Early implant placement with soft tissue healing (type 2) is the most frequently used treatment approach, in particular in the anterior maxilla but also in premolar sites of both jaws. This approach offers good treatment outcomes from the functional and esthetic points of view, meeting the primary objectives of high predictability and a low risk of complications. In addition, the overall treatment time from extraction to implant restoration is about 14 to 16 weeks in most cases, which is quite attractive to patients.

If primary implant stability cannot be expected with type 2 placement because of bone defects in the periapical area, type 3 placement with 12 to 16 weeks of healing postextraction is used. This approach is also preferred in molar sites because it allows a less demanding implant surgery without bone augmentation in most patients and is more cost effective. This approach will extend the treatment time but not significantly.

Immediate and late implant placements are much less frequently used and then are used only in specific clinical situations. In esthetic sites, to avoid the risk of mucosal recession, immediate implants are only recommended in low-risk patients presenting with ideal clinical conditions. Clinicians without routine experience in postextraction implant placement should avoid using this approach at all. With carefully selected clinical conditions, flapless immediate implant placement can be considered.

Late implant placement is used even more rarely, because this is the least attractive of the different time points for treatment after extraction. This approach always involves an extended treatment time from extraction to implant restoration. To avoid severe collapse of the crest width, a ridge preservation technique that incorporates a low-substitution bone filler is highly recommended in such situations. This requires an additional surgical procedure separate from implant placement. Because of these disadvantages, this approach is only used when absolutely necessary, for example, in adolescent patients.

References

1. Schulte W, Kleineikenscheidt H, Linder K, Schareyka R. The Tübingen immediate implant in clinical studies. Dtsch Zahnärztl Z 1978;33:348–359.
2. d'Hoedt B. 10 Jahre Tübinger Implantat aus Frialit—Eine Zwischenauswertung der Implantatdatei. Z Zahnärztl Implantol 1986;2:6–10.
3. Lazzara RJ. Immediate implant placement into extraction sites: Surgical and restorative advantages. Int J Periodontics Restorative Dent 1989;9:332–343.
4. Nyman S, Lang NP, Buser D, Bragger U. Bone regeneration adjacent to titanium dental implants using guided tissue regeneration: A report of two cases. Int J Oral Maxillofac Implants 1990;5:9–14.
5. Mayfield LJA. Immediate, delayed and late submerged and transmucosal implants. In: Lang NP, Karring T, Lindhe J (eds). Proceedings of the 3rd European Workshop on Periodontology: Implant Dentistry. Berlin: Quintessence, 1999:520–534.
6. Gelb DA. Immediate implant surgery: Three-year retrospective evaluation of 50 consecutive cases. Int J Oral Maxillofac Implants 1993;8:388–399.
7. Rosenquist B, Grenthe B. Immediate placement of implants into extraction sockets: Implant survival. Int J Oral Maxillofac Implants 1996;11:205–209.
8. Schwartz-Arad D, Chaushu G. Placement of implants into fresh extraction sites: 4 to 7 years retrospective evaluation of 95 immediate implants. J Periodontol 1997;68:1110–1116.
9. Becker W, Dahlin C, Lekholm U, et al. Five-year evaluation of implants placed at extraction and with dehiscences and fenestration defects augmented with ePTFE membranes: Results from a prospective multicenter study. Clin Implant Dent Relat Res 1999;1:27–32.
10. Hammerle CH, Chen ST, Wilson TG Jr. Consensus statements and recommended clinical procedures regarding the placement of implants in extraction sockets. Int J Oral Maxillofac Implants 2004;19 (suppl):26–28.
11. Chen ST, Wilson TG Jr, Hammerle CH. Immediate or early placement of implants following tooth extraction: Review of biologic basis, clinical procedures, and outcomes. Int J Oral Maxillofac Implants 2004;19(suppl):12–25.
12. Chen ST, Buser D. Implants in post-extraction sites: A literature update. In: Buser D, Belser U, Wismeijer D (eds). ITI Treatment Guide, vol 3. Implants in Extraction Sockets. Berlin: Quintessence, 2008: 9–16.
13. Chen ST, Buser D. Clinical and esthetic outcomes of implants placed in postextraction sites. Int J Oral Maxillofac Implants 2009;24(suppl) (in press).
14. Schropp L, Wenzel A, Kostopolous L, Karring T. Bone healing and soft tissue contour changes following single-tooth extraction: A clinical and radiographic 12-month prospective study. Int J Periodontics Restorative Dent 2003;23:313–323.

15. Berglundh T, Lindhe J. Dimension of the periimplant mucosa. Biological width revisited. J Clin Periodontol 1996;23:971–973.
16. Cochran DL, Hermann JS, Schenk RK, Higginbottom FL, Buser D. Biologic width around titanium implants. A histometric analysis of the implanto-gingival junction around unloaded and loaded nonsubmerged implants in the canine mandible. J Periodontol 1997;68:186–198.
17. Kan JY, Rungcharassaeng K, Umezu K, Kois JC. Dimensions of peri-implant mucosa: An evaluation of maxillary anterior single implants in humans. J Periodontol 2003;74:557–562.
18. Botticelli D, Berglundh T, Lindhe J. Hard-tissue alterations following immediate implant placement in extraction sites. J Clin Periodontol 2004;31: 820–828.
19. Araujo MG, Sukekava F, Wennstrom JL, Lindhe J. Ridge alterations following implant placement in fresh extraction sockets: An experimental study in the dog. J Clin Periodontol 2005;32:645–652.
20. Araujo MG, Sukekava F, Wennstrom JL, Lindhe J. Tissue modeling following implant placement in fresh extraction sockets. Clin Oral Implants Res 2006;17:615–624.
21. Araujo MG, Wennstrom JL, Lindhe J. Modeling of the buccal and lingual bone walls of fresh extraction sites following implant installation. Clin Oral Implants Res 2006;17:606–614.
22. Chen ST, Darby IB, Adams GG, Reynolds EC. A prospective clinical study of bone augmentation techniques at immediate implants. Clin Oral Implants Res 2005;16:176–184.
23. Lindeboom JA, Tjiook Y, Kroon FH. Immediate placement of implants in periapical infected sites: A prospective randomized study in 50 patients. Oral Surg Oral Med Oral Pathol Oral Radiol Endod 2006;101:705–710.
24. Chen ST, Darby IB, Reynolds EC. A prospective clinical study of non-submerged immediate implants: Clinical outcomes and esthetic results. Clin Oral Implants Res 2007;18:552–562.
25. Evans CJD, Chen ST. Esthetic outcomes of immediate implant placements. Clin Oral Implants Res 2008;19:73–80.
26. Cordaro L, Torsello F, Roccuzzo M. Clinical outcome of submerged versus non-submerged implants placed in fresh extraction sockets. Clin Oral Implants Res 2009 (in press).
27. Chen ST, Darby I, Reynolds EC, Clement JG. Immediate implant placement post-extraction without flap elevation: A case series. J Periodontol 2009;80:163–172.
28. Kan JYK, Rungcharassaeng K, Sclar A, Lozada JL. Effects of the facial osseous defect morphology on gingival dynamics after immediate tooth replacement and guided bone regeneration: 1-year results. J Oral Maxillofac Surg 2007;65:13–19.
29. Dawson T, Chen ST. The SAC Classification in Implant Dentistry. Berlin: Quintessence, 2009.
30. Martin WC, Morton D, Buser D. Diagnostic factors for esthetic risk assessment. In: Buser D, Belser U, Wismeijer D (eds). ITI Treatment Guide, vol 1. Implant Therapy in the Esthetic Zone for Single-Tooth Replacements. Berlin: Quintessence, 2006: 11–20.
31. Langer B. Spontaneous in situ gingival augmentation. Int J Periodontics Restorative Dent 1994;14: 524–535.
32. Wood DL, Hoag PM, Donnenfeld OW, Rosenfeld LD. Alveolar crest reduction following full and partial thickness flaps. J Periodontol 1972;43:141–144.
33. Fickl S, Zuhr O, Wachtel H, Bolz W, Huerzeler M. Tissue alterations after tooth extraction with and without surgical trauma: A volumetric study in the beagle dog. J Clin Periodontol 2008;35:356–363.
34. Buser D, Chen ST, Weber HP, Belser UC. Early implant placement following single-tooth extraction in the esthetic zone: Biologic rationale and surgical procedures. Int J Periodontics Restorative Dent 2008;28:441–451.
35. Buser D, Bornstein MM, Weber HP, Grutter L, Schmid B, Belser UC. Early implant placement with simultaneous guided bone regeneration following single-tooth extraction in the esthetic zone: A cross-sectional, retrospective study in 45 subjects with a 2- to 4-year follow-up. J Periodontol 2008;79:1773–1781.
36. Buser D, Hart C, Bornstein M, Grütter L, Chappuis V, Belser UC. Early implant placement with simultaneous GBR following single-tooth extraction in the esthetic zone: 12-month results of a prospective study with 20 consecutive patients. J Periodontol 2009;80:152–162.
37. Jovanovic SA, Spiekermann H, Richter EJ. Bone regeneration around titanium dental implants in dehisced defect sites: A clinical study. Int J Oral Maxillofac Implants 1992;7:233–245.
38. Buser D, Hoffmann B, Bernard JP, Lussi A, Mettler D, Schenk RK. Evaluation of filling materials in membrane-protected bone defects. A comparative histomorphometric study in the mandible of miniature pigs. Clin Oral Implants Res 1998;9: 137–150.
39. Jensen SS, Broggini N, Hjørting-Hansen E, Schenk R, Buser D. Bone healing and graft resorption of autograft, anorganic bovine bone and beta-tricalcium phosphate. A histologic and histomorphometric study in the mandibles of minipigs. Clin Oral Implants Res 2006;17:237–243.
40. Jensen SS, Yeo A, Dard M, Hunziker E, Schenk R, Buser D. Evaluation of a novel biphasic calcium phosphate in standardized bone defects. A histologic and histomorphometric study in the mandibles of minipigs. Clin Oral Implants Res 2007;18:752–760.
41. Jensen SS, Bornstein MM, Dard M, Bosshardt DD, Buser D. Comparative study of biphasic calcium phosphates with different HA/TCP ratios in mandibular bone defects. A long-term histo-morphometric study in minipigs. J Biomed Mater Res B Appl Biomater 2009;90B:171–181.

42. Buser D, Broggini N, Wieland M, et al. Enhanced bone apposition to a chemically modified SLA titanium surface. J Dent Res 2004;83:529–533.
43. Ferguson SJ, Broggini N, Wieland M, et al. Biomechanical evaluation of the interfacial strength of a chemically modified sandblasted and acid-etched titanium surface. J Biomed Mater Res A 2006;78:291–297.
44. Schwarz F, Wieland M, Schwartz Z, et al. Potential of chemically modified hydrophilic surface characteristics to support tissue integration of titanium dental implants. J Biomed Mater Res B Appl Biomater 2009;88:544–557.
45. Bornstein MM, Valderrama P, Jones AA, Wilson TG, Seibl R, Cochran DL. Bone apposition around two different sandblasted and acid-etched titanium implant surfaces: A histomorphometric study in canine mandibles. Clin Oral Implants Res 2008; 19:233–241.
46. Bornstein MM, Hart CN, Halbritter SA, Morton D, Buser D. Early loading of nonsubmerged titanium implants with a chemically modified sand-blasted and acid-etched surface: 6-month results of a prospective case series study in the posterior mandible focusing on peri-implant crestal bone changes and implant stability quotient (ISQ) values. Clin Implant Dent Relat Res 2009 Apr 23 [Epub ahead of print].
47. Morton D, Bornstein MM, Wittneben J, Martin WC, Ruskin JD, Buser D. Early loading after 21-days of healing of non-submerged titanium implants with a chemically modified sandblasted and acid-etched surface: 2-year results of a prospective 2-center study. Clin Implant Dent Relat Res (in press).
48. Schwarz F, Herten M, Sager M, Wieland M, Dard M, Becker J. Bone regeneration in dehiscence-type defects at chemically modified (SLActive) and conventional SLA titanium implants: A pilot study in dogs. J Clin Periodontol 2007;34:78–86.
49. Schwarz F, Sager M, Ferrari D, Herten M, Wieland M, Becker J. Bone regeneration in dehiscence-type defects at non-submerged and submerged chemically modified (SLActive) and conventional SLA titanium implants: An immunohistochemical study in dogs. J Clin Periodontol 2008;35:64–75.
50. Cochran DL, Buser D, ten Bruggenkate CM, et al. The use of reduced healing times on ITI implants with a sandblasted and acid-etched (SLA) surface: Early results from clinical trials on ITI SLA implants. Clin Oral Implants Res 2002;13:144–153.
51. Bornstein MM, Lussi A, Schmid B, Belser UC, Buser D. Early loading of nonsubmerged titanium implants with a sandblasted and acid-etched (SLA) surface: 3-year results of a prospective study in partially edentulous patients. Int J Oral Maxillofac Implants 2003;18:659–666.
52. Bornstein MM, Schmid B, Belser UC, Lussi A, Buser D. Early loading of non-submerged titanium implants with a sandblasted and acid-etched surface. 5-year results of a prospective study in partially edentulous patients. Clin Oral Implants Res 2005;16:631–638.
53. Cochran D, Oates T, Morton D, Jones A, Buser D, Peters F. Clinical field trial examining an implant with a sand-blasted, acid-etched surface. J Periodontol 2007;78:974–982.
54. Chen ST, Buser D. Clinical and esthetic outcomes of implants placed in post-extraction sites. Int J Oral Maxillofac Implants 2009;24(suppl) (in press).
55. Darby IB, Chen ST, Buser D. Ridge preservation techniques for implant therapy. Int J Oral Maxillofac Implants 2009;24(suppl) (in press).

CHAPTER 8

Guided Bone Regeneration and Autogenous Block Grafts for Horizontal Ridge Augmentation: A Staged Approach

Thomas von Arx
Daniel Buser

The correct three-dimensional placement of dental implants requires a certain bone volume that is often less than ideal following bone loss because of ridge alterations following extraction, infection, trauma, or malformation. If the bone deficiency precludes primary implant stability or results in an inadequate implant positioning with possible compromised function or esthetics, horizontal ridge augmentation prior to implant placement should be considered. A variety of surgical techniques and materials have been described to establish a sufficient bony structure for supporting dental implants, including particulate graft augmentation with guided bone regeneration (GBR), block graft augmentation (with or without GBR), ridge splitting, or distraction osteogenesis. A recent systematic review[1] has assessed which hard tissue augmentation techniques are the most successful in furnishing bony support for implant placement. With regard to increase of alveolar ridge width, the greatest implant survival rate (95.5%) was found for the GBR technique.

The present chapter focuses on horizontal ridge augmentation using autogenous block grafts in conjunction with barrier membranes. The use of veneer or onlay grafting to improve alveolar bone width prior to implant placement has a long tradition in implant dentistry.[2] Brånemark and coworkers[3] introduced the use of an autogenous bone graft for bone reconstruction of defective mandibles, and in 1980 Breine and Brånemark[4] published the first information about endosseous implants placed in grafted bone as a part of the reconstructive procedure. However, these augmentation procedures used bone grafts harvested extraorally, mainly from the iliac crest. In the early 1990s, the first reports on block grafts from intraoral donor sites for localized alveolar ridge augmentation were published.[5,6]

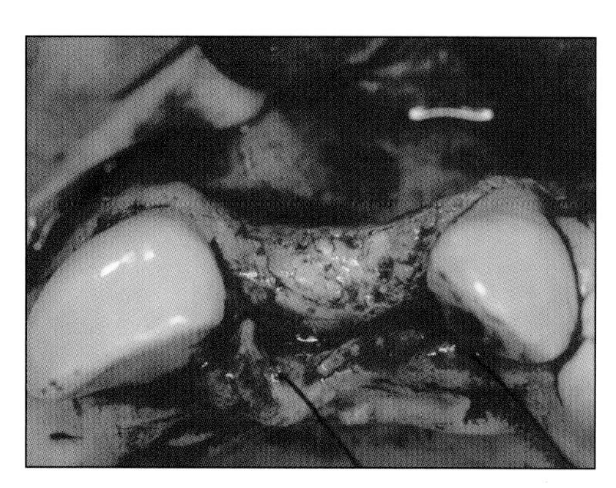

Fig 8-1a A single-tooth gap with a narrow crest of less than 4 mm requires ridge augmentation to allow implant placement.

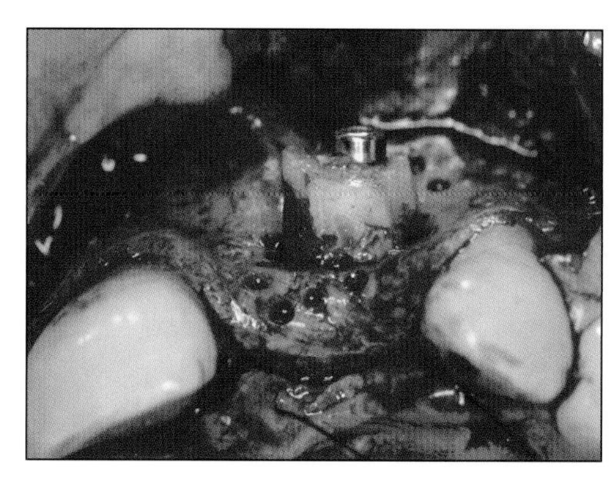

Fig 8-1b An autogenous block graft is placed and stabilized with a fixation screw.

Following the introduction of GBR in 1988,[7] barrier membranes and/or bone replacement materials (bone fillers) were gradually and increasingly applied in combination with block graft augmentation techniques. In the first 10 years of GBR application, bioinert, nonresorbable expanded polytetrafluoroethylene (ePTFE) membranes were predominantly used for horizontal ridge augmentation in combination with bone grafts.[8–10] This surgical technique offered successful outcomes with high predictability (Fig 8-1). However, this surgical technique was clinically demanding and showed an increased risk for complications in case of a soft tissue dehiscence.[11]

Thus, in the late 1990s, efforts were made to simplify the surgical procedure and to reduce the risk of complications. It was decided to replace the bioinert, nonresorbable ePTFE membrane with a resorbable collagen membrane made of pork skin (Bio-Gide, Geistlich). This membrane showed favorable results in various preclinical and clinical studies, mainly for simultaneous GBR applications to regenerate peri-implant bone defects.[12,13] This membrane is hydrophilic and easy to handle during surgery and has a much lower risk of complication in case of a soft tissue dehiscence. A prospective case series study of the use of Bio-Gide for horizontal ridge augmentation in 42 patients showed excellent outcomes with high predictability.[14]

Recently, the use of bone substitute block material instead of autogenous block grafts for horizontal ridge augmentation has been advocated to avoid block graft harvesting.[15–18] These techniques, however, are not routine yet in daily practice and need to be evaluated further.

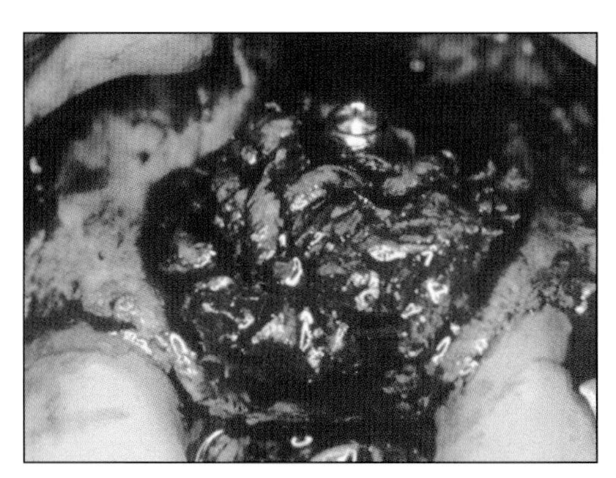

Fig 8-1c The surrounding voids are filled with autogenous bone chips to round off the augmentation site.

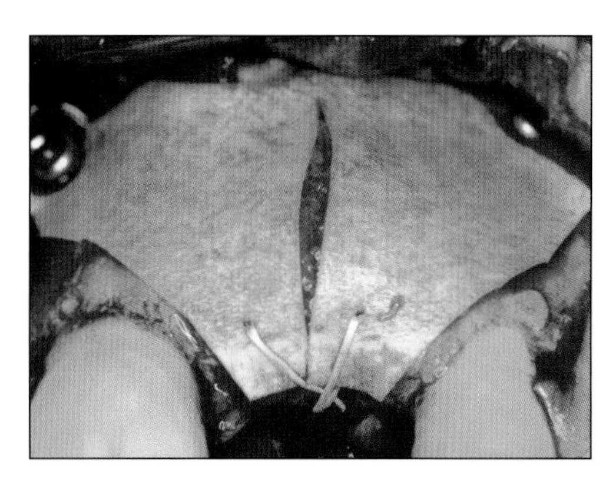

Fig 8-1d A bioinert ePTFE membrane is placed to serve as barrier. The membrane is stabilized with a mattress suture toward the palate and with two miniscrews on the facial aspect.

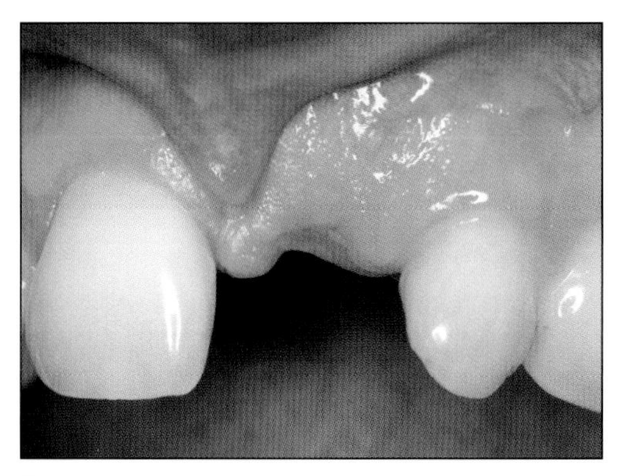

Fig 8-1e Following primary wound closure, uneventful soft tissue healing has taken place over the 6-month healing period.

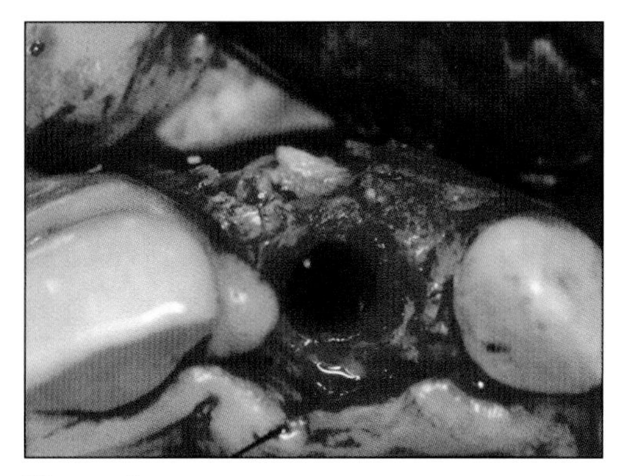

Fig 8-1f At the second surgical procedure, the crest width measures more than 7 mm, allowing implant placement in a correct three-dimensional position.

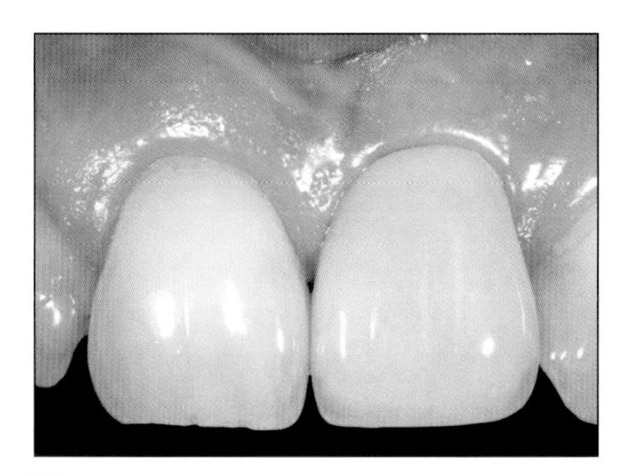

Fig 8-1g The 10-year follow-up examination reveals a pleasing esthetic outcome with stable peri-implant soft tissues.

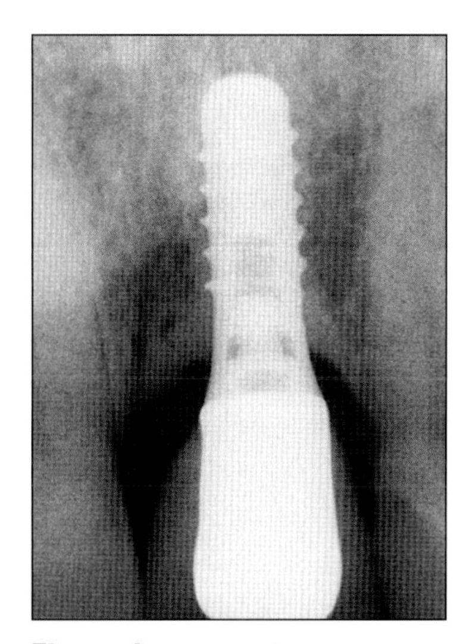

Fig 8-1h The 10-year follow-up radiograph reveals stable bone crest levels.

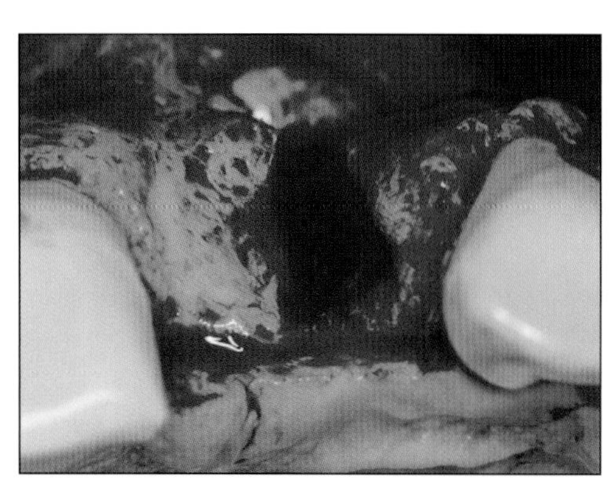

Fig 8-2a Eight weeks following tooth extraction, the ridge shows a craterlike, two-wall defect and a crest width of more than 6 mm. This allows implant placement with simultaneous GBR.

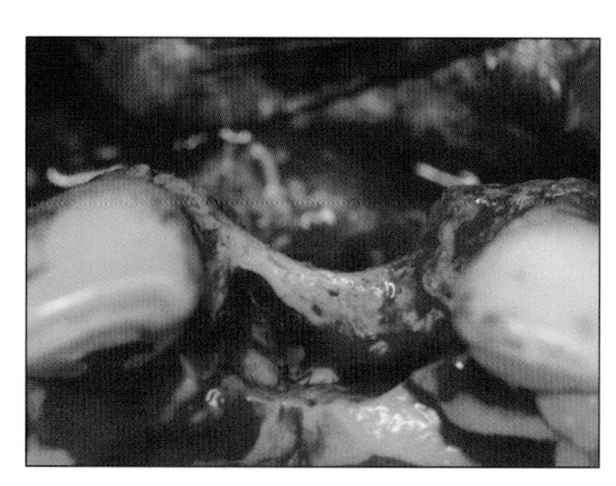

Fig 8-2b An extended, one-wall bone defect with facial flattening and a crest width of less than 4 mm requires an initial ridge augmentation procedure followed by implant placement using a staged approach.

Rationale for Horizontal Block Graft Augmentation

Insertion of an endosseous implant requires sufficient bone volume to achieve correct three-dimensional implant positioning. Crestal bone dehiscences or facial undercuts may be managed with implant placement and simultaneous peri-implant bone augmentation, provided that the implant can be inserted with sufficient primary stability in a restorable position and that the peri-implant bone defect has a morphology with at least two bone walls (Fig 8-2a). In many instances, however, alveolar resorption following extraction, trauma, or pathologic conditions results in a ridge form that precludes implant insertion without prior augmentation. In these clinical situations, the crest width often measures less than 4 mm, which would lead to an exposed implant surface outside the alveolar ridge if an implant were inserted. This anatomical situation results in a one-wall defect morphology, which is much more demanding to treat successfully than a two-wall defect (Fig 8-2b). In addition, high esthetic demands by the patient, with or without a high smile line, may be further indications for a staged approach using block grafts to enhance a deficient alveolar ridge before staged implant placement.

In the posterior mandible, tooth loss resulting from periodontal or endodontic infections may result in compromise of the buccal plate and a reduction in alveolar width. This bone resorption continues in a medial direction until a knife-edged ridge forms. Implants cannot be anchored in the basal bone because of the mandibular canal; therefore, block graft augmentation is a viable treatment option prior to staged implant placement.

Autogenous block graft augmentation is able to increase bone volume and improve bone quality prior to implant placement, ensuring better primary implant stability and improved three-dimensional implant positioning.[19] Finally, greater bone density is obtained when symphyseal bone or ramus buccal shelf bone is used, and crestal bone with increased density can withstand implant loading in a more favorable biomechanical manner.[20]

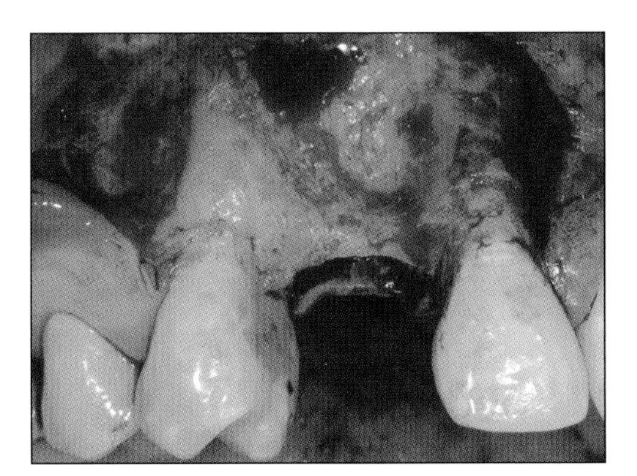

Fig 8-3a A mucoperiosteal flap is raised to access the surgical site (maxillary right canine).

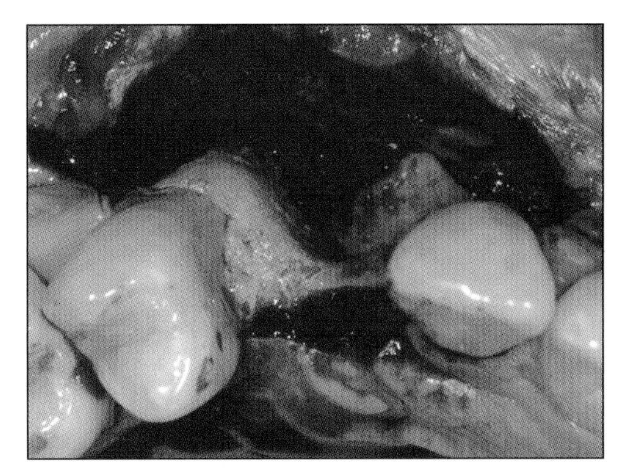

Fig 8-3b The occlusal view clearly shows a knife-edged thin alveolar ridge with a large horizontal defect on the facial aspect of the alveolar process.

Considerations in Horizontal Augmentation Procedures

Surgical technique

Localized horizontal ridge augmentation by means of intraorally harvested block grafts can normally be performed under local anesthesia on an outpatient basis; however, because of the length of surgery with two surgical sites (donor and recipient sites), sedation is highly recommended. Patients should also be premedicated with antibiotics to reduce the risk of a postsurgical infection, as described in the next section.

The recipient site is prepared with a midcrestal incision (in anterior maxillary sites, the incision is shifted slightly palatally on the crest) that is continued into the facial and lingual sulci at the adjacent teeth and includes vestibular divergent releasing incisions. Mucoperiosteal flaps are raised on the facial and lingual aspects and retracted with sutures (Figs 8-3a and 8-3b). Important anatomical landmarks should be located at this time to avoid damage to neurovascular structures such as the mental foramen or the incisive foramen. The bony crest is curetted to remove all soft tissues. The geometry of the recipient site is carefully examined, and the size of the block graft required for bone augmentation is determined using a periodontal probe.

Subsequently, the facial cortex is perforated with a small round bur to open the bone marrow cavity to optimize vascular supply of the recipient bed. Caution must be exercised to avoid touching adjacent roots or perforating knife-edged thin ridges when these bony holes are drilled. To prevent desiccation of the recipient bed, wet gauze can be placed, or the flap can be temporarily repositioned. The harvesting procedure for autogenous block grafts (Fig 8-3c) is described in chapter 5.

To allow intimate contact of the block graft with the recipient bed, the bone block might be slightly adapted to the defect site morphology, or the recipient bed might be modified with bone drills. Subsequently, the block graft is stabilized with one or two fixation screws

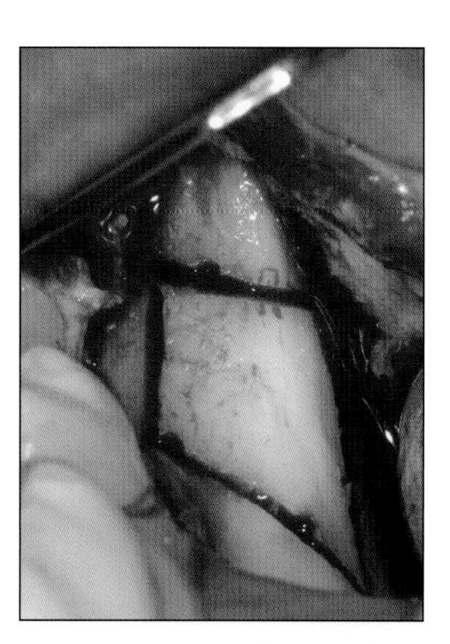

Fig 8-3c An autogenous block graft is outlined in the left ramus area by means of piezoelectric surgery.

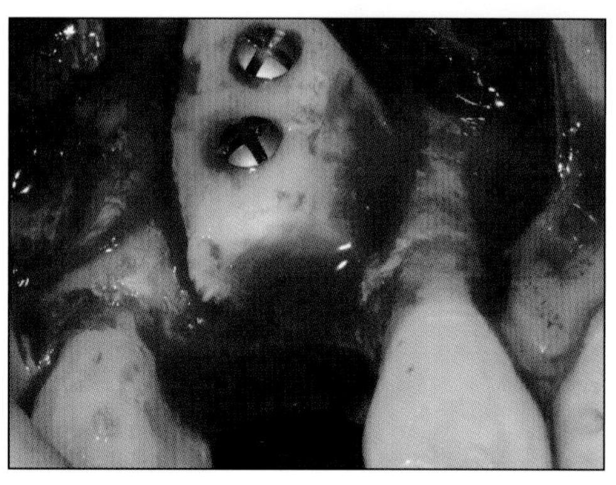

Fig 8-3d The corticocancellous block graft is secured with two fixation screws that anchor in the palatal bone wall.

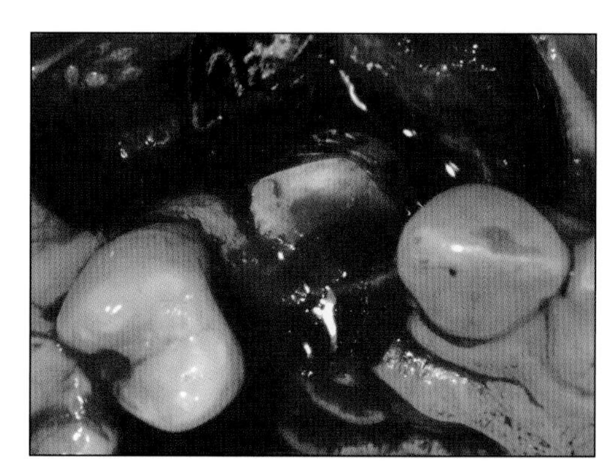

Fig 8-3e The facial contour has been reestablished by means of the block graft.

that engage the residual lingual or palatal bone wall (Figs 8-3d and 8-3e). Sharp edges of the block graft may be rounded with a large diamond bur to prevent mucosal irritation.

Voids around the block graft can be filled with cancellous bone grafts or bone chips harvested from the donor site or from adjacent cortical bone surfaces (or from the anterior nasal spine in the anterior maxilla). A deproteinized bovine bone mineral (DBBM) particulate graft (Bio-Oss, Geistlich) is mixed with blood obtained from the surgical site. This mixture is applied to entirely cover the block graft to prevent surface resorption and to contour the augmented site (Figs 8-3f and 8-3g). A collagen membrane (Bio-Gide) is placed to prevent displacement of the DBBM particles (Fig 8-3h). The membrane is adapted in a double-layer fashion to improve its stability.

A periosteal releasing incision is made to allow flap mobilization and tension-free primary wound closure. Wound adaptation is accomplished with single interrupted sutures, but horizontal mattress sutures are recommended in the crestal area to prevent wound dehiscence (Fig 8-3i).

Patients are recalled after 3 days, and sutures are removed 10 to 14 days postoperatively. Removable and provisional prostheses must be carefully adapted and may not be worn during the first 3 days when wound swelling is most prominent. Measures

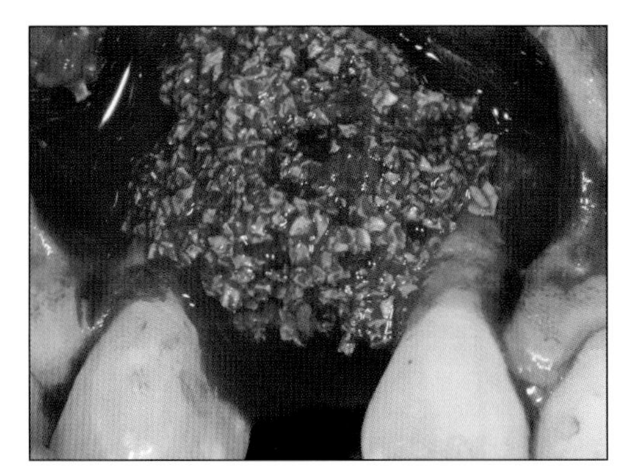

Fig 8-3f The block graft is fully covered with DBBM particles.

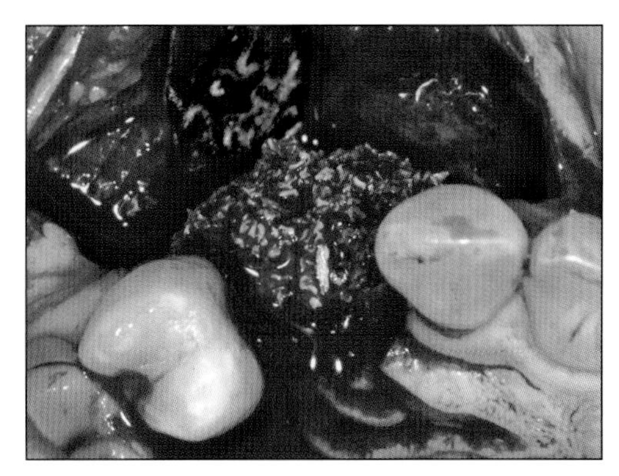

Fig 8-3g Voids between the block graft and adjacent bony structures are filled with DBBM particles.

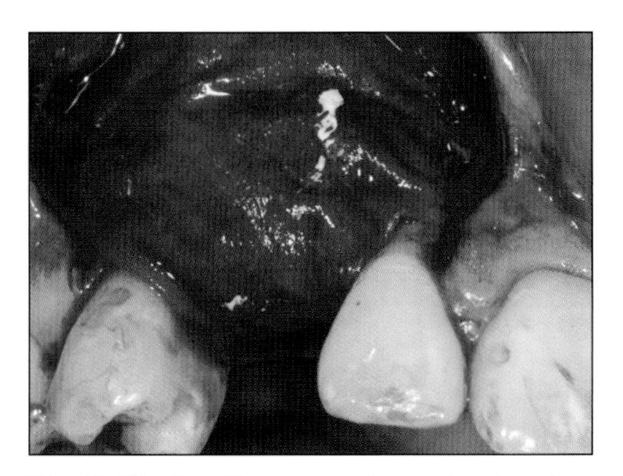

Fig 8-3h A collagen membrane is placed to completely cover the augmented site.

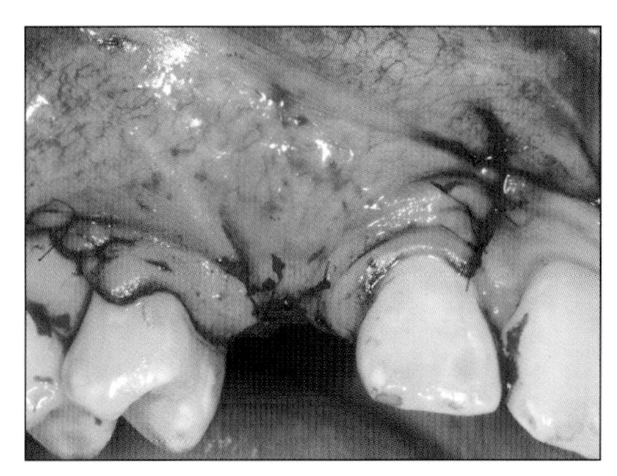

Fig 8-3i After a periosteal releasing incision is made, the flap is coronally advanced to assure primary and tension-free wound closure.

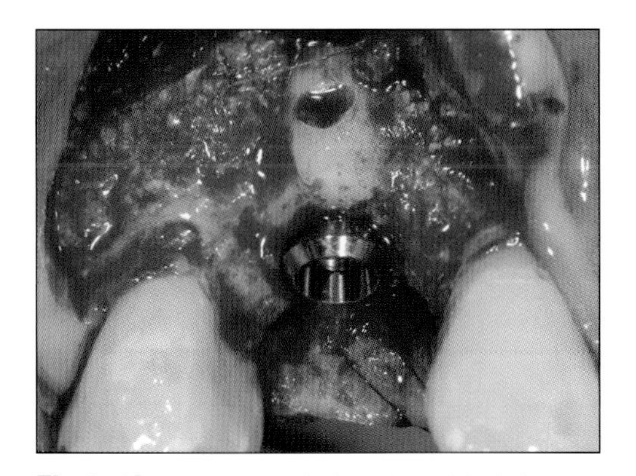

Fig 8-3j After removal of the bone block fixation screws, the implant is placed.

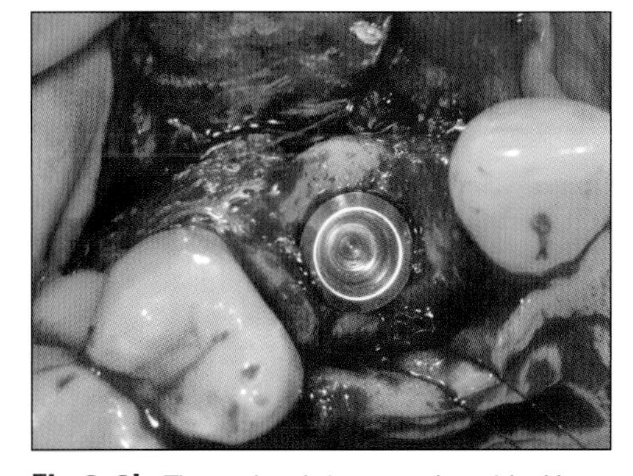

Fig 8-3k The occlusal view reveals an ideal bony contour at the facial aspect of the implant shoulder.

to reduce postsurgical swelling include short-term steroid medication, anti-inflammatory agents, cold packs, and extraoral pressure dressings. If healing is uneventful, patients are scheduled for reentry and implant placement 5 months after ridge augmentation. At this time, the bone fixation screws are removed, and the implant bed is prepared (Figs 8-3j and 8-3k). It is recommended that the implant bed be tapped before implant insertion to avoid lateral forces that may detach the formerly placed block graft.

Antimicrobial prophylaxis

Any implant surgery or bone graft surgery is considered a clean-contaminated surgery, because the intraoral surgical access inevitably entails contamination of the surgical wound with the facultative pathogenic mixed flora of the oral cavity.[21] A postoperative infection might have a significant effect on postsurgical morbidity and may result in a compromised outcome, particularly in bone augmentation procedures. Following wound infection, a block graft may undergo considerable resorption, making subsequent implant insertion impossible. Potential measures to avoid wound infection include administration of topical or systemic antimicrobial agents.

Many surgeons advocate the use of an antiseptic mouthwash before surgery to reduce the occurrence of wound infection. Chlorhexidine digluconate is considered one of the best documented antiseptic agents. In 1970, Löe and Schiott[22] showed that rinsing with 10 mL of 0.2% chlorhexidine for 1 minute twice a day inhibited plaque regrowth and the development of gingivitis, even in the absence of normal oral hygiene. Clinical studies have shown that immediate preoperative chlorhexidine rinsing or irrigation reduced the bacterial load and contamination of the surgical area.[23,24]

Chlorhexidine should also be used postoperatively because it offers the advantage of reducing plaque formation when mechanical cleaning may be difficult because of trismus, pain, or discomfort or because oral hygiene may be discontinued to avoid mechanical damage to the surgical wound. Regimens vary, but chlorhexidine should be used immediately posttreatment and until the patient can resume normal oral hygiene.

With regard to systemic antimicrobial prophylaxis, the debate regarding overprescription of antibiotics raises the need for a critical evaluation of proper antibiotic coverage in association with implant treatment. Indiscriminate use of antibiotics is unacceptable, and surgeons should adhere to basic principles to gain the most benefit from the use of prophylactic antibiotics. Although the authors of the present chapter also advocate the use of a single-dose, preoperative antibiotic regimen for standard implant placement without bone augmentation,[25,26] a different approach is recommended in GBR cases. All patients with an increased risk of postsurgical hematoma formation and subsequent bacterial contamination, such as those with block grafts, extended flaps, or periosteal releasing incisions, should be reexamined no later than 3 to 4 days postsurgery, and systemic antimicrobial coverage should be continued for that period. A clinical study of 20 patients who underwent an onlay graft procedure for lateral ridge augmentation prior to implant placement clearly demonstrated the benefit of oral antibiotic administration: No infections were observed in patients with antibiotic coverage, whereas 50% of the patients of the placebo group developed infections, in either the donor or receptor site or both sites.[21]

Block versus particulate grafts

The clinical situation of an alveolar ridge with a more or less intact height but knife-edged thin crest is a challenging situation for horizontal augmentation, particularly because of the geometry of the site, which often only has a one-wall configuration.

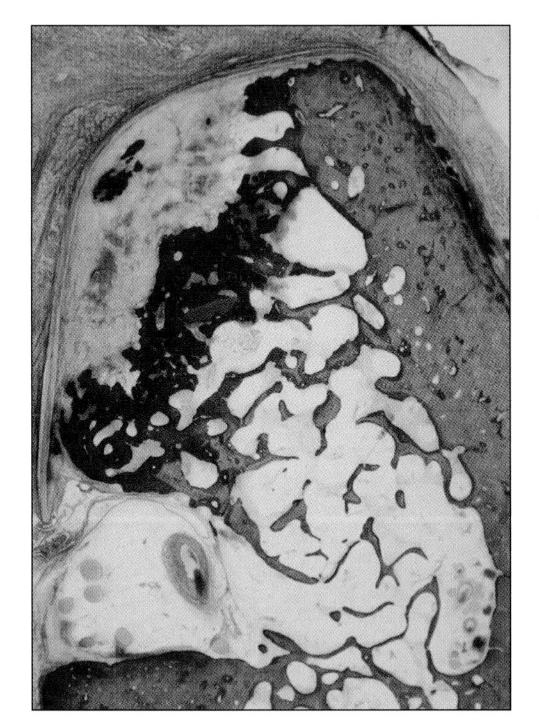

Fig 8-4a Histology of a site 6 months after lateral ridge augmentation with β-tricalcium phosphate particles and ePTFE membrane coverage. The β-tricalcium phosphate particles are only integrated into newly formed bone close to the bone marrow space, but soft tissue has formed within the lateral aspect of the membrane-confined space (toluidine blue–basic fuchsin stain). (Reprinted from von Arx et al[27] with permission.)

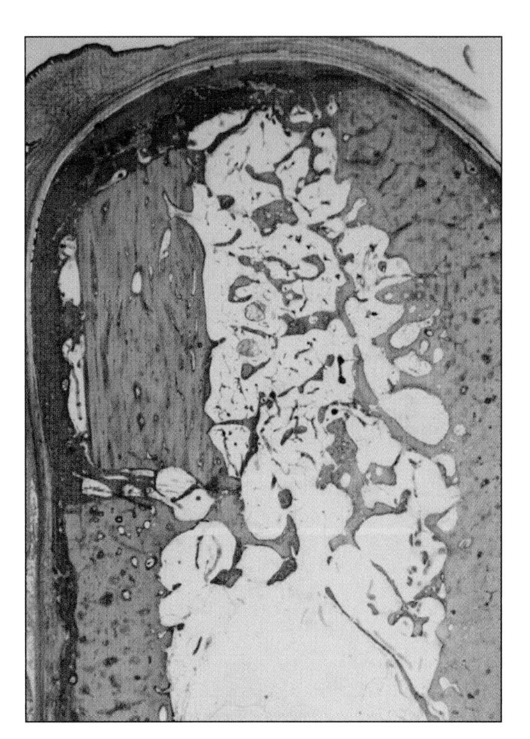

Fig 8-4b Histology of a site 6 months after block graft augmentation with ePTFE-membrane coverage. The block graft shows complete maintenance of the ridge expansion with an ideal ridge profile for implant placement (toluidine blue–basic fuchsin stain). (Reprinted from von Arx et al[27] with permission.)

Such a narrow alveolar ridge may be horizontally augmented with a block or a particulate graft. Although a block graft can be securely stabilized with one or more fixation screws, a particulate graft (either a bone substitute material or a composite of such material and locally harvested bone chips) may be more difficult to stabilize firmly. An experimental study in dogs revealed that particulate bone substitutes (β-tricalcium phosphate and demineralized freeze-dried bone allograft) resulted in considerably less new bone formation and inadequate volume maintenance compared with autogenous block grafts used for lateral ridge augmentation of extended one-wall defects[27] (Fig 8-4).

Similarly, two clinical studies described greater gain of bone width obtained with securely fixed bone blocks compared with that obtained with a particulate graft used for horizontal augmentation of a deficient alveolar ridge.[17,28] Both studies also reported that large areas of the particulate graft were encapsulated by connective tissue.

Rigid skeletal fixation appears to be a key factor for bone graft augmentation.[29–31] Particulate grafting material, irrespective of its source, cannot be securely fixed to the recipient site and hence might be more susceptible to initial micromotion than a block graft stabilized with fixation screws. Intermittent micromotion has been shown to inhibit bone ingrowth.[32] In addition, it has been found that, although revascularization is a necessary precondition for bone resorption and deposition, biomechanical and structural factors may be more decisive in the maintenance of bony volume, favoring a block versus a particulate graft.[33]

Bone marrow perforation

The rationale for bone marrow perforation (localized decortication) is twofold: *(1)* to allow bone marrow cells to populate the augmentation site and *(2)* to facilitate angiogenesis. Both aspects are important requirements in GBR.[34] Conflicting information has been reported with regard to bone marrow perforation and block graft integration in experimental animal studies of block grafts used for lateral ridge augmentation.[35,36] No clinical studies have assessed the advantage of recipient bed perforation with regard to block graft healing in horizontal ridge augmentation. An interesting finding was recently reported by Adeyemo et al[36]; the excision of the host periosteum overlying the block grafts was accompanied by rapid absorption of block grafts and partial or complete replacement with fibrous connective tissue.

Similarly, conflicting results have also been reported about skeletal or extraskeletal GBR with or without decortication. While some researchers[37–39] observed more bone formation in titanium chambers, cylinders, or domes with decortication than in those without, no such effect was found by other researchers.[40,41] However, because these studies were performed either in rats or rabbits, such data can only be extrapolated cautiously to the clinical situation in humans.

Block graft protection

Several experimental studies[27,42–46] and clinical studies[10,14,28,47–50] have shown that "unprotected" autogenous bone blocks will undergo surface resorption to various extents; in contrast, coverage of block grafts with nonresorbable membranes or nonresorbable bone substitute particles may limit surface resorption and therefore may largely preserve the volume of the block graft (Table 8-1 and Fig 8-5).

The elevation of a full-thickness flap results in the detachment of the periosteum from the recipient site. Following block graft fixation for ridge augmentation, the mucoperiosteal flap is repositioned over the "nude" block graft. In many instances, a periosteal releasing incision is necessary to advance the flap over the augmented ridge to accomplish tension-free, primary wound closure. Multiple factors may play a role in subsequent surface resorption of the block graft: mechanical load applied to the graft surface by a removable provisional prosthesis, mucosal pressure resulting from overcontouring, resorptive activities of exposed subperiosteal tissues following periosteal releasing incision, limited nutrition of the peripheral zone of the block graft, remodeling process of the block graft, and structural composition and size of the block graft.

Table 8-1 Reported loss of width (surface resorption) of autogenous bone block grafts from time of block graft placement to reentry

Type of graft used in study	Resorption (%)
Unprotected	
Widmark et al[47]	25*
Chiapasco et al[28]	25
Antoun et al[48]	43
Proussaefs and Lozada[49]	17
Maiorana et al[50]	25
Protected with ePTFE membrane	
Buser et al[10]	0
Antoun et al[48]	7
Protected with DBBM particles	
Maiorana et al[50]	12
von Arx and Buser[14]	7†

*60% at abutment connection.
†DBBM particles were covered with collagen membrane.

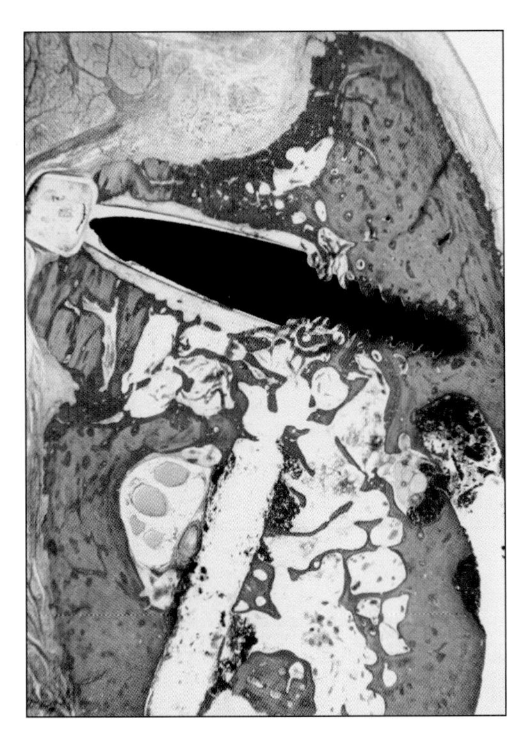

Fig 8-5a Histology of a site 6 months after block graft augmentation without membrane coverage. The buccocrestal portion of the block graft has undergone substantial resorption (toluidine blue-basic fuchsin stain). (Reprinted from von Arx et al[27] with permission.)

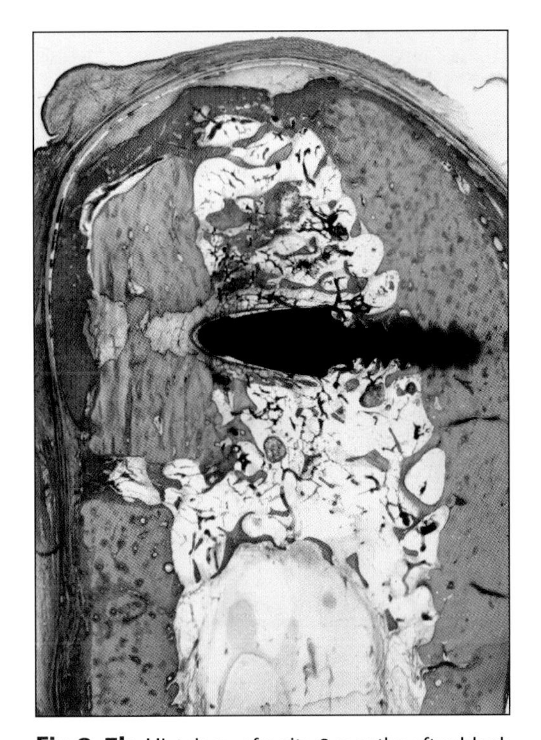

Fig 8-5b Histology of a site 6 months after block graft augmentation with ePTFE-membrane coverage. The block graft has fully maintained its contour, and the formation of a neocortex can be seen immediately below the membrane (toluidine blue-basic fuchsin stain). (Reprinted from von Arx et al[27] with permission.)

The thought that the embryologic origin of the graft may play a role has been refuted because it has been shown that the revascularization is not dependent on the embryologic origin but rather on the cancellous compartment within the graft.[51]

Two clinical studies have directly compared the fate of protected and unprotected block grafts. One study reported that significantly ($P < .01$) less surface resorption occurred when the block had been covered with an ePTFE membrane (7% loss of graft width) than when the block graft was unprotected (43% loss of graft width).[48] The other study calculated a 12% loss of graft width for DBBM-protected block grafts versus a 25% loss in unprotected block grafts, as measured at reentry for implant placement.[50]

The antiresorptive protective effect of DBBM has recently been confirmed in a clinical study.[14] A collagen membrane was additionally placed to fully cover the block grafts and to stabilize the thin layer of DBBM particles shielding the block grafts. The clinical measurements taken at augmentation sites before and after placement of the block grafts and after a mean healing period of 5.8 months during reentry for implant placement yielded a mean loss of graft width of only 0.36 mm (7%). The calculated mean gain of horizontal bone thickness was 4.6 mm (range of 2.0 to 7.0 mm), which is comparable to previously reported data.[10,48,50]

Incorporation and Remodeling of Block Grafts

Several factors have been identified or suggested that may influence the integration of autogenous bone grafts and their ultimate maintenance, such as the rate and extent of revascularization, structural composition, biologic differences between graft types, rigid fixation, inclusion of periosteum as a component of the graft, graft orientation, and contents of local growth factors.[52] Cortical bone largely dies after disruption of its blood supply except for a superficial layer of cells.[53] Cancellous bone, on the other hand, contains many osteogenic cells that are more easily nourished by diffusion and survive direct transfer within the host.[54] A tendency for superficial osteocytes to survive and contribute to bone formation has been observed, although the contribution of the endosteal lining cells and possibly the stromal cells of the marrow appears to be most important.[54,55]

While the majority of investigations focus on the graft and its handling, less attention has been directed toward the recipient milieu. Burchardt[56] emphasized that the recipient bed plays a fundamental role in the graft integration process. Among the morphologic aspects of autogenous bone graft repair, one of the most relevant is creeping substitution. Burchardt and Enneking[57] described it as a dynamic reconstructive and healing process of the graft, ie, a mechanism in which necrotic bone within the graft is gradually resorbed and replaced by new viable bone. Creeping substitution is only possible because of the presence of adequate nourishment from the recipient bed and graft surroundings.

With regard to integration and remodeling, the fate of autogenous block grafts placed for ridge augmentation has been examined in experimental studies[58–60] and in clinical studies.[49,61–63] The majority of osteocytes within the block graft did not survive grafting, and the nonvital bone was progressively remodeled into new vital bone. Depending on the healing period of the evaluated block graft biopsy specimens, vitality (lacunae with viable osteocytes) within the cortical component varied to a great extent.

A minimum healing period of 5 months is suggested between horizontal ridge augmentation using autogenous block grafts and implant placement. It is also recommended that the implant bed, in dense bone in particular, be tapped before using threaded implants. This precaution will diminish compression forces on the bone and may prevent loosening of the formerly placed block graft.

Outcomes for Implants in Block Grafts

Several clinical studies have reported the successful outcome of implants that were placed in a staged procedure in sites that had previously been horizontally augmented with block grafts.[64–67]

Buser and coworkers[68] evaluated the 5-year survival and success rates of 66 titanium implants placed in bone that had been previously augmented with autogenous block grafts and ePTFE membranes. During the observation period, three patients with five implants dropped out of the study. None of the remaining 61 implants were lost during the follow-up period. One implant exhibited a peri-implant infection, whereas 60 implants were considered clinically and radiographically successful at the 5-year examination, resulting in a 5-year success rate of 98.3%.

In general, clinical and radiographic data from these studies show that good long-term results can be expected when titanium dental implants are placed in augmented bone in a staged approach and that these implants do not differ in their behavior from implants placed in pristine host bone.

Case Reports

Case 1

A 47-year-old woman was referred by her private dentist for implant restoration in the left side of the mandible (Fig 8-6a). The missing teeth had been absent for 30 years; therefore, the alveolar process showed a marked lateral deficiency because of horizontal bone resorption. However, the height of the (lingual) crest was intact. The cone-beam computed tomogram confirmed the presence of a knife-edged thin alveolar ridge with good vertical dimension (Fig 8-6b). The plan was first to augment the deficient ridge in the area of the second premolar and first molar with a block graft from the right side of the symphysis (because the mandibular right lateral incisor and canine both were endodontically treated) and second to insert two implants in a staged procedure.

A full-thickness flap was raised in the left side of the mandible (Fig 8-6c), and the incision was continued to the contralateral side below the mucogingival line to access the symphysis. A corticocancellous block graft was prepared with piezoelectric surgery in the right side of the chin (Fig 8-6d). The autogenous bone block was placed at the

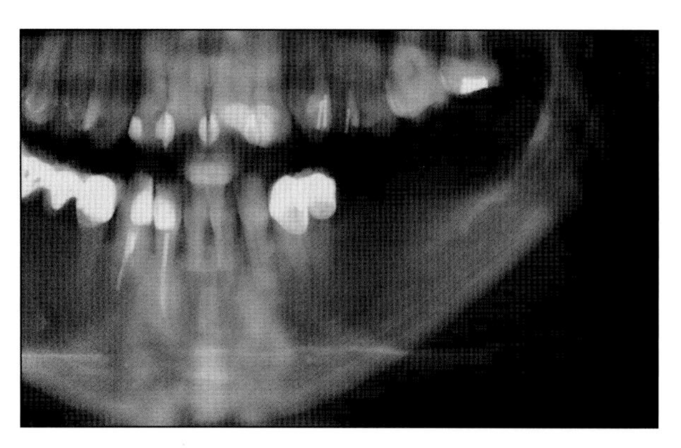

Fig 8-6a The panoramic radiograph shows the edentulous area in the posterior left mandible.

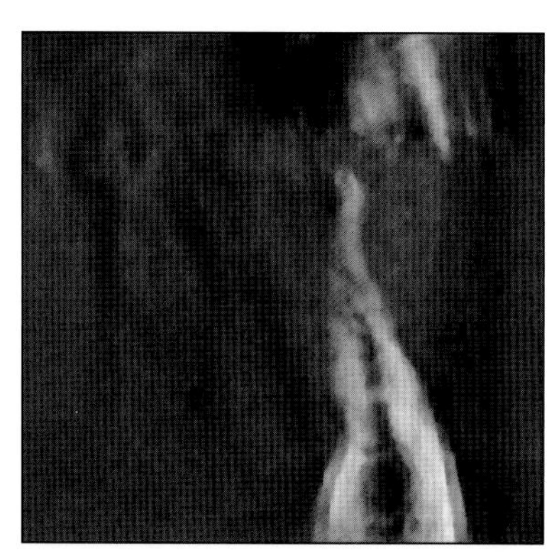

Fig 8-6b The cross-cut image (cone-beam computed tomogram, coronal view) demonstrates the intact bony height, but the alveolar ridge shows substantial loss of width.

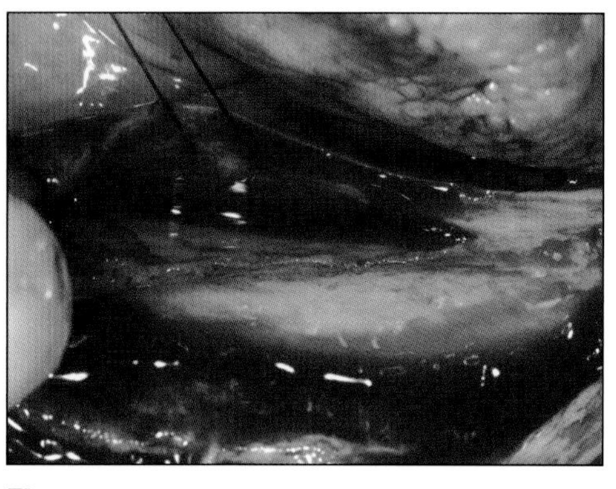

Fig 8-6c A knife-edged thin crest is visible following flap elevation.

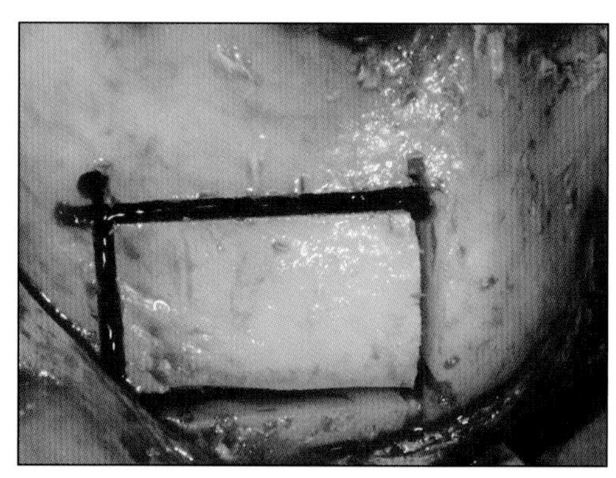

Fig 8-6d A block graft is cut in the symphysis via piezoelectric surgery.

desired location for horizontal augmentation and secured with two fixation screws (Figs 8-6e to 8-6g). A mixture of DBBM particles and blood was placed around and on top of the block graft, and the augmentation site was fully covered with a collagen membrane (Fig 8-6h). A periosteal releasing incision was made, and primary, tension-free wound closure was accomplished with multiple interrupted and mattress sutures.

The radiograph taken 6 months after augmentation surgery showed uneventful healing of the grafted and donor sites (Figs 8-6i and 8-6j). At the reentry surgery, the left side of the mandibular alveolar ridge presented with a width of 6.0 mm compared to a width of 1.5 mm at baseline (Fig 8-6k). Two dental implants were inserted in the region of the second premolar and first molar (Figs 8-6l and 8-6m).

After a healing period of 4 months (Figs 8-6n and 8-6o), the patient was sent back to her private dentist for implant restoration. He inserted a fixed three-unit prosthesis, including a distal cantilever (Figs 8-6p and 8-6q).

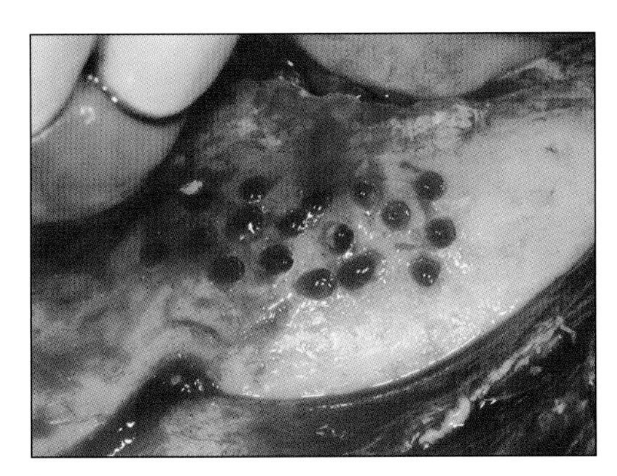

Fig 8-6e Multiple bone marrow perforations are prepared with a small round bur. Note the mental foramen at the bottom.

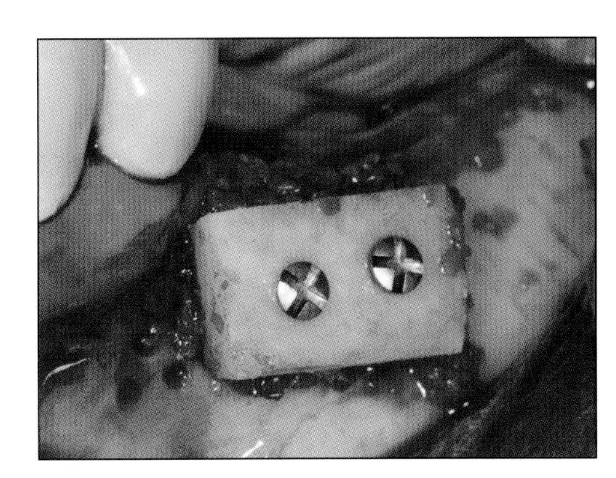

Fig 8-6f The corticocancellous block graft is oriented in a mesiodistal direction and secured with two fixation screws.

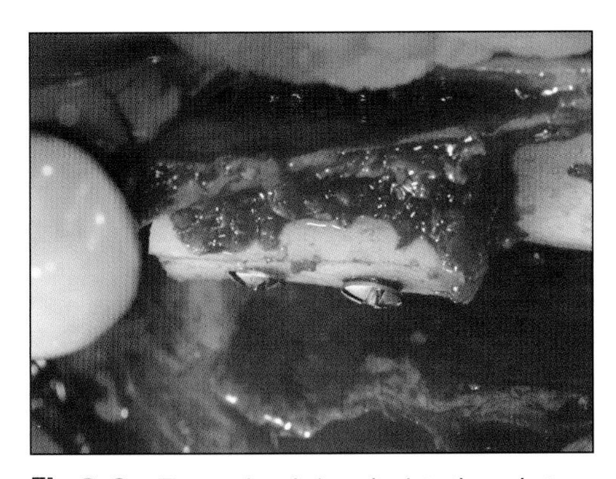

Fig 8-6g The occlusal view depicts the substantial gain in ridge width.

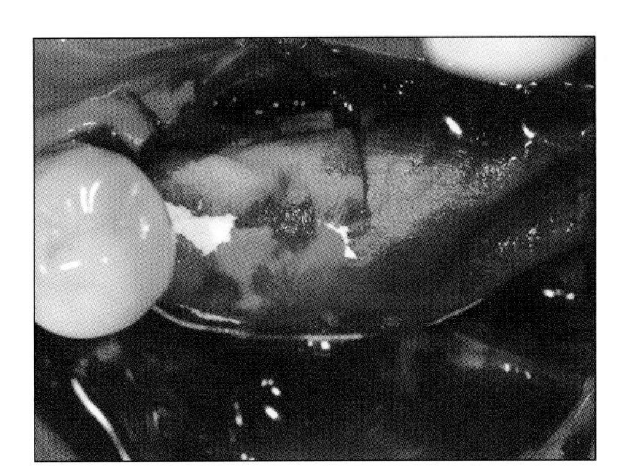

Fig 8-6h Following application of DBBM particles around the block graft, the augmented site is covered with a collagen membrane.

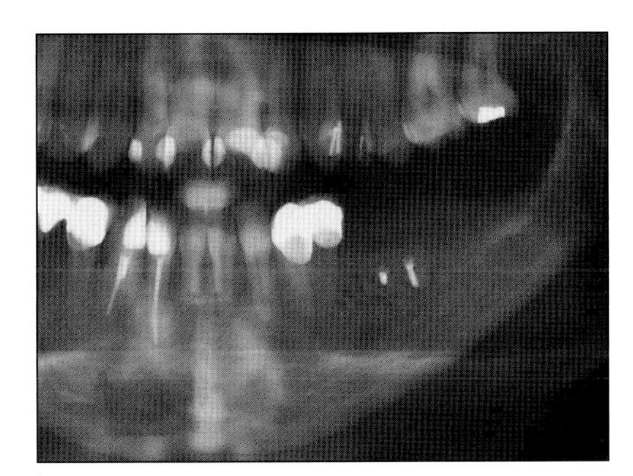

Fig 8-6i The postoperative panoramic radiograph shows the donor and receptor sites in the mandible.

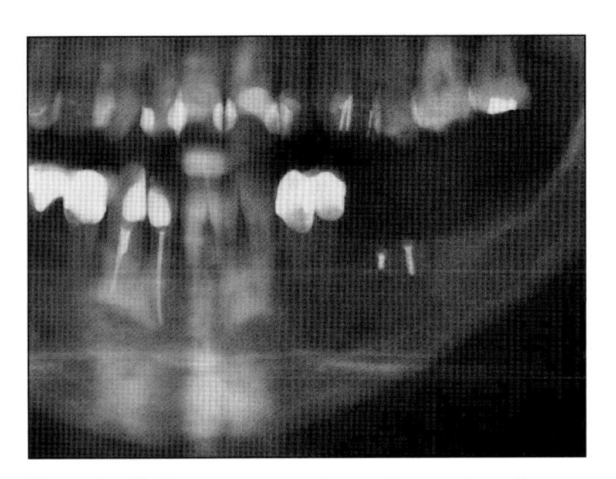

Fig 8-6j The panoramic radiograph taken 6 months after surgery demonstrates the healing of the donor and receptor sites.

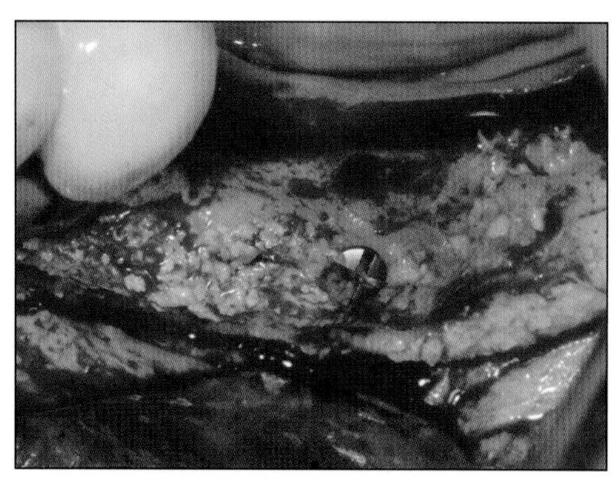

Fig 8-6k Flap elevation at the reentry procedure reveals that the volume of the augmented site has been fully maintained.

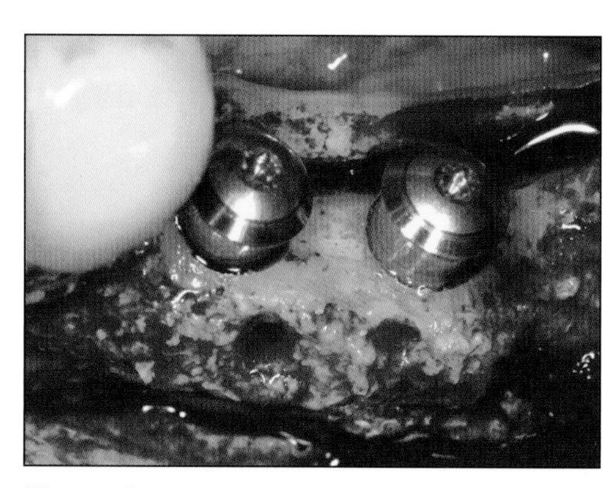

Fig 8-6l Two dental implants are placed in the horizontally augmented ridge.

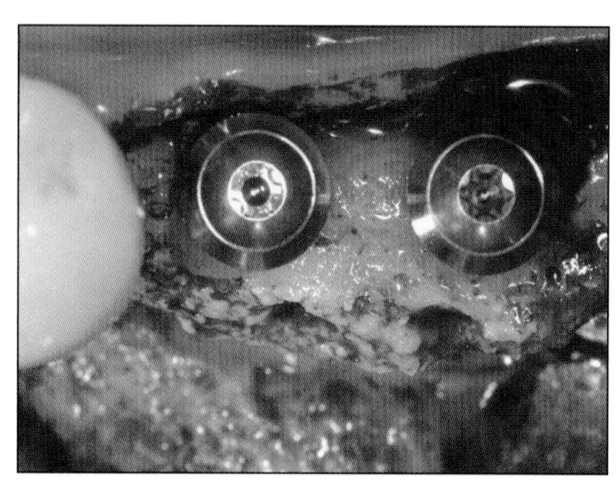

Fig 8-6m Sufficient width of bone is present on the facial aspect of both implants.

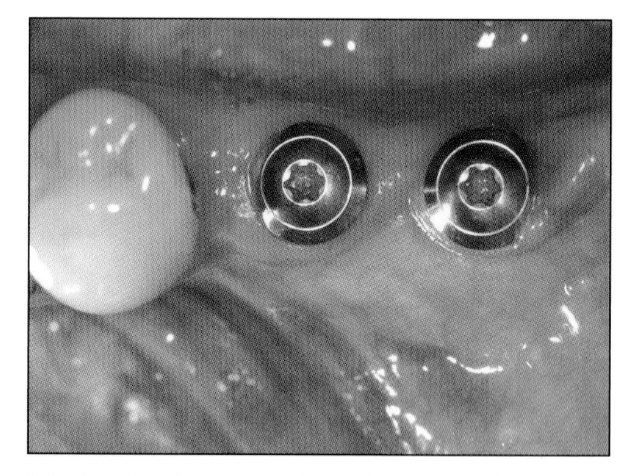

Fig 8-6n At completion of the wound healing, both implants are well integrated.

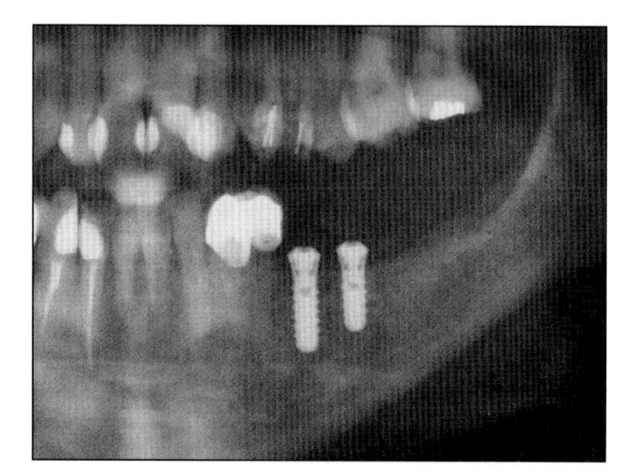

Fig 8-6o The radiograph confirms tissue integration of both implants.

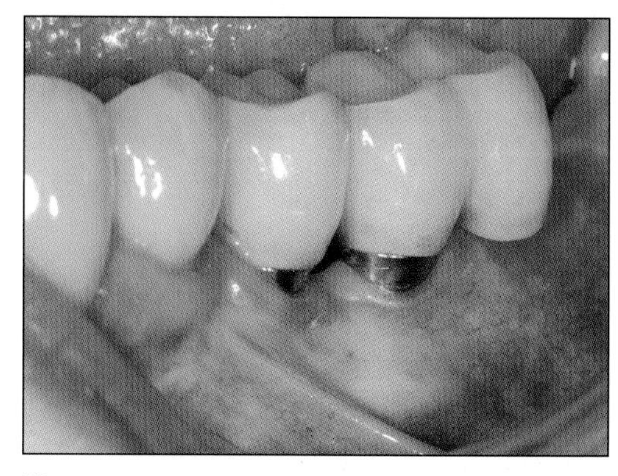

Fig 8-6p The three-unit fixed dental prosthesis is surrounded by healthy peri-implant soft tissues.

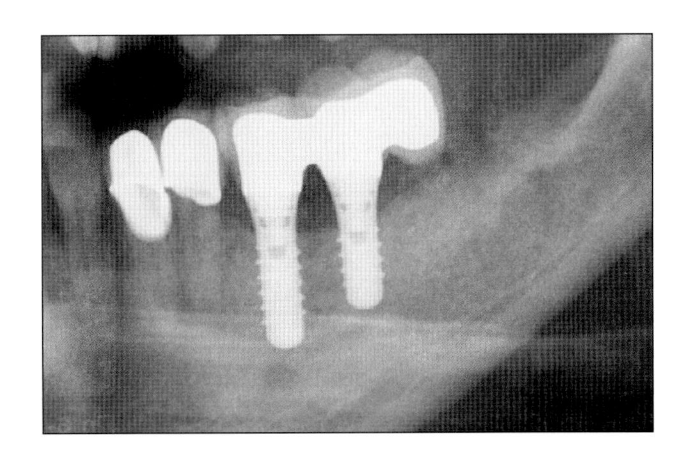

Fig 8-6q A radiograph taken at the 3-year follow-up examination shows stable levels of peri-implant bone.

Case 2

A 31-year-old woman was referred for ridge augmentation and implant reconstruction. The patient had been involved in a car accident 4 years previously with injury to her maxillary left incisors. Both teeth had to be extracted later. The alveolar ridge in the area of the left central and lateral incisors presented with atrophy of the facial aspect but with good vertical dimension. The plan included horizontal ridge augmentation with a mandibular block graft and staged implant placement.

The edentulous space was accessed with mucoperiosteal vestibular and palatal flap elevation (Figs 8-7a and 8-7b). Subsequently, a corticocancellous block graft was harvested from the midsymphyseal region. The rectangular bone block was placed in a mesiodistal direction for horizontal bone augmentation in the crestal area of the edentulous space (Figs 8-7c and 8-7d). The block graft was secured with two fixation screws and fully covered with a thin layer of DBBM particles mixed with blood (Fig 8-7e). A collagen membrane was adapted to the augmentation site to keep the DBBM particles in place (Fig 8-7f). A periosteal releasing incision was made, and the flap was slightly advanced in a coronal direction. Primary tension-free wound closure was accomplished with one mattress and multiple interrupted sutures (Fig 8-7g).

Healing was uneventful (Figs 8-7h and 8-7i). Because of pregnancy, the patient did not return until 14 months after the augmentation surgery for implant placement. At the reentry surgery, the block graft showed no surface resorption and was fully integrated (Fig 8-7j). Two implants were inserted, a regular-neck implant in the central incisor site and a narrow-neck implant in the lateral incisor site (Figs 8-7k and 8-7l). After an implant healing period of 3 months, two implant crowns were placed (Figs 8-7m to 8-7o).

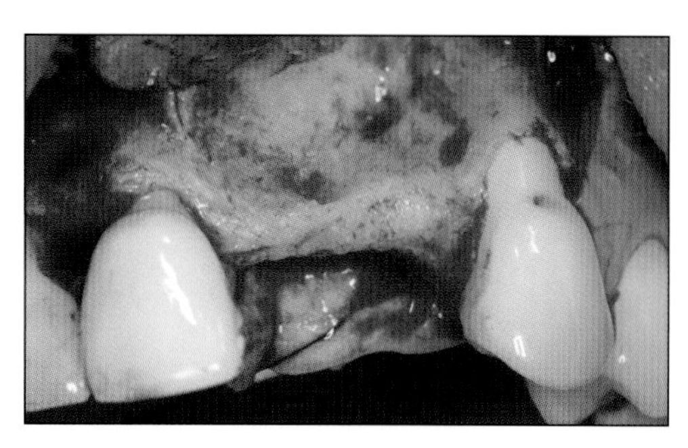

Fig 8-7a The edentulous space is accessed with a mucoperiosteal flap incision. The height of the alveolar ridge is intact.

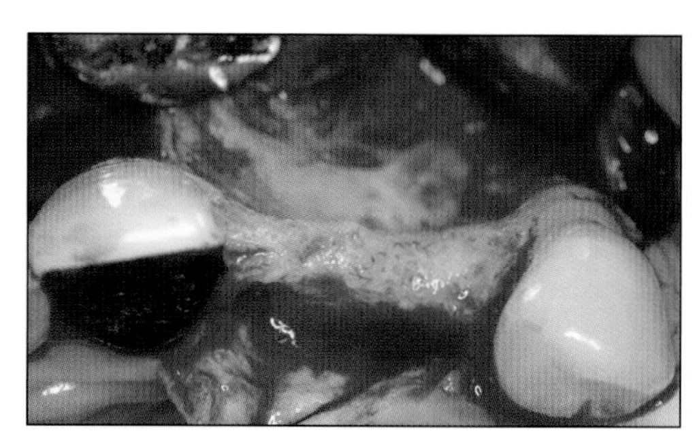

Fig 8-7b The occlusal view demonstrates marked resorption of the facial bony wall, resulting in a concave geometry of the crest.

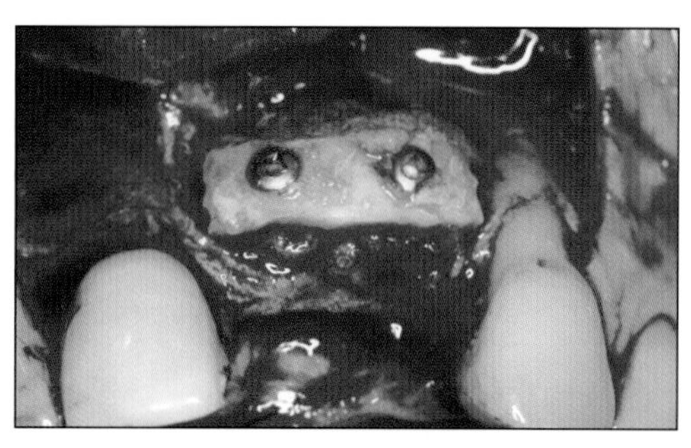

Fig 8-7c A symphyseal corticocancellous block graft is placed in the recipient bed and stabilized with two fixation screws.

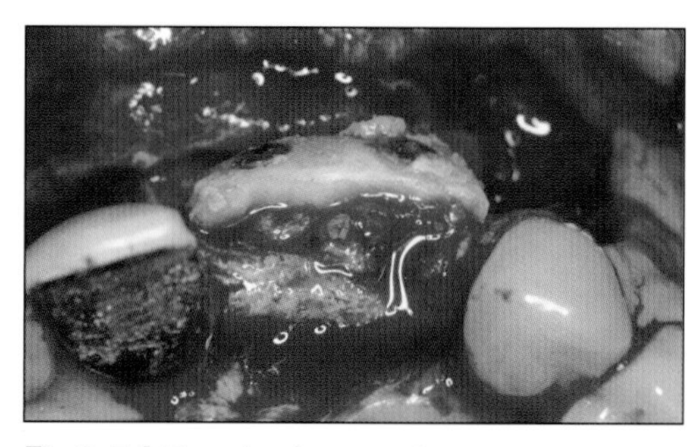

Fig 8-7d There has been a substantial gain in ridge width with overcontouring of the former defect.

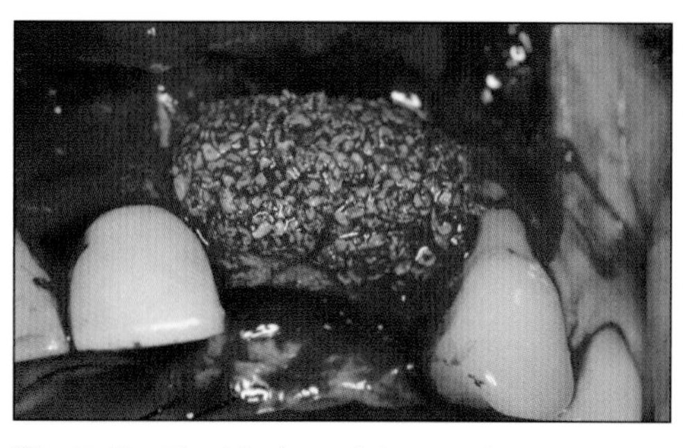

Fig 8-7e The block graft is completely covered with DBBM particles.

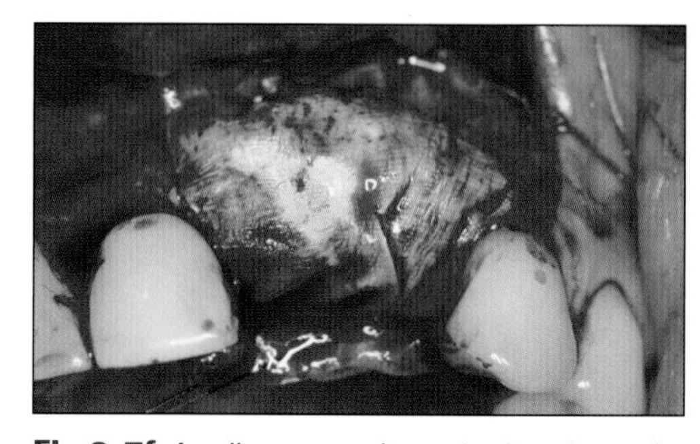

Fig 8-7f A collagen membrane is placed over the augmented site.

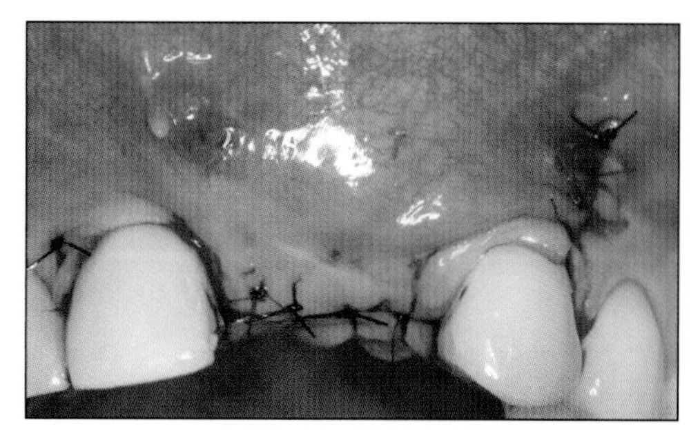

Fig 8-7g Primary wound closure is accomplished following placement of a periosteal releasing incision.

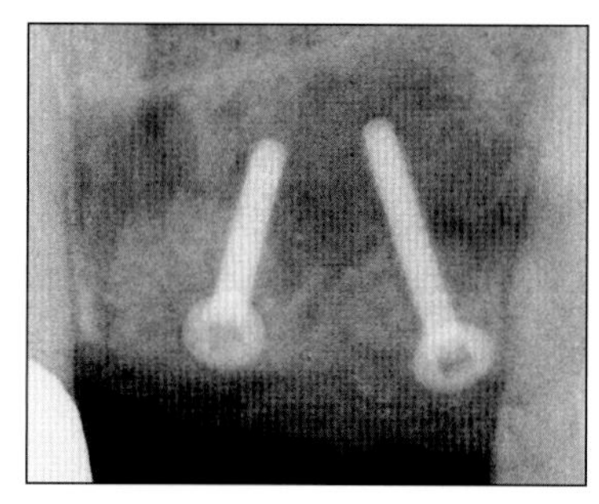

Fig 8-7h The postoperative periapical radiograph reveals the block graft with the two fixation screws.

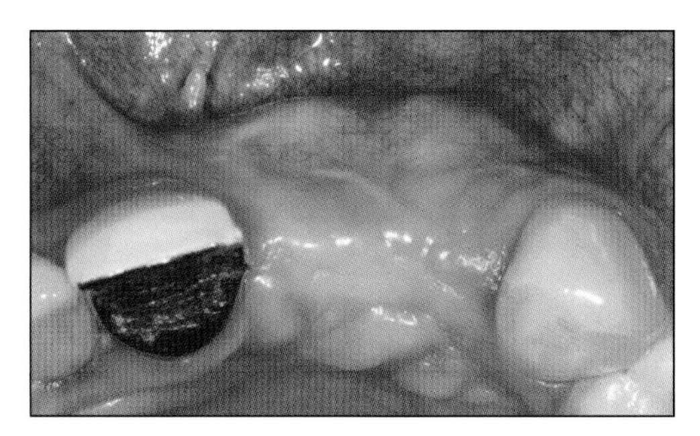

Fig 8-7i The clinical situation immediately before reentry, 14 months after the augmentation surgery, indicates the uneventful healing period.

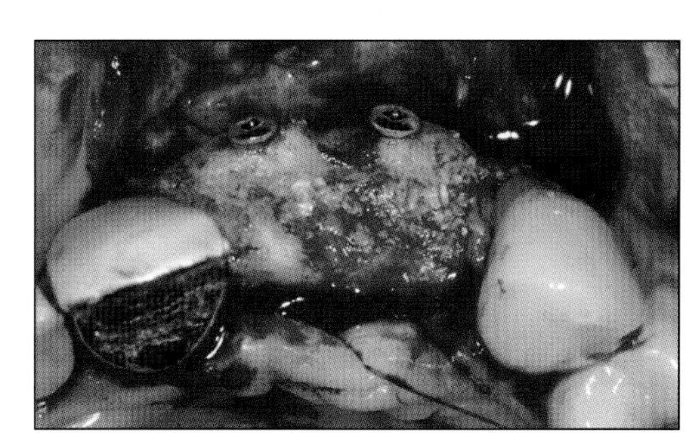

Fig 8-7j The occlusal view following flap elevation demonstrates the well-preserved augmentation site. The screw heads at the surface of the former block graft indicate that no bone resorption has occurred between the first surgery and the reentry.

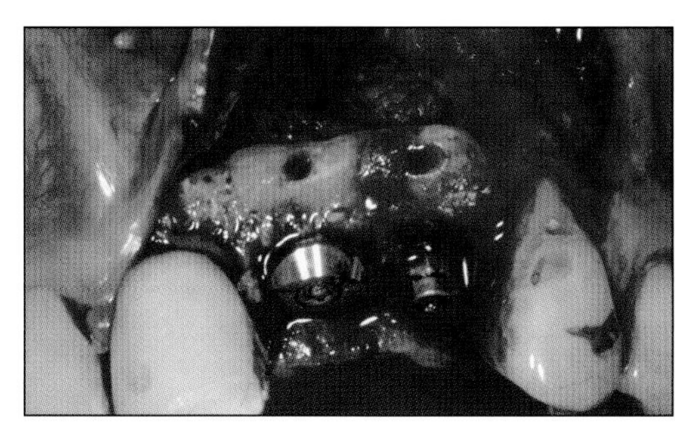

Fig 8-7k A regular-neck implant and a narrow-neck implant are placed in the augmented ridge.

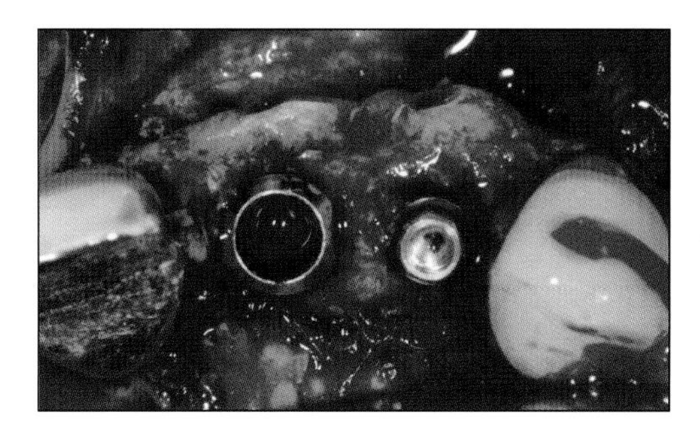

Fig 8-7l A sufficient width of bone is present at the facial aspect of both implants.

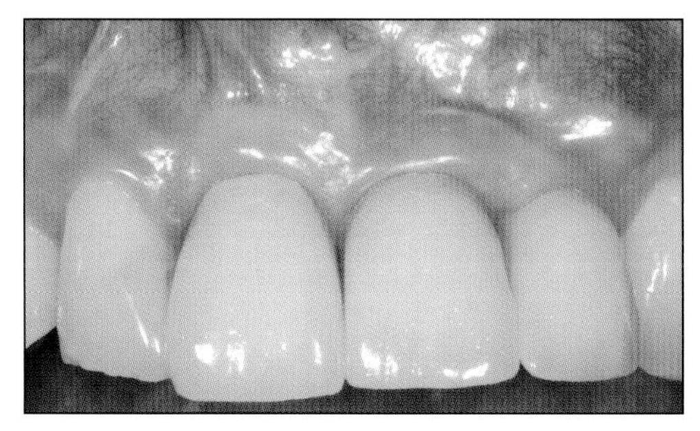

Fig 8-7m Clinical status at the 5-year follow-up examination demonstrates a pleasing esthetic treatment outcome with healthy soft tissue at both implants.

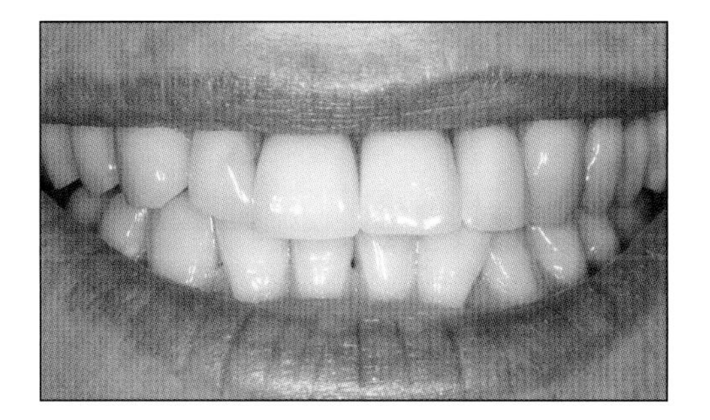

Fig 8-7n The patient yields a medium lip line.

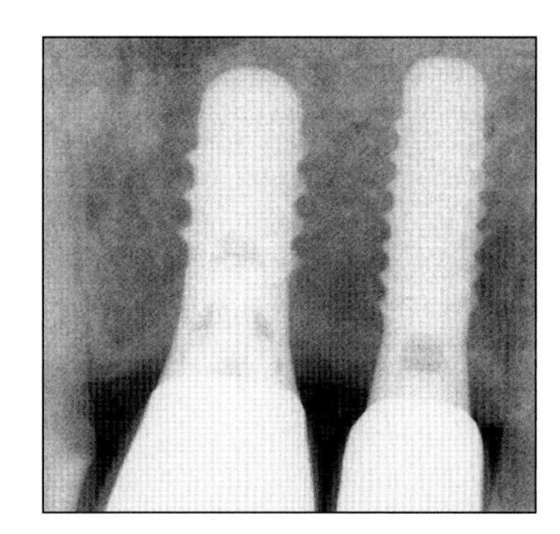

Fig 8-7o The 5-year periapical radiograph shows stable peri-implant bone crest levels.

Case 3

A 27-year-old man was referred to the department with a posttraumatic situation. The patient presented with a high smile line and a disharmonious esthetic situation in the anterior maxilla (Fig 8-8a). The left central incisor was ankylosed and apically malpositioned, leading to the appearance of a longer clinical crown and gingival recession compared with the contralateral tooth (Fig 8-8b). The root ankylosis and partial root resorption were confirmed by a periapical radiograph (Fig 8-8c). It was decided to surgically remove the ankylosed tooth and to place an implant-borne restoration.

Removal of the ankylosed tooth required flap elevation with a papilla-sparing incision and a local osteotomy. As expected, a large bone deficiency resulted, including a through-and-through defect on the palatal aspect (Fig 8-8d). The wound was closed to establish well-healed soft tissues in the future augmentation site (Fig 8-8e).

After a healing period of 3 months, the clinical status showed facial flattening and some scar tissue formation (Fig 8-8f). Following flap elevation, the occlusal view clearly showed a large facial defect with a crest width of less than 3 mm (Fig 8-8g). A corticocancellous block was harvested from the chin, vertically applied in the augmentation site, and stabilized with a fixation screw (Fig 8-8h). Autogenous bone chips were used to fill the voids lateral to the block graft. A superficial layer of DBBM particles was applied for graft protection (Fig 8-8i). Following membrane application with a double-layer technique (Fig 8-8j) and an incision of the periosteum, the augmentation surgery was completed with a tension-free primary wound closure (Fig 8-8k).

Soft tissue healing was uneventful. Following 5 months of healing (Fig 8-8l), the reopening procedure revealed successful horizontal ridge augmentation and no graft resorption (Figs 8-8m to 8-8o), which allowed implant placement in a correct three-dimensional position (Fig 8-8p). Primary wound closure was performed to achieve submerged implant healing (Fig 8-8q).

Two months later, the implant site was reopened with a punch technique (Fig 8-8r) to initiate prosthetic restoration. In addition to preparation for a single crown on the implant, the contralateral tooth was prepared for a ceramic veneer (Fig 8-8s). The esthetic treatment outcome was quite pleasing considering the demanding initial clinical situation with the soft tissue defect, although the implant crown was slightly longer than the contralateral tooth (Fig 8-8t).

The periapical radiograph at the 1-year examination showed a well-integrated screw-type implant (Fig 8-8u). The 8-year follow-up examination revealed stable peri-implant soft tissues and bone crest levels (Figs 8-8v to 8-8x).

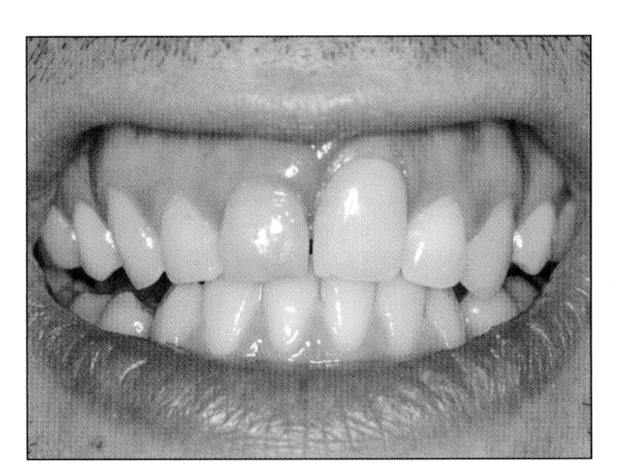

Fig 8-8a A 27-year-old man displays a high smile line and a disharmonious esthetic situation in the anterior maxilla.

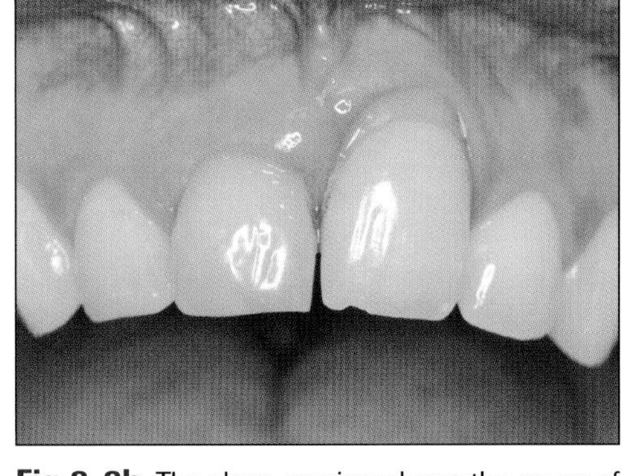

Fig 8-8b The close-up view shows the cause of the esthetic problem. The maxillary left central incisor is ankylosed in an apical malposition, displaying a longer clinical crown and gingival recession compared with the contralateral tooth.

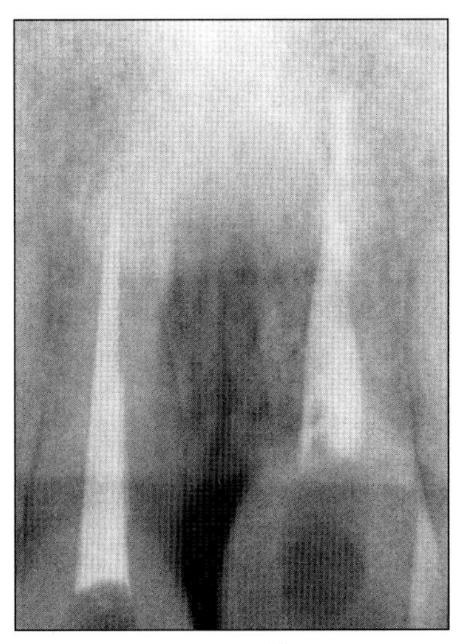

Fig 8-8c The periapical radiograph reveals the ankylosed root with signs of root resorption.

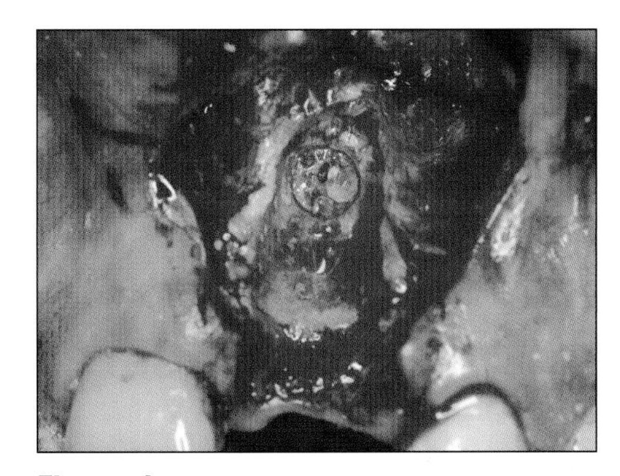

Fig 8-8d To remove the ankylosed root, flap elevation with a papilla-sparing incision was necessary. Following osteotomy and root removal, an extended through-and-through bone defect to the palatal aspect is visible.

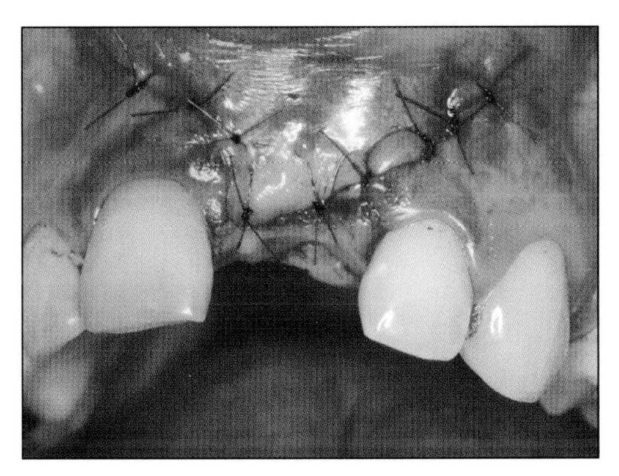

Fig 8-8e The first surgery is completed with a primary flap closure to achieve intact soft tissues in the future augmentation site.

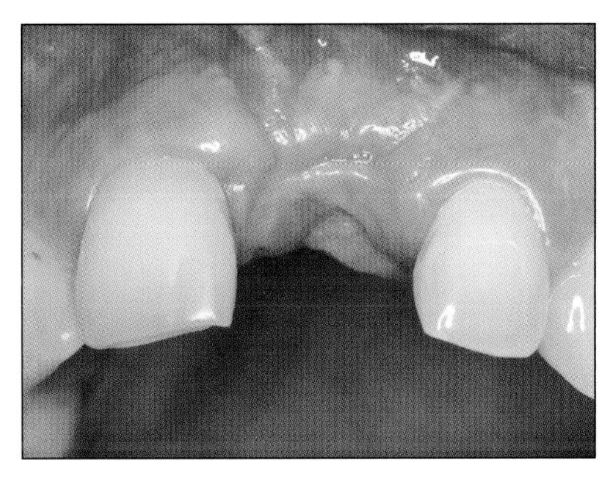

Fig 8-8f Six months following tooth removal, the soft tissues are intact. The scar lines caused by the papilla-sparing incision technique are clearly visible.

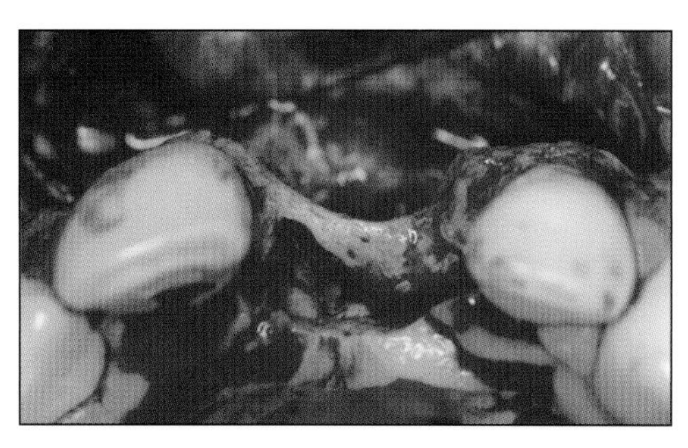

Fig 8-8g The surgical occlusal view reveals the narrow alveolar crest with a facial flattening. The crest width of less than 3 mm requires horizontal ridge augmentation with a block graft and GBR.

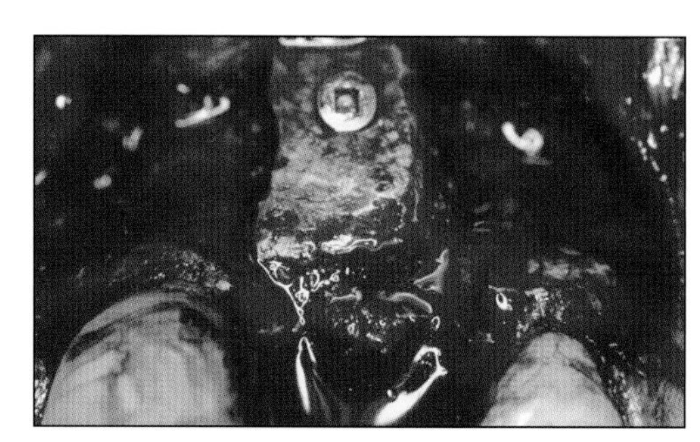

Fig 8-8h A 5 × 10-mm block graft harvested from the chin is applied in a vertical direction. The graft is stabilized with a fixation screw. Autogenous bone chips will be used to fill the voids lateral to the block graft.

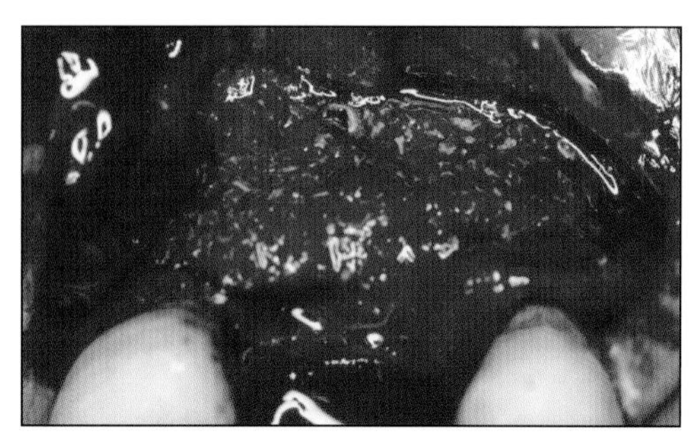

Fig 8-8i The augmentation material is covered with a superficial layer of DBBM particles for graft protection. DBBM, with its low substitution rate, is used to better maintain the created volume.

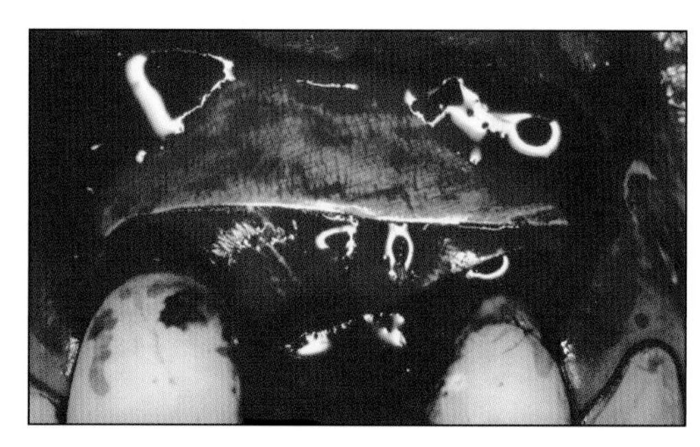

Fig 8-8j The augmentation material is covered with a collagen membrane to act as a temporary barrier. The membrane is applied with a double-layer technique to improve membrane stability.

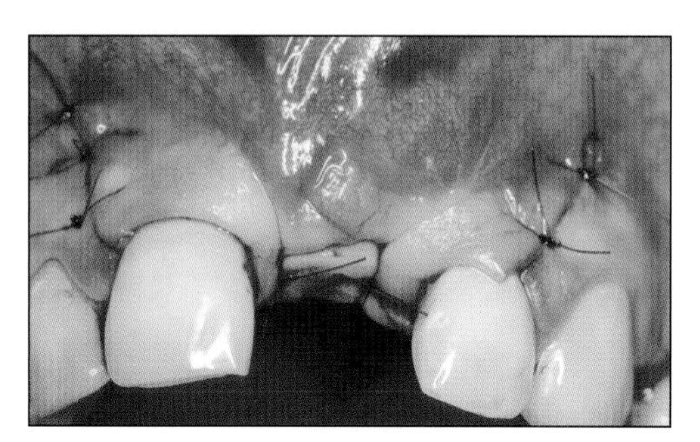

Fig 8-8k The surgery is completed with tension-free primary wound closure following the release of the periosteum.

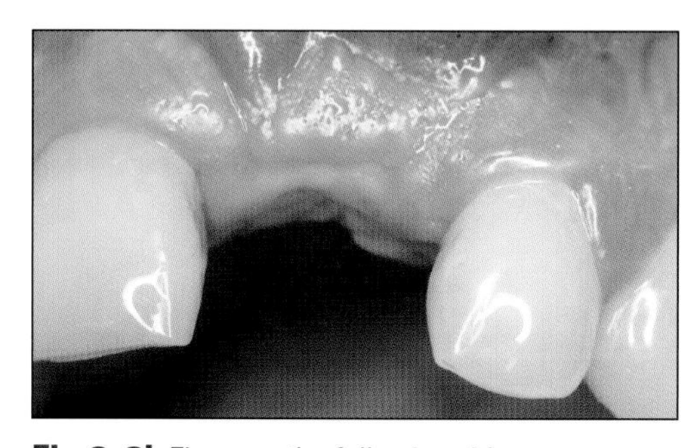

Fig 8-8l Five months following ridge augmentation, the soft tissues have healed well without complications.

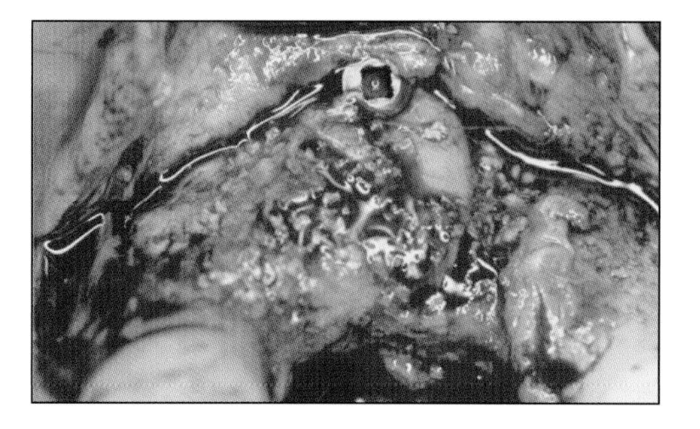

Fig 8-8m The position of the fixation screw head indicates that the volume of the block graft has been well maintained.

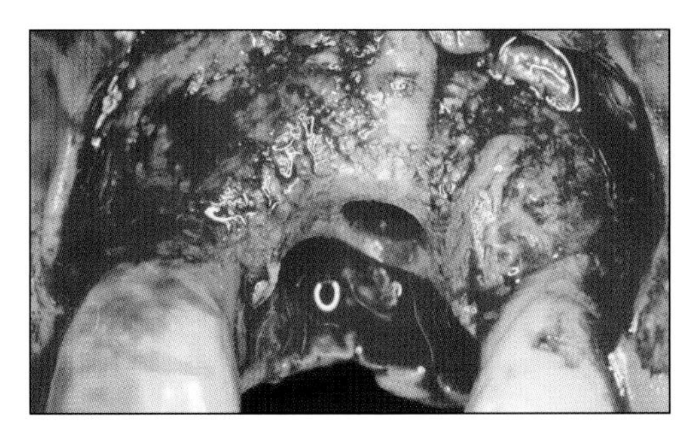

Fig 8-8n The facial view of the surgical site demonstrated that there was still a vertical deficiency of about 2 mm.

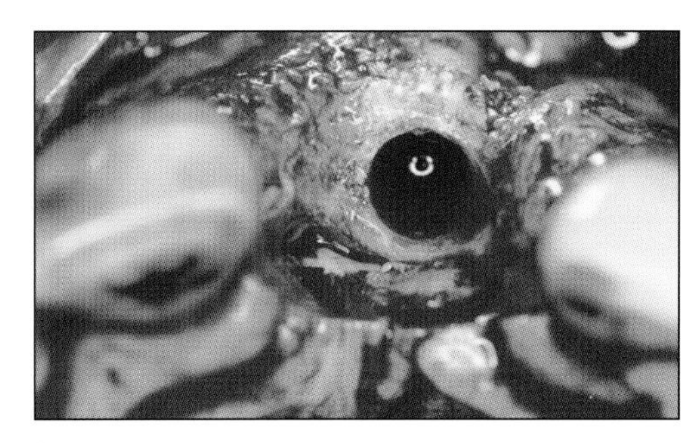

Fig 8-8o The occlusal view confirms successful horizontal augmentation that will allow implant placement. Following implant bed preparation, the facial bone wall measures roughly 3 mm.

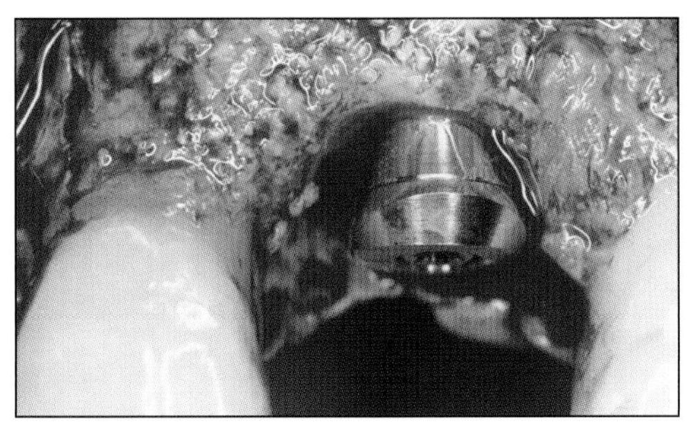

Fig 8-8p The implant is placed in a correct three-dimensional position, and a 2-mm beveled healing cap is applied.

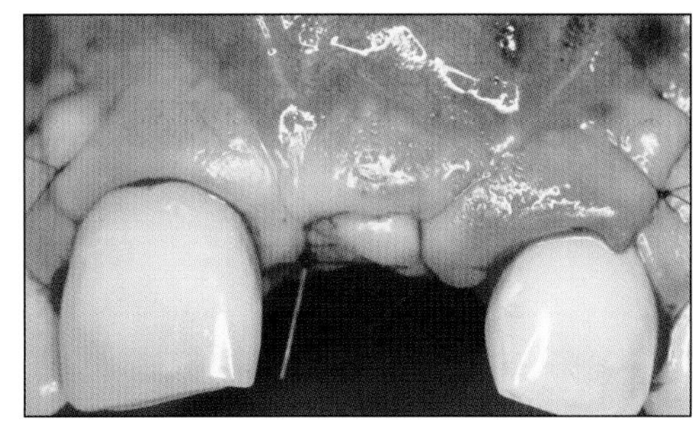

Fig 8-8q Primary wound closure is achieved to allow submerged healing.

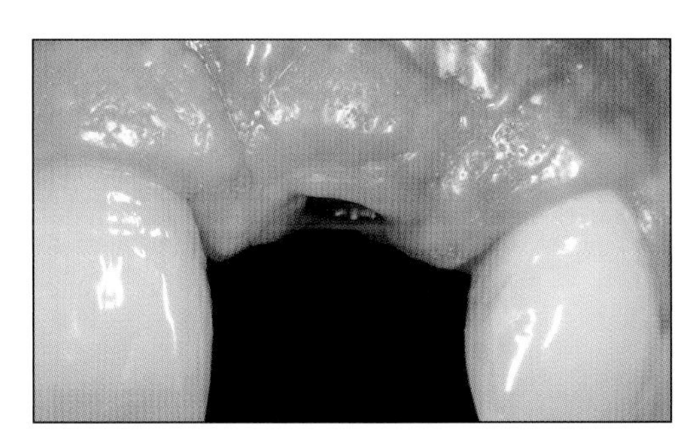

Fig 8-8r Two months later, the implant site is reopened to initiate prosthetic restoration.

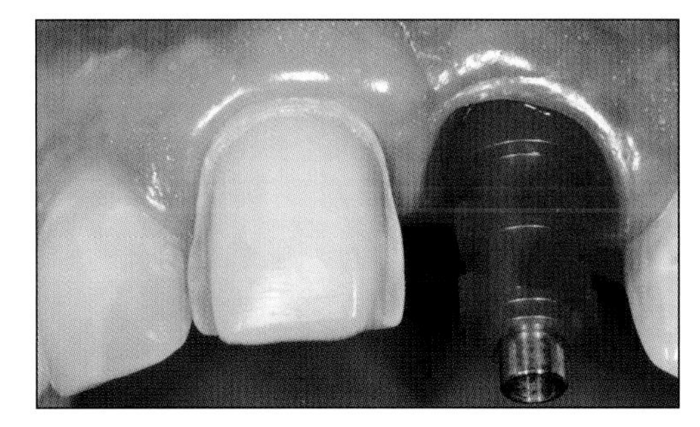

Fig 8-8s An impression is taken with a transfer coping. The right central incisor is prepared for a ceramic veneer.

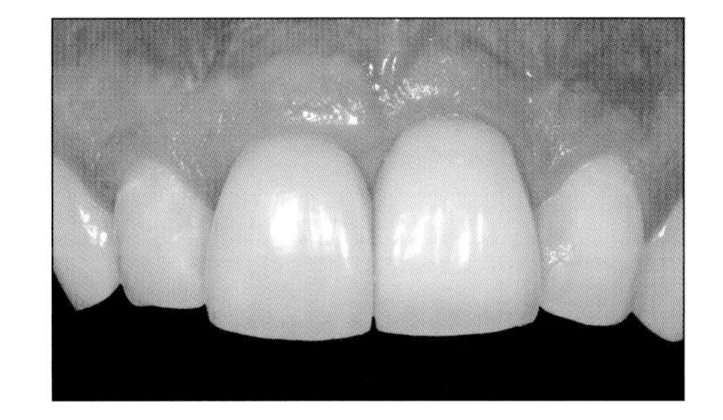

Fig 8-8t A ceramic veneer is on the right central incisor, and an implant-borne metal-ceramic crown is on the left central incisor. There is still a slight discrepancy in crown lengths.

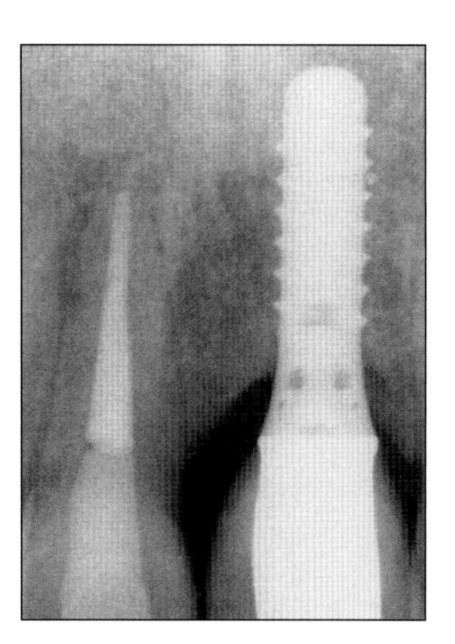

Fig 8-8u The periapical radiograph 1 year following implant insertion indicates that bone crest levels around the implant-supported single crown are stable.

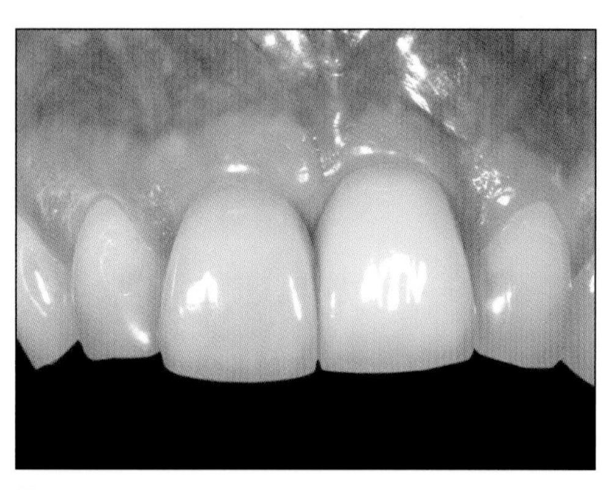

Fig 8-8v At the 8-year follow-up examination, although there is a slight difference in tissue height at the facial mucosa of both incisors, the esthetic outcome is very pleasing compared with the initial clinical status.

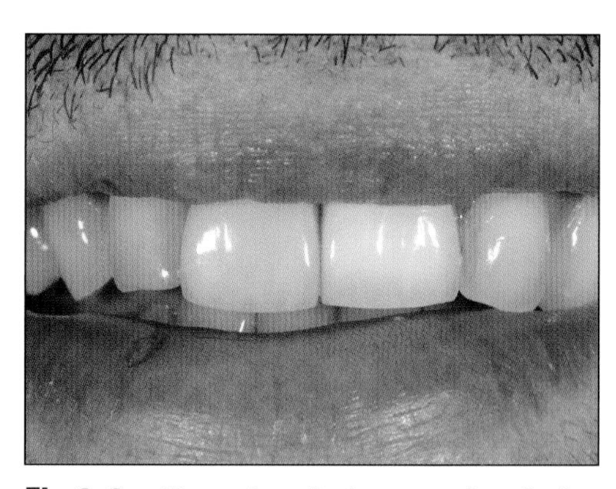

Fig 8-8w The patient displays a medium lip line when smiling.

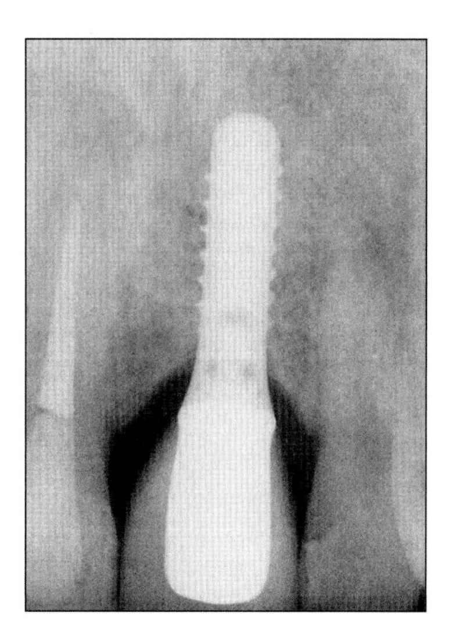

Fig 8-8x The 8-year radiographic follow-up examination confirms that peri-implant bone crest levels are stable.

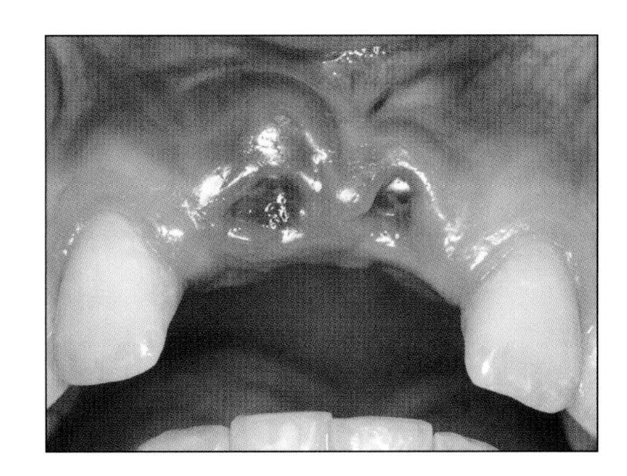

Fig 8-9a Fifteen years following implant placement in the areas of the maxillary central incisors, both crowns have been removed by the referring dentist because of a chronic infection. The right central incisor implant has increased probing depths and shows signs of inflammation and suppuration.

Case 4

A 29-year-old woman had a chronic infection around two adjacent implants in the anterior maxilla (Fig 8-9a). Both implants had been inserted 15 years earlier, in the mid-1980s. The radiograph showed a peri-implant radiolucency that extended close to the root surface of the adjacent lateral incisor (Fig 8-9b). It was obvious that both implants had to be removed.

The implant removal surgery was initiated with a papilla-sparing flap. Following flap elevation, the implants showed no facial bone wall on the exposed implant surface, and a facial malpositioning of the oversized, wide-platform implants (Fig 8-9c). Both implants were carefully removed, leaving the palatal bone wall intact (Fig 8-9d), and primary wound closure was obtained (Fig 8-9e).

Soft tissue healing was uneventful (Fig 8-9f), but at 3 months the edentulous space with two missing teeth demonstrated a large horizontal bone defect in the alveolar crest (Figs 8-9g and 8-9h). To augment the bone deficiency, a large block graft was harvested from the chin area (Fig 8-9i) and grafted in place with two fixation screws (Figs 8-9j and 8-9k). The voids around the applied block graft were filled with autogenous bone chips and covered with a layer of DBBM particles for graft protection (Fig 8-9l). Following application of a collagen membrane using a double-layer technique (Fig 8-9m), primary tension-free wound closure was achieved to complete the surgery (Fig 8-9n).

Eight months following a complication-free wound healing, the reopening procedure demonstrated an excellent augmentation outcome that allowed the placement of two implants in a favorable position (Figs 8-9o to 8-9q). Prior to wound closure, the facial bone wall again was covered with a layer of DBBM particles for bone protection (Figs 8-9r and 8-9s).

Three months following implant placement and uneventful healing, prosthetic restoration was initiated with a reopening procedure (Figs 8-9t and 8-9u). The two implants were first restored with provisional single crowns (Figs 8-9v and 8-9w). The 5-year follow-up examination revealed final metal-ceramic crowns with successful tissue integration (Figs 8-9x to 8-9z).

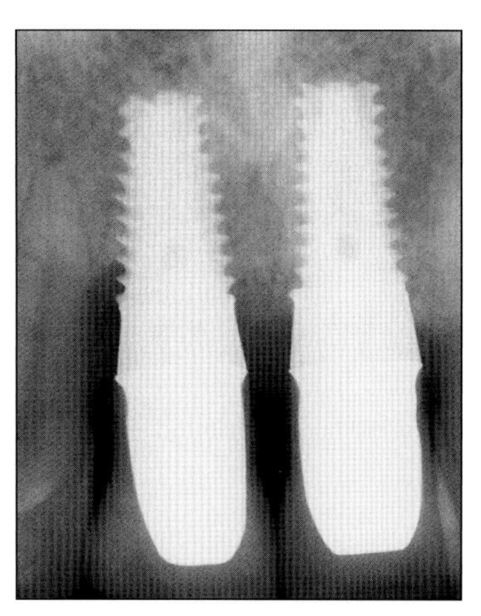

Fig 8-9b The periapical radiograph demonstrates that oversized implants had been inserted in the mid-1980s. The peri-implant infection around the right central incisor implant also affected the adjacent right lateral incisor.

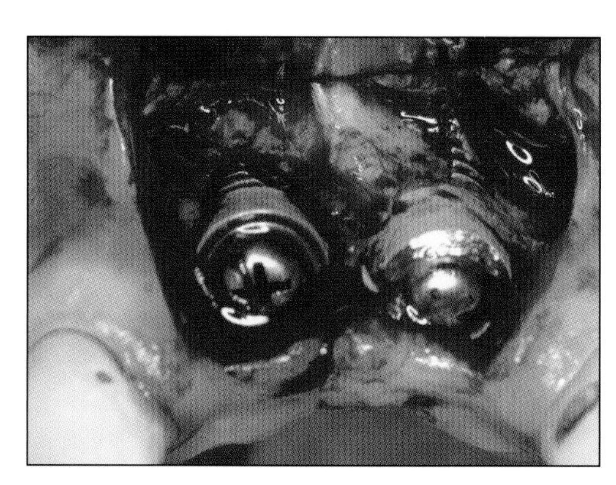

Fig 8-9c Following flap elevation with a papilla-sparing incision, it is evident that the platform diameter of the chosen implants was too large. Neither implant shows a facial bone wall.

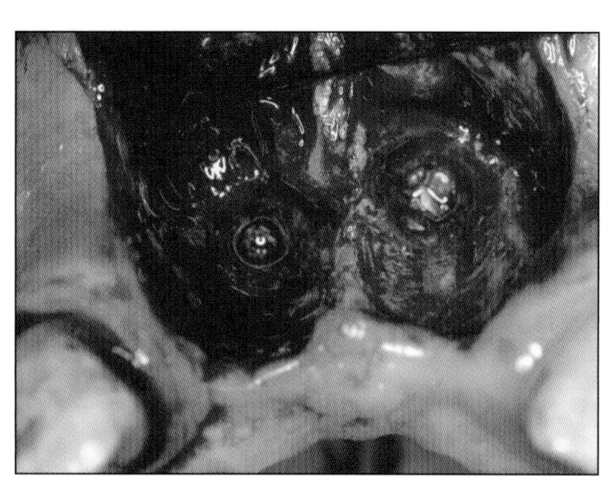

Fig 8-9d The removal of both implants has caused an extensive bone defect in the area of the central incisors.

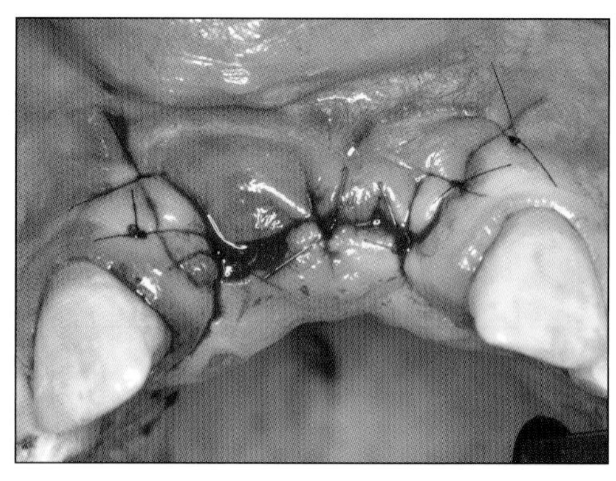

Fig 8-9e The surgery is completed with primary wound closure using interrupted single sutures.

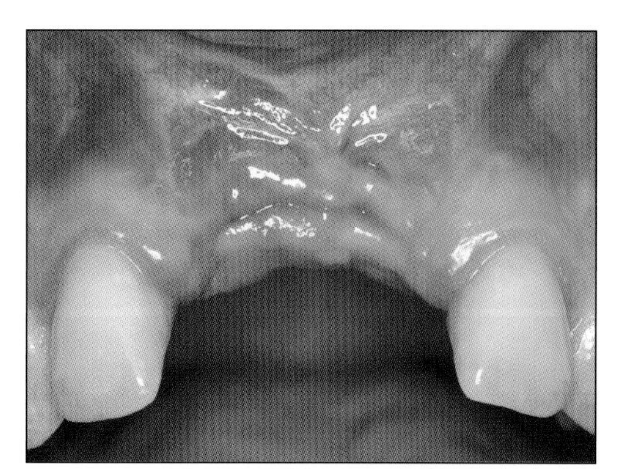

Fig 8-9f Three months following implant removal, the area is well healed but shows scar tissue formation.

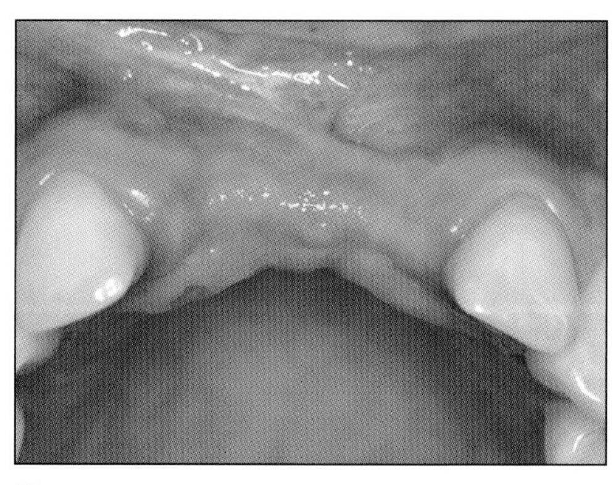

Fig 8-9g The extensive facial flattening necessitates a ridge augmentation procedure prior to implant placement using a staged approach.

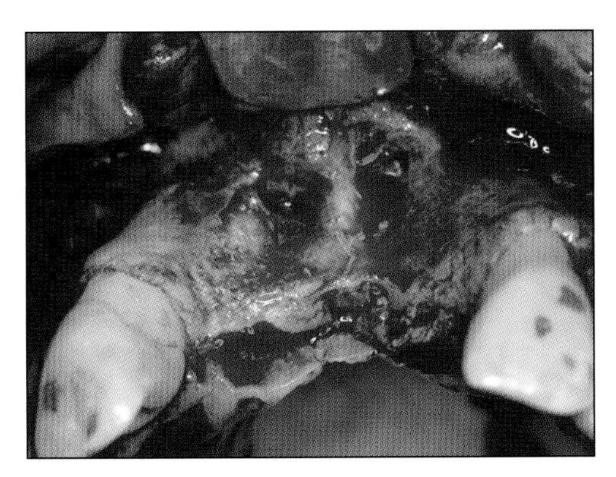

Fig 8-9h Following flap elevation, the large bone defect in the area of the central incisors is evident. However, the alveolar bone is intact at the adjacent right lateral incisor root.

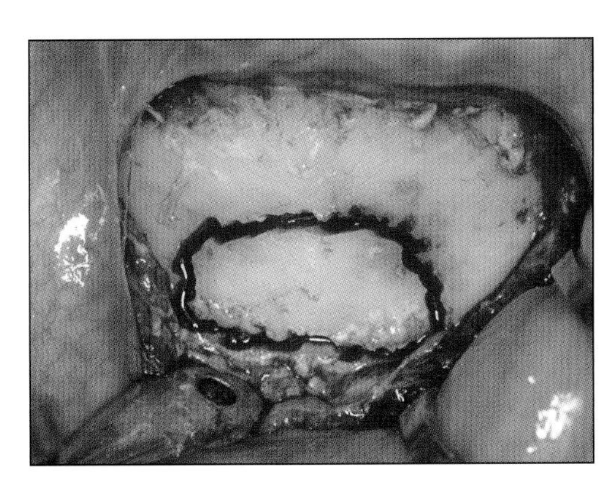

Fig 8-9i A donor site in the chin is used to harvest a large corticocancellous block graft.

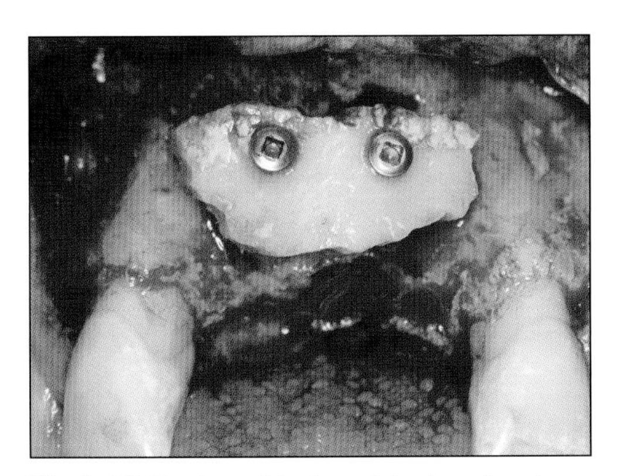

Fig 8-9j The large block graft is placed and stabilized with two fixation screws.

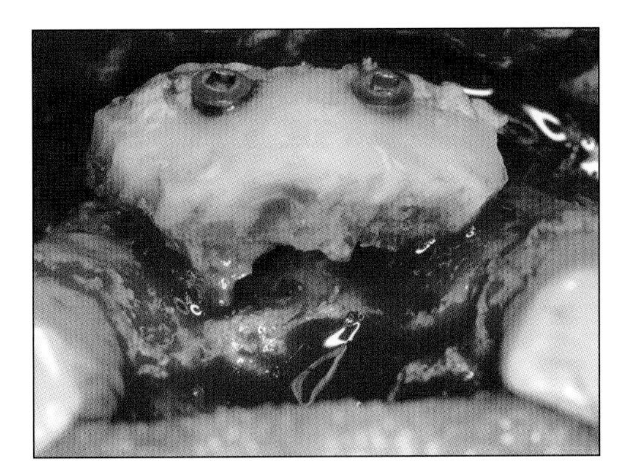

Fig 8-9k The cortical portion of the block graft is used to reestablish a new facial cortex. The cancellous portion is in contact with the perforated host bed. The voids between the bone surface and the block graft will be filled with autogenous bone chips.

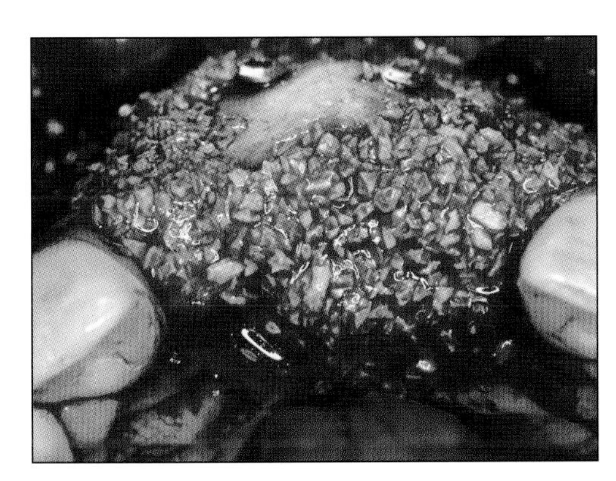

Fig 8-9l The augmentation site is covered with a layer of DBBM particles to round off the ridge contour and to protect the block graft.

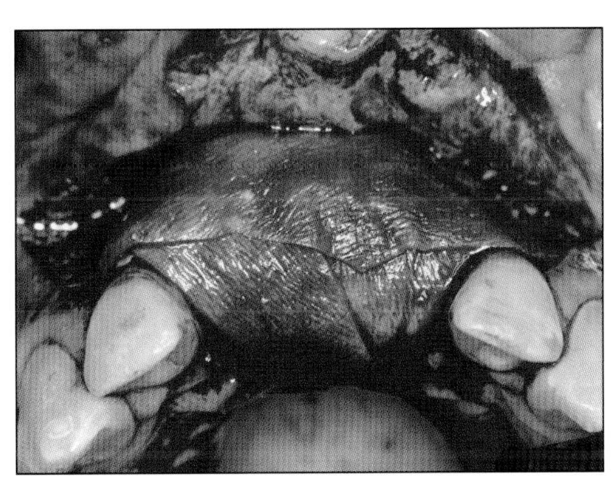

Fig 8-9m The augmentation material is covered with a large collagen membrane (30 × 40 mm) using a double-layer technique.

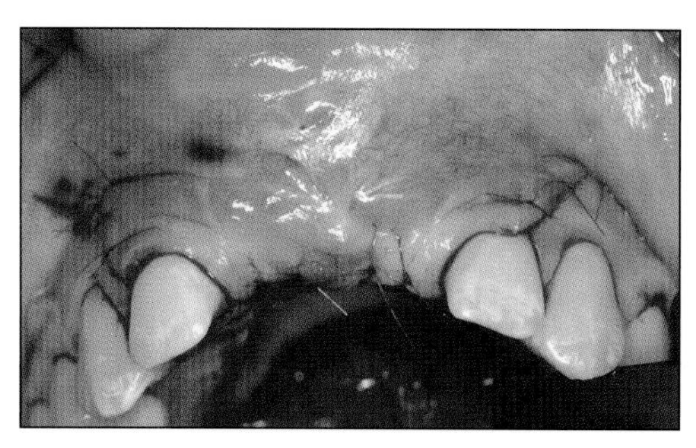

Fig 8-9n Following incision of the periosteum, the surgery is completed with tension-free primary wound closure.

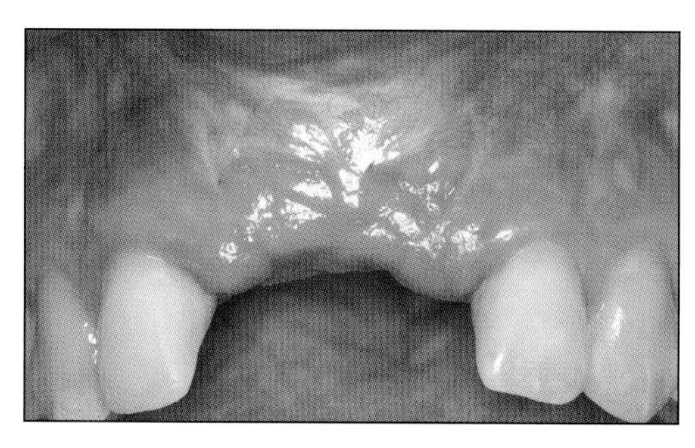

Fig 8-9o Eight months following ridge augmentation, the site demonstrates complication-free healing.

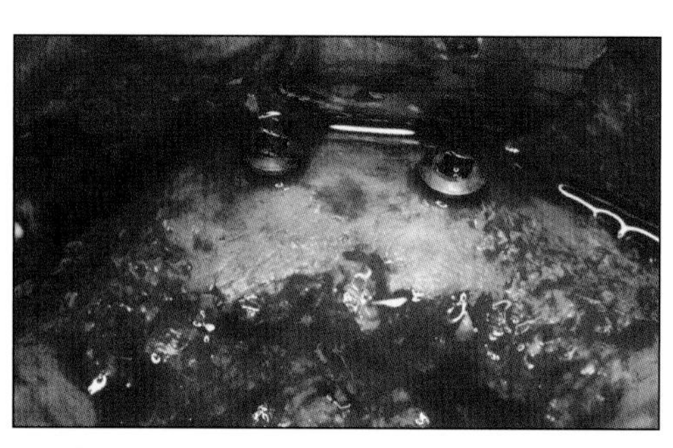

Fig 8-9p An excellent regenerative outcome is apparent following flap elevation. The heads of the fixation screws indicate that no significant surface resorption of the block graft took place during healing.

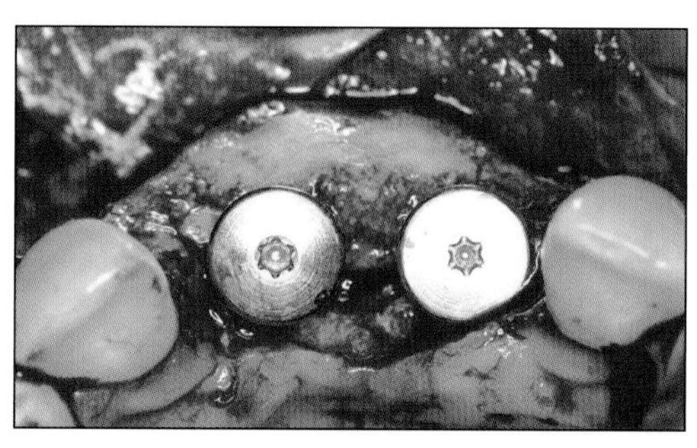

Fig 8-9q The regenerative outcome has allowed implant placement in a correct three-dimensional position.

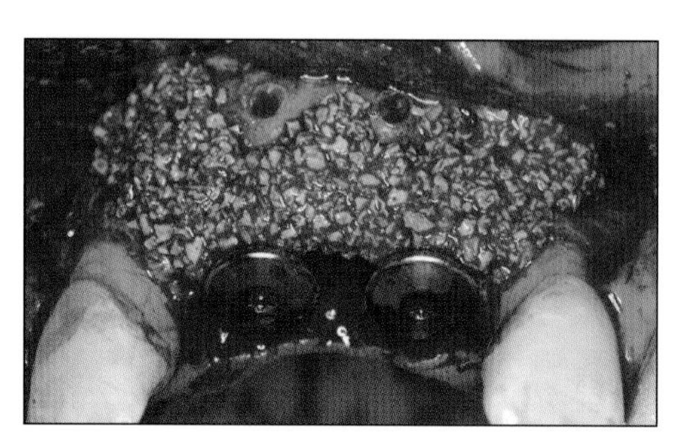

Fig 8-9r To protect the newly established facial bone wall against resorption, a layer of DBBM particles again is applied prior to wound closure.

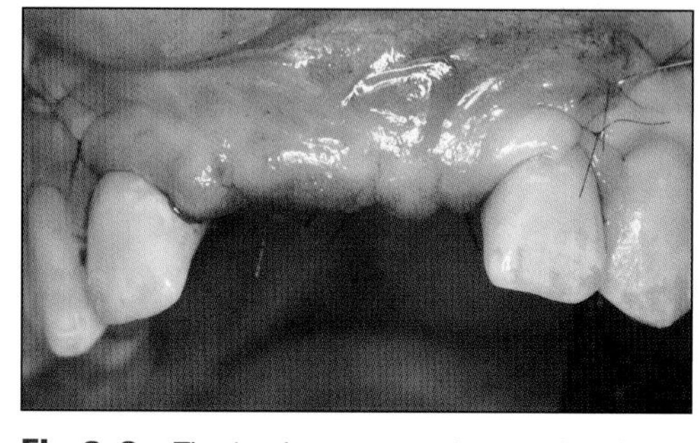

Fig 8-9s The implant surgery is completed with primary wound closure to allow submerged implant healing.

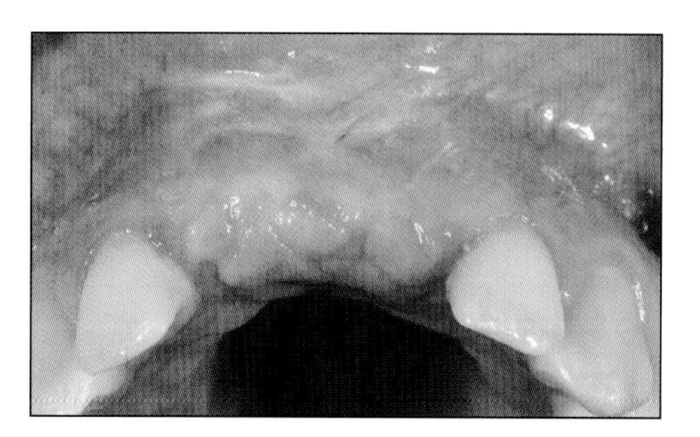

Fig 8-9t After 3 months of healing, examination of the clinical status revealed uneventful healing of the soft tissues.

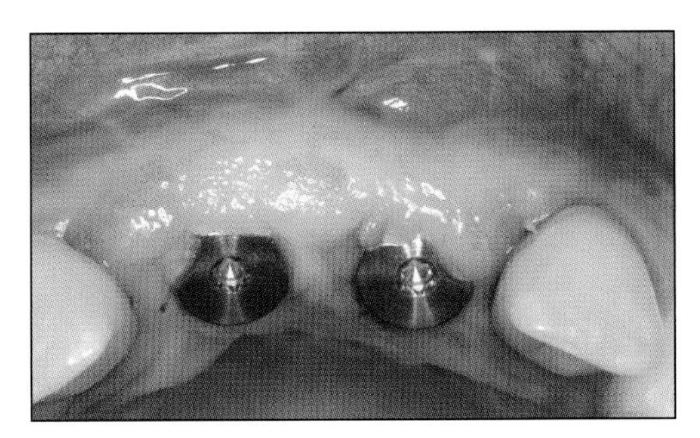

Fig 8-9u To initiate prosthetic restoration, a reopening procedure is performed with a punch technique. Longer titanium healing abutments are inserted. The blanching of the mucosa indicates the pressure deliberately applied to move the keratinized mucosa toward the facial aspect.

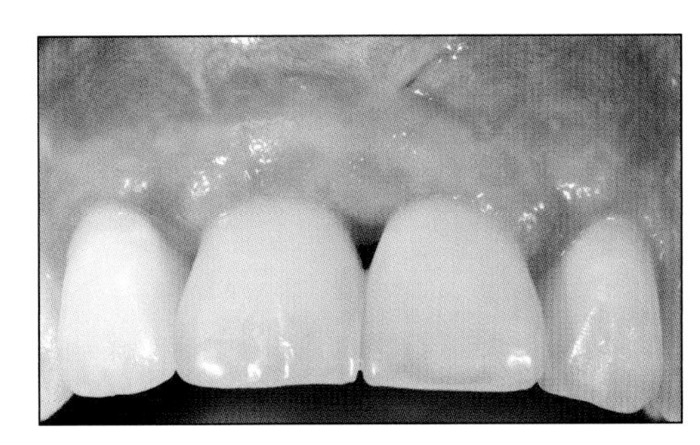

Fig 8-9v Two provisional crowns are placed to initiate the important phase of soft tissue conditioning.

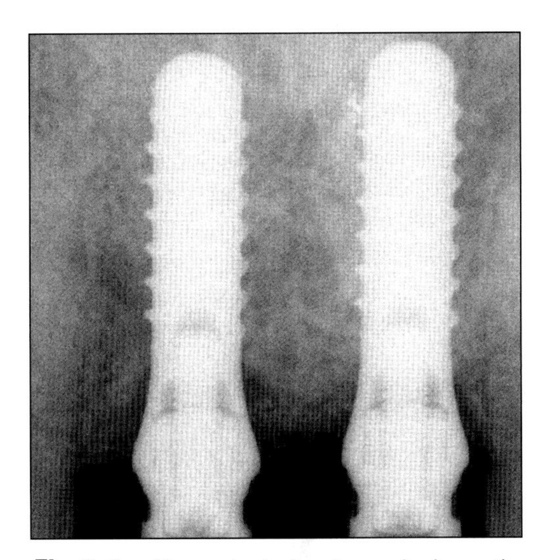

Fig 8-9w The periapical radiograph shows the two implants and the surrounding bone tissue. The two implants were restored with titanium copings and acrylic resin provisional crowns.

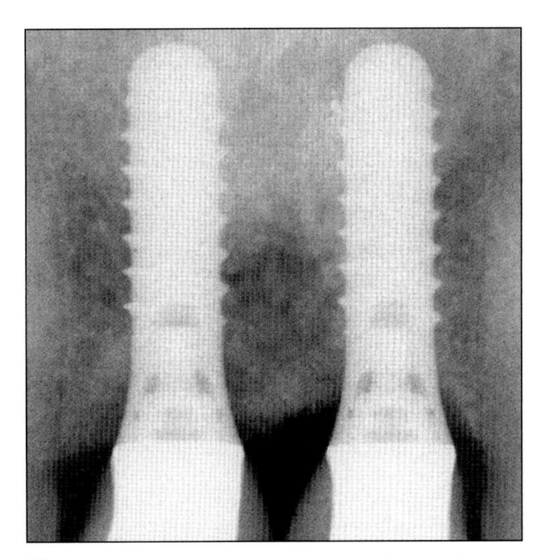

Fig 8-9x The 5-year follow-up radiograph confirms that peri-implant bone crest levels are stable.

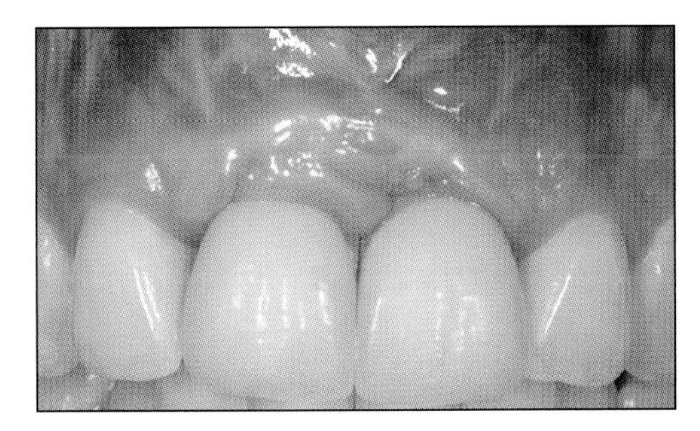

Fig 8-9y At 5 years, both implants have been restored with metal-ceramic crowns by the referring dentist. The soft tissue levels are quite pleasing, but scar tissue formation is evident.

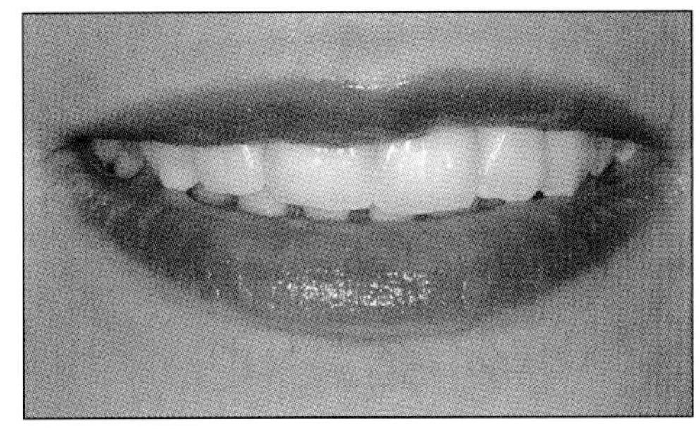

Fig 8-9z Because of the patient's low lip line, the esthetic outcome is pleasing.

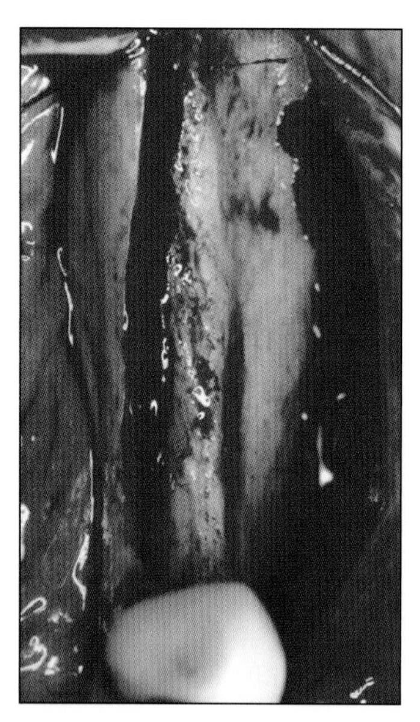

Fig 8-10a A distal-extension situation in the left side of the mandible is complicated by a narrow crest. The crest width measures less than 3 mm, requiring horizontal ridge augmentation using a staged approach.

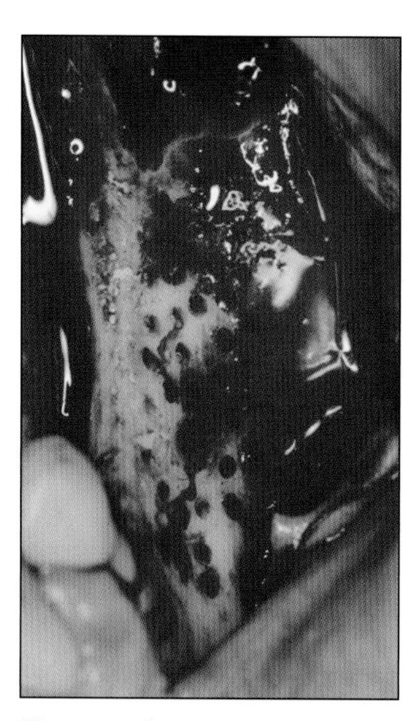

Fig 8-10b The cortical bone surface is perforated with a small round bur to open the marrow cavity of the host bone.

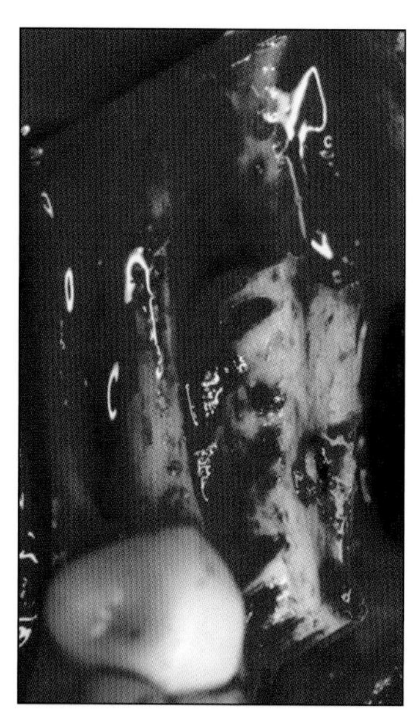

Fig 8-10c A corticocancellous block graft is harvested from the retromolar area within the same flap and appropriately positioned to increase the crest width. The graft is stabilized with a fixation screw.

Case 5

A 54-year-old woman had a distal-extension situation in the left side of the mandible and a narrow alveolar crest of less than 3 mm (Fig 8-10a). This necessitated horizontal ridge augmentation using a block graft harvested from the retromolar area. The same surgical procedure described previously was used (Figs 8-10b to 8-10f).

Postoperatively, a hematoma developed and caused a soft tissue dehiscence in the surgical area, leading to exposure of the collagen membrane (Fig 8-10g). The patient was prescribed antibiotic medication and local rinsing with chlorhexidine digluconate (0.1%), and weekly follow-up examinations ensured that the soft tissues healed by secondary wound healing. Within 4 weeks, the soft tissues had healed without development of an infection in the membrane site (Fig 8-10h). This case confirmed the low risk for complications in the case of a soft tissue dehiscence.

Healing continued without complications, and the soft tissues were satisfactory 6 months postgrafting (Fig 8-10i). The uneventful bone healing was also confirmed with panoramic radiographs (Figs 8-10j and 8-10k). The reopening procedure confirmed an excellent regenerative outcome, despite the initial soft tissue dehiscence (Fig 8-10l), allowing the placement of two implants (Fig 8-10m). The 5-year follow-up examination revealed that both implants were successfully integrated without signs of peri-implant inflammation or bone loss (Figs 8-10n and 8-10o).

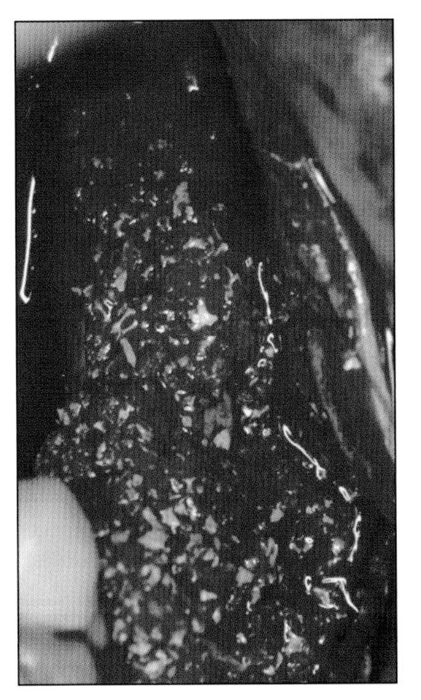

Fig 8-10d The applied block graft is covered with a layer of DBBM particles as graft protection.

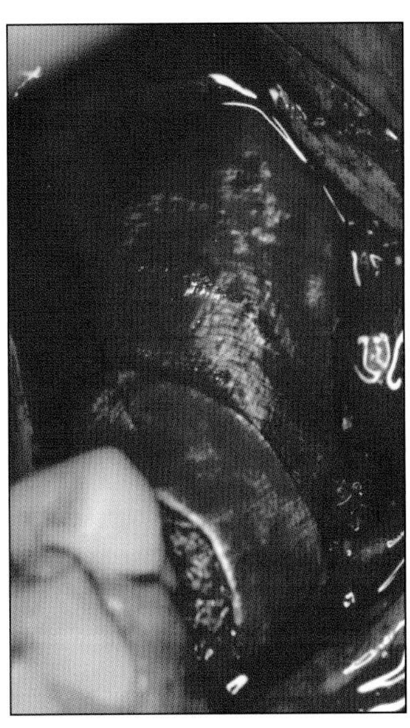

Fig 8-10e A collagen membrane is applied to serve as a barrier and to keep applied bone fillers in place.

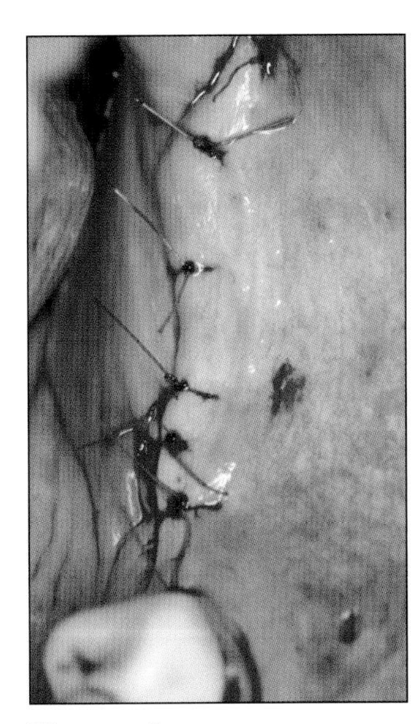

Fig 8-10f The surgery is completed with primary wound closure using interrupted single sutures. In retrospect, the distance between the posterior sutures is too great, which ultimately caused a soft tissue dehiscence when a hematoma developed.

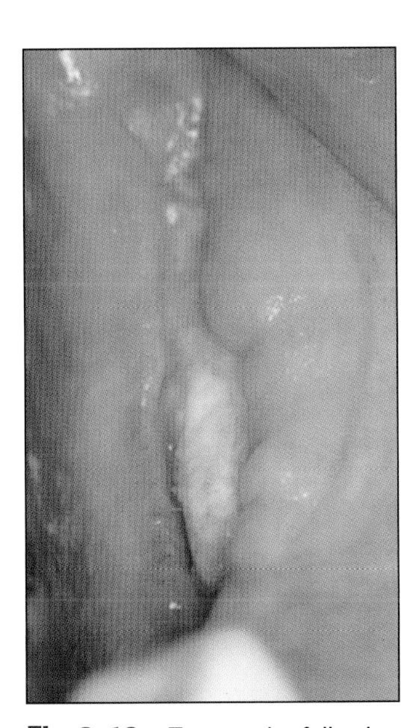

Fig 8-10g Two weeks following augmentation, an extended soft tissue dehiscence is evident with the collagen membrane largely exposed. The patient continued local rinsing with chlorhexidine digluconate and returned weekly for local cleaning.

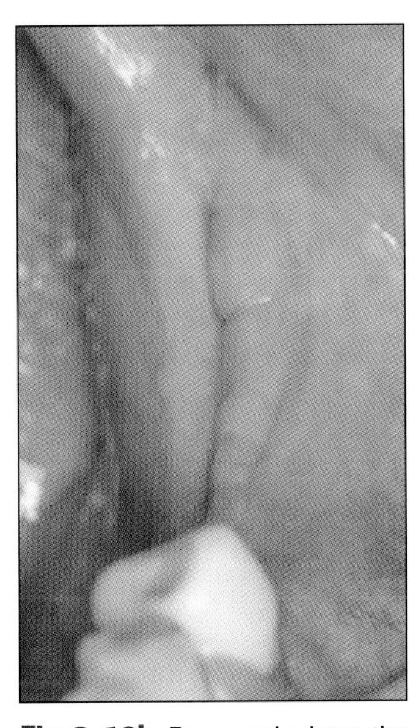

Fig 8-10h Four weeks later, the situation is significantly improved. By secondary wound healing, the dehiscence has closed without development of an infection.

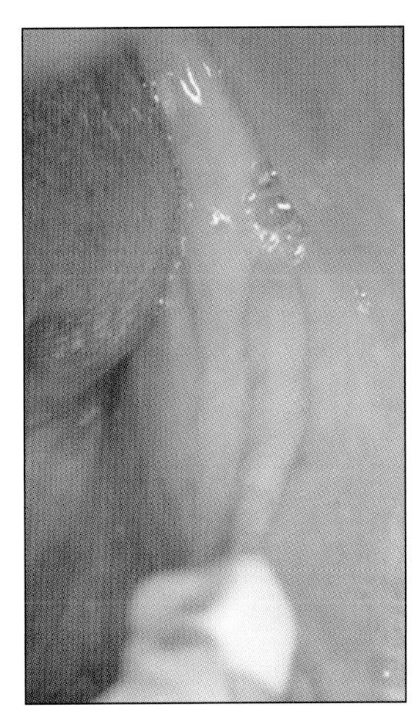

Fig 8-10i Six months following augmentation, soft tissues in the surgical site are well healed.

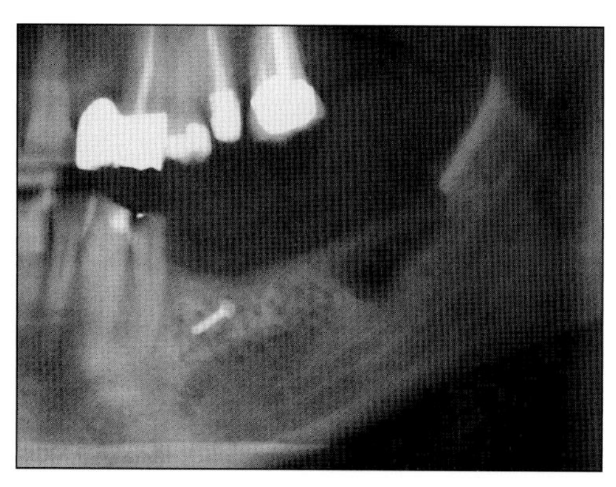

Fig 8-10j The postsurgical radiograph reveals the donor site and the augmentation site with the applied perforations of the cortical bone surface.

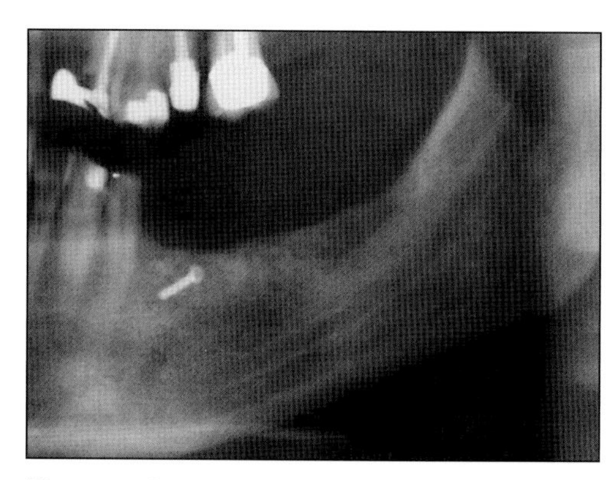

Fig 8-10k A radiograph taken 6 months later demonstrates clear signs of bone regeneration in both sites.

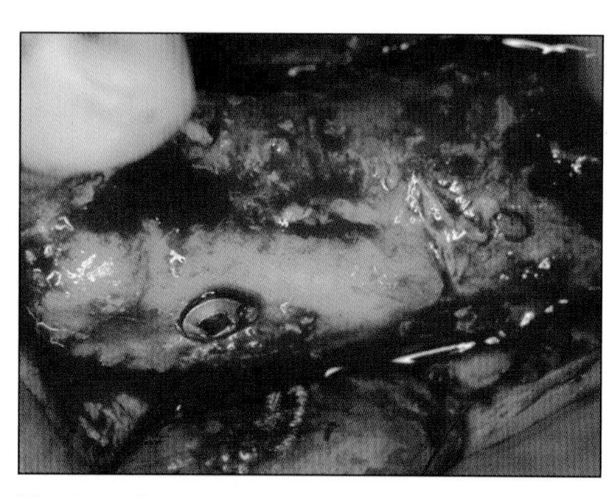

Fig 8-10l During the second surgery, the applied block is clearly recognizable. Its volume has been well maintained.

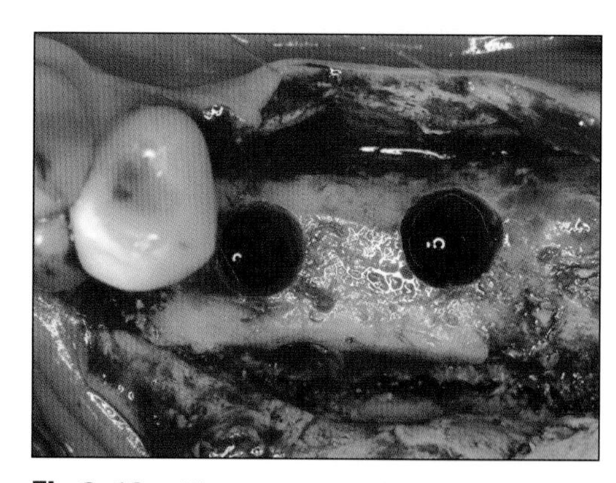

Fig 8-10m The new crest width of roughly 7 mm allows implant placement with a thick facial bone wall at both implant sites.

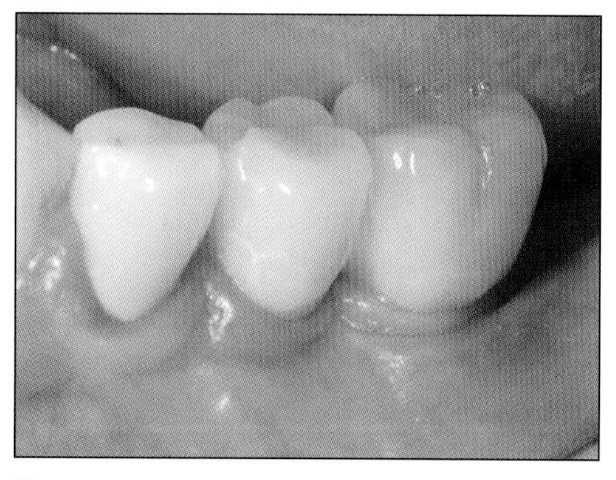

Fig 8-10n At the 5-year follow-up examination, the sites demonstrate healthy peri-implant soft tissues.

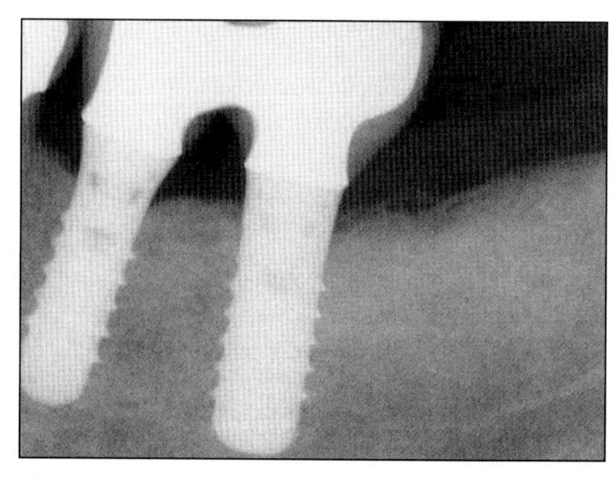

Fig 8-10o The 5-year follow-up radiograph reveals excellent peri-implant bone levels.

Conclusion

In many instances, alveolar resorption following tooth extraction, trauma, or pathologic conditions results in a ridge form that precludes implant insertion without prior augmentation. Autogenous block graft augmentation can increase bone volume and improve bone quality prior to implant placement, ensuring better primary implant stability and improving three-dimensional implant positioning. This chapter discussed the surgical techniques and conditions that are known to enhance the predictability of success for horizontal ridge augmentation.

References

1. Aghaloo TL, Moy PK. Which hard tissue augmentation techniques are the most successful in furnishing bony support for implant placement? Int J Oral Maxillofac Implants 2007;22(suppl):49–70.
2. Tolman DE. Reconstructive procedures with endosseous implants in grafted bone: A review of the literature. Int J Oral Maxillofac Implants 1995;10:275–294.
3. Brånemark PI, Lindström J, Hallén O, Breine U, Jeppson PH, Ohman A. Reconstruction of the defective mandible. Scand J Plast Reconstr Surg 1975;9:116–128.
4. Breine U, Brånemark PI. Reconstruction of alveolar jaw bone. Scand J Plast Reconstr Surg 1980;14:23–48.
5. Ten Bruggenkate CM, Kraaijenhagen HA, van der Kwast WA, Krekeler G, Oostenbeek HS. Autogenous maxillary bone grafts in conjunction with placement of ITI endosseous implants. Int J Oral Maxillofac Surg 1992;21:81–84.
6. Misch CM, Misch CE, Resnik RR, Ismail YH. Reconstruction of maxillary alveolar defects with mandibular symphysis grafts for dental implants: A preliminary procedural report. Int J Oral Maxillofac Implants 1992;7:360–366.
7. Dahlin C, Linde A, Gottlow J, Nyman S. Healing of bone defects by guided tissue regeneration. Plast Reconstr Surg 1988;81:672–676.
8. Buser D, Dula K, Belser U, Hirt HP, Berthold H. Localized ridge augmentation using guided bone regeneration. 1. Surgical procedure in the maxilla. Int J Periodontics Restorative Dent 1993;13:29–45.
9. Nevins M, Mellonig JT. The advantages of localized ridge augmentation prior to implant placement. A staged event. Int J Periodontics Restorative Dent 1994;14:97–111.
10. Buser D, Dula K, Hirt HP, Schenk RK. Lateral ridge augmentation using autografts and barrier membranes: A clinical study with 40 partially edentulous patients. J Oral Maxillofac Surg 1996;54:420–432.
11. Augthun M, Yildirim M, Spiekermann H, Biesterfeld S. Healing of bone defects in combination with immediate implants using the membrane technique. Int J Oral Maxillofac Implants 1995;10:421–428.
12. Hürzeler MB, Strub JR. Guided bone regeneration around exposed implants: A new bioresorbable device and bioresorbable membrane pins. Pract Periodontics Aesthet Dent 1995;7:37–47; quiz 50.
13. Zitzmann NU, Naef R, Schärer P. Resorbable versus nonresorbable membranes in combination with Bio-Oss for guided bone regeneration. Int J Oral Maxillofac Implants 1997;12:844–852.
14. von Arx T, Buser D. Horizontal ridge augmentation using autogenous block grafts and the guided bone regeneration technique with collagen membranes: A clinical study with 42 patients. Clin Oral Implants Res 2006;17:359–366.
15. Hising P, Bolin A, Branting C. Reconstruction of severely resorbed alveolar ridge crests with dental implants using a bovine bone mineral for augmentation. Int J Oral Maxillofac Implants 2001;16:90–97.
16. Friedmann A, Strietzel FP, Maretzki B, Pitaru S, Bernimoulin JP. Histological assessment of augmented jaw bone utilizing a new collagen barrier membrane compared to a standard barrier membrane to protect a granular bone substitute material. A randomized clinical trial. Clin Oral Implants Res 2002;13:587–594.
17. Meijndert L, Raghoebar GM, Schüpbach P, Meijer HJ, Vissink A. Bone quality at the implant site after reconstruction of a local defect of the maxillary anterior ridge with chin bone or deproteinised cancellous bovine bone. Int J Oral Maxillofac Surg 2005;34:877–884.
18. Hämmerle CH, Jung RE, Yaman D, Lang NP. Ridge augmentation by applying bioresorbable membranes and deproteinized bovine bone mineral: A report of twelve consecutive cases. Clin Oral Implants Res 2008;19:19–25.
19. Pikos MA. Block autografts for localized ridge augmentation. 1. The posterior maxilla. Implant Dent 1999;8:279–285.
20. Pikos MA. Block autografts for localized ridge augmentation. 2. The posterior mandible. Implant Dent 2000;9:67–75.

21. Lindeboom JAH, van den Akker HP. A prospective placebo-controlled double-blind trial of antibiotic prophylaxis in intraoral bone grafting procedures: A pilot study. Oral Surg Oral Med Oral Pathol Oral Radiol Endod 2003;96:669–672.
22. Löe H, Schiott CR. The effect of mouth rinses and topical application of chlorhexidine on the development of dental plaque and gingivitis in man. J Periodontal Res 1970;5:79–83.
23. Worral SF, Knibbs PJ, Glenwright HD. Methods of reducing contamination of the atmosphere from use of an air polisher. Br Dent J 1987;163:118–119.
24. Balbuena L, Stambaugh KI, Ramirez SG, Yeager C. Effects of topical oral antiseptic rinses on bacterial counts of saliva in healthy human subjects. Otolaryngol Head Neck Surg 1998;118:625–629.
25. Binahmed A, Stoykewych A, Peterson L. Single preoperative dose versus long-term prophylactic antibiotic regimens in dental implant surgery. Int J Oral Maxillofac Implants 2005;20:115–117.
26. Kashani H, Dahlin C, Alse'n B. Influence of different prophylactic antibiotic regimens on implant survival rate: A retrospective clinical study. Clin Implant Dent Relat Res 2005;7:32–35.
27. von Arx T, Cochran DL, Hermann JS, Schenk RK, Buser D. Lateral ridge augmentation using different bone fillers and barrier membrane application. Clin Oral Impl Res 2001;12:260–269.
28. Chiapasco M, Abati S, Romeo E, Vogel G. Clinical outcome of autogenous bone blocks or guided bone regeneration with ePTFE membranes for the reconstruction of narrow edentulous ridges. Clin Oral Implants Res 1999;10:278–288.
29. Phillips JH, Rahn BA. Fixation effects on membranous and endochondral onlay bone-graft resorption. Plast Reconstr Surg 1988;82:872–877.
30. LaTrenta GS, McCarthy JG, Breitbart AS, May M, Sissons HA. The role of rigid skeletal fixation in bone-graft augmentation of the craniofacial skeleton. Plast Reconstr Surg 1989;84:578–588.
31. Lin KY, Bartlett SP, Yaremchuk MJ, Fallon M, Grossman RF, Whitaker LA. The effect of rigid fixation on the survival of onlay bone grafts: An experimental study. Plast Reconstr Surg 1990:86:449–456.
32. Aspenberg P, Goodman S, Toksvig-Larsen S, Ryd L, Albrektsson T. Intermittent micromotion inhibits bone ingrowth. Titanium implants in rabbits. Acta Orthop Scand 1992;63:141–145.
33. Phillips JH, Rahn BA. Fixation effects on membranous and endochondral onlay bone graft revascularization and bone deposition. Plast Reconstr Surg 1990;85:891–897.
34. Schenk RK, Buser D, Hardwick WR, Dahlin C. Healing pattern of bone regeneration in membrane-protected defects: A histologic study in the canine mandible. Int J Oral Maxillofac Implants 1994;9: 13–29.
35. de Carvalho PS, Vasconcellos LW, Pi J. Influence of bed preparation on the incorporation of autogenous bone grafts: A study in dogs. Int J Oral Maxillofac Implants 2000;15:565–570.
36. Adeyemo WL, Reuther T, Bloch W, et al. Influence of host periosteum and recipient bed perforation on the healing of onlay mandibular bone graft: An experimental pilot study in the sheep. Oral Maxillofac Surg 2008;12:19–28.
37. Majzoub Z, Berengo M, Giardino R, Aldini N, Cordioli G. Role of intramarrow penetration in osseous repair: A pilot study in the rabbit calvaria. J Periodontol 1999;70:1501–1510.
38. Rompen EH, Biewer R, Vanheusden A, Zahedi S, Nusgens B. The influence of cortical perforations and of space filling with peripheral blood on the kinetics of guided bone generation. A comparative histometric study in the rat. Clin Oral Implants Res 1999;10:85–94.
39. Min S, Sato S, Murai M, et al. Effects of marrow penetration on bone augmentation within a titanium cap in rabbit calvarium. J Periodontol 2007;78: 1978–1984.
40. Lundgren AK, Lundgren D, Hämmerle CH, Nyman S, Sennerby L. Influence of decortication of the donor bone on guided bone augmentation. An experimental study in the rabbit skull bone. Clin Oral Implants Res 2000;11:99–106.
41. Slotte C, Lundgren D. Impact of cortical perforations of contiguous donor bone in a guided bone augmentation procedure: An experimental study in the rabbit skull. Clin Implant Dent Relat Res 2002;4:1–10.
42. Donos N, Kostopoulos L, Karring T. Augmentation of the mandible with GTR and onlay cortical bone grafting. An experimental study in the rat. Clin Oral Implants Res 2002;13:175–184.
43. Donos N, Kostopoulos L, Karring T. Alveolar ridge augmentation by combining autogenous mandibular bone grafts and non-resorbable membranes. An experimental study in the rat. Clin Oral Implants Res 2002;13:185–191.
44. Donos N, Kostopoulos L, Karring T. Augmentation of the rat jaw with autogeneic cortico-cancellous bone grafts and guided tissue regeneration. Clin Oral Implants Res 2002;13:192–202.
45. Donos N, Kostopoulos L, Karring T. Alveolar ridge augmentation using a resorbable copolymer membrane and autogenous bone grafts. An experimental study in the rat. Clin Oral Implants Res 2002;13: 203–213.
46. Busenlechner D, Kantor M, Tangl S, et al. Alveolar ridge augmentation with a prototype trilayer membrane and various bone grafts: A histomorphometric study in baboons. Clin Oral Implants Res 2005;16:220–227.
47. Widmark G, Andersson B, Ivanoff CJ. Mandibular bone graft in the anterior maxilla for single-tooth implants. Int J Oral Maxillofac Surg 1997;26:106–109.
48. Antoun H, Sitbon JM, Martinez H, Missika P. A prospective randomized study comparing two techniques of bone augmentation: Onlay graft alone or associated with a membrane. Clin Oral Implants Res 2001;12:632–639.
49. Proussaefs P, Lozada J. The use of intraorally harvested autogenous block grafts for vertical alveolar ridge augmentation: A human study. Int J Periodontics Restorative Dent 2005;25:351–363.

50. Maiorana C, Beretta M, Salina S, Santoro F. Reduction of autogenous bone graft resorption by means of Bio-Oss coverage: A prospective study. Int J Periodontics Restorative Dent 2005;25:19–25.
51. Pinholt EM, Solheim E, Talsnes O, Larsen TB, Bang GB, Kirkeby OJ. Revascularization of calvarial, mandibular, tibial, and iliac bone grafts in rats. Ann Plast Surg 1994;33:193–197.
52. Alberius P, Gordh M, Lindberg L, Johnell O. Influence of surrounding soft tissues on onlay bone graft incorporation. Oral Surg Oral Med Oral Pathol Oral Radiol Endod 1996;82:22–33.
53. Ham AW. Some histophysiological problems peculiar to calcified tissues. J Bone Joint Surg Am 1952;34:701–728.
54. Burwell RG. Studies in the transplantation of bone. 8. The fresh composite homograft-autograft of cancellous bone. J Bone Joint Surg Br 1964;46:110–140.
55. Gray CJ, Elves MW. Early osteogenesis in compact bone isografts: A quantitative study of the contributions of the different graft cells. Calcif Tissue Int 1979;29:225–237.
56. Burchardt H. The biology of bone graft repair. Clin Orthop 1983;174:28–42.
57. Burchardt H, Enneking WF. Transplantation of bone. Surg Clin North Am 1978;58:403–427.
58. Nathanson A. The early vascularization of an autogenous bone inlay into an artificial defect in the rabbit mandibula. Acta Otolaryngol 1978;85:135–148.
59. de Marco AC, Jardini MA, Lima LA. Revascularization of autogenous block grafts with or without an ePTFE membrane. Int J Oral Maxillofac Implants 2005;20:867–874.
60. Jardini MA, de Marco AC, Lima LA. Early healing pattern of autogenous bone grafts with and without ePTFE membranes: A histomorphometric study in rats. Oral Surg Oral Med Oral Pathol Oral Radiol Endod 2005;100:666–673.
61. Lorenzetti M, Mozzati M, Campanino PP, Valente G. Bone augmentation of the inferior floor of the maxillary sinus with autogenous bone or composite bone grafts: A histologic-histomorphometric preliminary report. Int J Oral Maxillofac Implants 1998;13:69–76.
62. Matsumoto MA, Filho HN, Francischone CE, Consolaro A. Microscopic analysis of reconstructed maxillary alveolar ridges using autogenous bone grafts from the chin and iliac crest. Int J Oral Maxillofac Implants 2002;17:507–516.
63. Zerbo IR, de Lange GL, Joldersma M, Bronckers AL, Burger EH. Fate of monocortical bone blocks grafted in the human maxilla: A histological and histomorphometric study. Clin Oral Implants Res 2003;14:759–766.
64. Raghoebar GM, Batenburg RH, Vissink A, Reintsema H. Augmentation of localized defects of the anterior maxillary ridge with autogenous bone before insertion of implants. J Oral Maxillofac Surg 1996;54:1180–1185.
65. Bedrossian E, Tawfilis A, Alijanian A. Veneer grafting: A technique for augmentation of the resorbed alveolus prior to implant placement. A clinical report. Int J Oral Maxillofac Implants 2000;15:853–858.
66. Sethi A, Kaus T. Ridge augmentation using mandibular block bone grafts: Preliminary results of an ongoing prospective study. Int J Oral Maxillofac Implants 2001;16:378–388.
67. McCarthy C, Patel RR, Wragg PF, Brook IM. Dental implants and onlay bone grafts in the anterior maxilla: Analysis of clinical outcome. Int J Oral Maxillofac Implants 2003;18:238–241.
68. Buser D, Ingimarsson S, Dula K, Lussi A, Hirt HP, Belser UC. Long-term stability of osseointegrated implants in augmented bone: A 5-year prospective study in partially edentulous patients. Int J Periodontics Restorative Dent 2002;22:108–117.

CHAPTER 9

Guided Bone Regeneration for Vertical Ridge Augmentation: Past, Present, and Future

Massimo Simion
Isabella Rocchietta

Successful osseointegration is predicated on the placement of dental implants in a sufficient volume of bone. When teeth are lost to trauma or periodontal disease, there is often a lack of adequate bone volume. Placement of implants in areas with limited bone height may not be possible. Such areas include the maxillary molar and premolar region, where only a reduced alveolar process may separate the maxillary sinus from the oral cavity, and the corresponding mandibular region with its mandibular nerve canal. Moreover, a large interarch space alters coronal length and form and produces an unfavorable crown-root ratio in the final prosthetic reconstruction.[1] The latter may result in an esthetically unacceptable final prosthetic restoration and/or lead to difficulties in performing adequate oral hygiene regimens, potentially jeopardizing the long-term prognosis.

A number of different techniques have been developed to reconstruct vertically deficient alveolar ridges to allow dental implant placement in either a simultaneous or staged approach. These include extraoral or intraoral autogenous onlay bone grafts, distraction osteogenesis, and guided bone regeneration (GBR). This chapter discusses the early development of GBR, describes the currently recommended surgical techniques for GBR in vertically deficient alveolar ridges, and considers possible future developments.

Past Research

GBR, a regenerative procedure derived from the principles of guided tissue regeneration around natural teeth, is used for ridge augmentation. The biologic principles of guided tissue regeneration were applied by Nyman et al[2] in the early 1980s. The surgical technique applied in GBR involves the placement of a cell-occlusive barrier membrane to protect the blood clot and to create a secluded space around the bone defect to allow bone regeneration without competition from other tissues. Schenk et al[3] demonstrated how the newly regenerated bone progresses in a programmed sequence through a series of biologic steps that closely parallel the pattern of normal bone growth and development.

Animal studies

The first animal studies reporting vertical bone regeneration around protruding implants date back to the 1990s. Schmid et al[4] presented an animal study on vertical ridge augmentation in which implants were placed in rabbit skulls. The implant portion that was left to protrude was covered by an expanded polytetrafluoroethylene (ePTFE) membrane. After 3 months of healing, some bone formation was detected under the membrane, demonstrating that osseointegration was possible with partially inserted implants. Similar findings were reported by Linde et al[5] in a rat calvaria study using dome-shaped ePTFE membranes.

Jovanovic et al[6] achieved supracrestal bone regeneration in five dogs with a submerged membrane technique, starting from a mean vertical mandibular defect of 2.7 mm. Jensen et al[7] chose to use the inferior mandibular border in four fox hounds as a model to simulate the chronic, corticalized human mandible. The protruding implants were grafted with demineralized freeze-dried bone allograft, corticocancellous iliac autograft, or blood clot. Some sites were covered with an ePTFE membrane, and others were left uncovered. Results showed that the barrier function improved graft volume and bone-to-implant contact. This was confirmed in a dog model a year later by Renvert et al,[8] who demonstrated the potential for alveolar bone growth in a protected space around screw implants with exposed threads.

In another dog model, attempts were made to use resorbable polylactic membranes for vertical ridge augmentation with and without an autogenous underlying graft.[9,10] Histologic and morphometric analyses performed after 3 and 5 months revealed that the membrane group did not exhibit greater bone-to-implant contact than the untreated controls. Thus, it was concluded that resorbable membranes did not fulfill the space-maintenance requirement for vertical ridge augmentation.

A recent report[11] described the placement of protruding implants in a canine mandible. The implants were covered with an ePTFE membrane, and peripheral venous blood was injected under the barrier. Histologic and histomorphometric analyses performed after 6 months revealed significant regeneration of bone volume. However, the bone did not appear to be in direct contact with the implants. This was due to the absence of a grafting material under the barrier membrane in a severe vertical alveolar defect.

Human studies

In 1994, Simion et al[12] reported the first human and histologic study of vertical bone regeneration of the atrophic edentulous ridge with the GBR technique. In five partially edentulous patients, 10 implants were inserted, left to protrude 4 to 7 mm from the original cortical bone level, and covered with ePTFE membranes secured with fixation screws. In addition, titanium miniscrews were placed for later histologic evaluation. The results demonstrated that vertical bone regeneration was possible to an extent of 4 mm in height. The histologic examination showed that all retrieved miniscrews were in direct contact with bone and that regenerated bone was able to osseointegrate with commercially pure titanium implants; the mean percentage of direct contact between the titanium surface and the newly regenerated bone was approximately 42%.

Tinti et al[13] tested this model in a clinical study in which 6 patients received 14 implants. Vertical bone regeneration extended up to 7 mm with the membrane technique when autogenous bone chips were added beneath the barrier. This technique for vertical augmentation was later confirmed by Simion et al[14] in 20 patients receiving 56 implants. Demineralized freeze-dried bone or autogenous bone chips were grafted under the ePTFE membranes. The study demonstrated highly successful and predictable vertical bone regeneration; the percentage of bone-to-implant contact varied from 39.1% to 63.2%, regardless of the allograft or autograft used.

Analogous results were reported the same year by Tinti and Parma-Benfenati,[15] who applied autogenous bone chips around protruding implants and covered them with a nonresorbable barrier membrane. A qualitative and quantitative histomorphometric analysis reported lower mean bone-to-implant contact values in the protruding threads than in the threads placed in native bone (22.0% ± 9.4% exposed vs 44.0% ± 7.8% unexposed).[16] At that time, there was clear evidence that significant volumes of vertical bone could be regenerated under titanium-reinforced ePTFE membranes since volume increased when a graft was positioned around the protruding implants. However, the predictability and long-term results of the newly regenerated bone were still questioned.

A retrospective multicenter study[17] evaluating 1 to 5 years of prosthetic loading was performed to answer this question. The study evaluated 123 implants inserted in atrophic alveolar ridges. The implants were allowed to protrude 2 to 7 mm from the bone crest, and a titanium-reinforced ePTFE membrane was positioned to protect either the blood clot (group A), an allograft (group B), or an autograft (group C). Mean bone loss of 1.35 mm for group A, 1.87 mm for group B, and 1.71 mm for group C was similar to that reported in previous long-term studies of implants placed in horizontally regenerated bone[18–20] or native bone.[21–23] Only 1 of 123 implants failed, and 2 demonstrated greater than normal bone loss, leading to an overall success rate of 97.5% according to the success criteria listed by Albrektsson et al.[24] On the basis of these results, the authors concluded that bone vertically regenerated with GBR techniques responds to implant placement like native, nonregenerated bone.[17]

Another retrospective study conducted in 2004 evaluated implant stability in regenerated bone after up to 7 years of prosthetic loading.[25] Severe atrophy of the posterior maxilla was treated by combining sinus floor elevation and vertical ridge augmentation. Implants were either placed simultaneously with the regenerative procedure using autogenous bone chips and an ePTFE membrane or at the stage-two surgery performed 6 to 13 months later. Examination of 38 implants consecutively placed in 16 surgical sites revealed mean crestal bone loss of 1.65 mm on the mesial side and 1.68 mm on the distal side between abutment connection and 1 to 7 years of follow-up.

Present Surgical Technique

A meticulous surgical technique is mandatory to achieve a successful functional and esthetic outcome.

Indications and prerequisites for surgery

The main indication for vertical ridge augmentation via GBR is a lack of adequate vertical bone height for implant placement in partially edentulous patients who have bone peaks present at the adjacent teeth. Patients must have adequate interarch space for the future prosthetic rehabilitation. In addition, patients whose loss of natural teeth in the anterior region of the maxilla has compromised esthetics are candidates for vertical augmentation.

Case selection and decision parameters

Soft and hard tissue assessments
The clinical examination should include a thorough assessment of the soft tissues because the presence of sufficient soft tissue is mandatory for correct tissue closure and site accessibility. Moreover, the patient's compliance and understanding of the procedure as well as his or her optimal health are necessary.

Preoperative planning requires clinical and radiographic examinations. Periapical radiographs, panoramic radiographs, and computed tomograms are mandatory to assess the alveolar ridge morphology.

Oral assessment
There must be no signs of active periodontitis or endodontic lesions in the oral cavity. All necessary treatments must be performed prior to any bone augmentation or implant placement procedure.

Bone peaks of adjacent teeth
The existing periodontium of the adjacent teeth should be the main consideration in selection of appropriate cases. The tooth or teeth should exhibit either moderate or no probing attachment loss. This prerequisite favors bone fill of the severe defect by allowing a natural blood supply from a vertical component other than the base of the defect. The adjacent tooth must have a bone peak, which will be the threshold of vertical bone gain, in order to predict the volume of bone that can be regenerated and to avoid involving adjacent periodontal regeneration.

Distance between the bone crest and the alveolar nerve/maxillary sinus cavity
The single-stage procedure involves simultaneous placement of the implants and performance of the augmentation procedure, leading to a healing period of 6 to 7 months prior to membrane removal and abutment connection. This procedure requires adequate bone height (minimum 6 to 7 mm) at baseline for primary stability of the dental implants.

The two-stage procedure involves the completion of the augmentation surgery alone as a first step because bone height is insufficient, followed by membrane removal and implant insertion 6 to 7 months later. The abutment connection is performed after 4 to 6 months of osseointegration, resulting in a total healing period of approximately 10 to 12 months.

Prosthetic margins of adjacent teeth
All fixed overhanging crowns have to be replaced with new removable provisional crowns (and subsequent abutment reconstruction) to avoid the creation of areas where oral hygiene is difficult, leading to bacterial colonization.

Third molar
In patients who are partially edentulous in the posterior segment, the presence of the third molar complicates the procedure and creates a possible area of infection risk other than the adjacent mesial tooth. Hence, if possible, extraction of the third molar in the area to be augmented is strongly recommended.

Graft selection

Autogenous bone grafts represent an ideal matrix to support new bone formation, providing an immunologically compatible source of bone complete with viable bone cells, an osteoconductive scaffold, and growth-modulating molecules required for optimal bone regeneration.[26,27] However, the pain and morbidity often reported at the donor site and the limited supply of autogenous graft material can negatively affect clinical outcomes and patient satisfaction.[28–31] Engineered bone graft materials provide an alternative treatment modality, supplying highly osteoconductive matrices with a chemical composition and crystalline structure similar to the mineral phase of natural bone.

Deproteinized bovine bone mineral (DBBM) is a xenogeneic graft material that has been widely used as a bone substitute in implant dentistry[32–35] and periodontology.[36] DBBM has osteoconductive properties, promoting cellular adhesion and the formation of new bone tissue.[37] It has a physicochemical structure similar to that of human cancellous bone, such as the calcium phosphorus index (2.03) and the isomeric crystalline dimension.[38,39]

Combining autogenous bone and a xenograft allows a reduction of the amount of autogenous bone harvested, decreasing the invasiveness of the technique and the patient's postoperative discomfort.[40] In addition, the combination of autogenous bone and DBBM adds the osteoconductive properties of the xenograft to the osteogenic properties of the autograft.

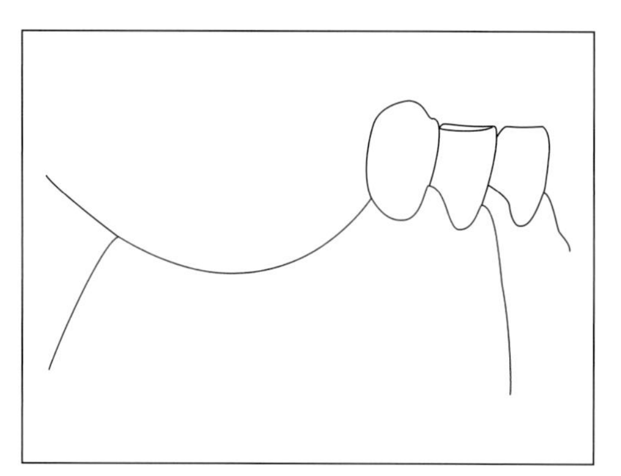

Fig 9-1 Buccal view of flap design. A J-shaped vertical releasing incision is made at the mesiobuccal line angle of the adjacent tooth.

Simion et al[41] evaluated the efficacy of a 1:1 mixture of DBBM and autogenous bone graft covered by an ePTFE membrane when applied for vertical ridge augmentation of atrophic jaws. Clinical results showed significant new hard tissue formation at the second-stage surgery, suggesting successful bone regeneration. Histologic analysis confirmed new bone formation and ongoing remodeling of the autogenous bone and the DBBM particles. These findings support the use of a graft mixture for vertical ridge augmentation.

Surgical procedure

The two-stage procedure provides vertical ridge augmentation of severely atrophic sites by means of tenting screws, a graft, and a nonresorbable barrier membrane.

Patient preparation

Presurgical medication consists of chlorhexidine digluconate 0.20% mouthrinse for 2 minutes (twice daily beginning 3 days in advance of surgery) and an extraoral scrub with povidone-iodine solution. Sedative premedication with diazepam is administered 30 minutes before the surgery. The local anesthetic consists of articaine 4% and epinephrine 1:100,000.

Flap design

A full-thickness crestal incision is performed in the center of the keratinized gingiva from the distal aspect of the last mesial residual tooth to the distal end of the edentulous ridge (or the mesial aspect of the last distal tooth, if present). The incision is extended intrasulcularly to the mesial aspect of one or two adjacent mesial teeth. Vertical releasing incisions are made at the mesiobuccal and mesiopalatal/mesiolingual line angles and at the distal aspect of the crestal incision (or at the distobuccal line angle of the last tooth, if present). Care is taken to create a J-shaped vertical mesial releasing incision to avoid damaging the interdental papilla or the buccal periodontium of the tooth (Fig 9-1).

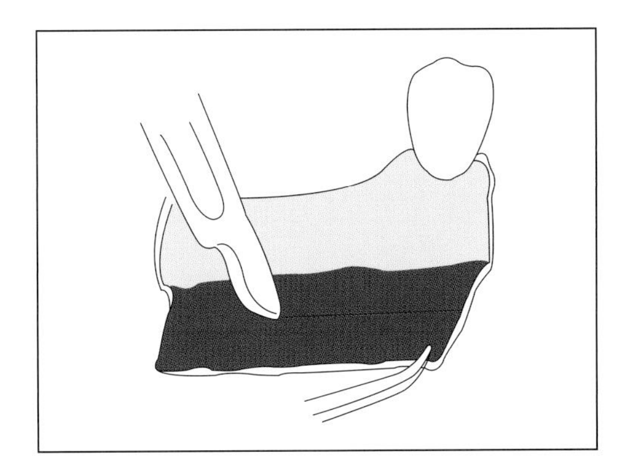

Fig 9-2 A periosteal releasing incision is made on the buccal elevated flap.

Recipient site preparation

The full-thickness buccal and palatal/lingual flaps are elevated to expose the atrophic ridge. All soft tissue remnants are discarded, and the adjacent teeth are root planed. Care is taken not to damage the palatine artery or the mental nerve in severely resorbed maxillae and mandibles. The flaps are handled gently to minimize soft tissue trauma and to strictly avoid soft tissue perforations. The tension of the buccal and palatal/lingual flaps is released by performing a delicate periosteal incision (Fig 9-2).

Graft and donor site preparation

The composite graft consists of autogenous bone mixed with DBBM in a 1:1 ratio. The autogenous bone is harvested in the proximity of the augmentation site with bone scrapers, when possible, or from the retromolar region with trephine burs. Bone harvesting from the mandibular ramus or the maxillary tuberosity is performed when the third molar is missing. A crestal incision is performed, starting 2 to 3 mm distal to the second molar and extending in the direction of the lateral margin of the ramus, followed by a short vertical mesial incision. After the elevation of a full-thickness flap, the osteotomy is accomplished with the use of trephines or thin carbide burs. Bone harvesting is carried out gently under copious irrigation. Care is taken to leave a minimum of 3 mm of bone over the mandibular alveolar nerve to avoid postoperative negative sequelae. After bone collection is completed, the flaps are sutured with interrupted 4-0 silk sutures.

Tenting screw placement

One or more tenting screws are placed, depending on the extent and severity of the atrophy. Care is taken not to surpass the existing bone level of the adjacent tooth or teeth. The exact height is measured by means of two perpendicular periodontal probes placed from the bone peak mesiodistally and from the bone crest apicocoronally. The screws are positioned to retain the graft and to prevent membrane collapse; hence the direction of insertion is vertical, horizontal, or both, according to the anatomy of the defect.

Cortical perforations are made to expose the medullary spaces and promote the bleeding process.

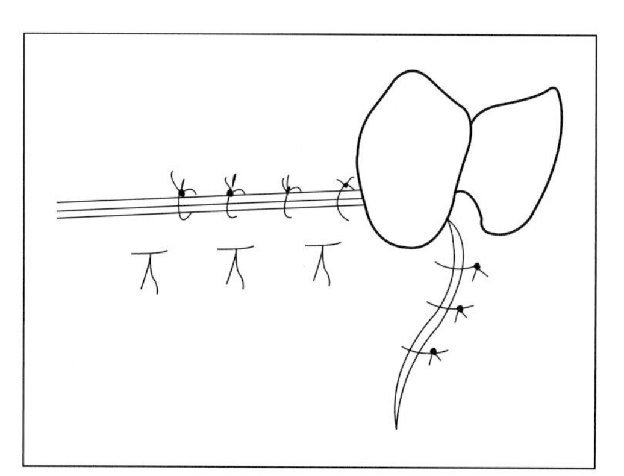

Fig 9-3 Horizontal mattress and interrupted sutures are used to achieve optimal soft tissue closure. Both techniques should be performed with 3- to 4-mm equidistant sutures.

Barrier membrane placement

Prior to membrane placement, the ePTFE barrier is shaped and trimmed to adapt to the defect area perfectly. The titanium structures of the membrane are bent with pliers to obtain the correct crest morphology, and the external portions are trimmed with scissors to extend at least 4 to 5 mm beyond the defect margin. Care is taken to ensure that the membrane is not in direct contact with the adjacent tooth or teeth to avoid bacterial contamination deriving from the sulcus (minimum 1-mm space from the tooth root to the membrane margin). The membrane is secured lingually or palatally by means of two fixation screws (one in a mesial position and one in a distal position).

The composite graft is then gently adapted and compacted in the area of interest around the tenting screws, and the membrane is closed buccally with two other fixation screws (again placed mesially and distally). Membrane stability is mandatory. Stability is assured by fixing the membrane with adequate tension.

Wound closure

GBR for vertical ridge augmentation requires excellent soft tissue management because the major and most frequent complication is premature membrane exposure resulting in bacterial contamination.[42,43] This complication is generally the result of insufficient periosteal releasing incisions and excessive tension in the sutures at closure.

Primary passive closure is ensured by placement of horizontal mattress sutures using nonresorbable ePTFE 4-0 sutures and overlying interrupted sutures. This ensures a double line of suture by everting the connective tissue of both flaps. The horizontal mattress sutures should be placed at least 3 to 4 mm apically from the gingival margin of the flap, and the interrupted sutures should be equally positioned 3 mm apart from each other (Fig 9-3). Sutures are removed 12 to 15 days postoperatively.

Postoperative care

No removable or fixed partial dentures are allowed to compress the augmented area throughout the healing period. In esthetic areas, fixed partial dentures can be applied as long as there is no compression of the surgical site. This is absolutely mandatory to avoid wound dehiscence with consequent membrane exposure that allows bacterial contamination and infection of the augmented site, thereby jeopardizing the overall result.

Prevention of complications

Adherence to the following recommendations will help to prevent surgical complications:

- In the case of tooth extraction, soft tissue maturation should be complete before the vertical ridge augmentation procedure is performed. A minimum time of 2.5 months from tooth extraction is required.
- One linear and precise midcrestal incision (in the middle of the keratinized tissue) should be performed with perfect right angles at the vertical releasing incisions.
- Tissues should be managed gently, and the full-thickness flap should be elevated without damaging the periosteum.
- A correct and continuous periosteal incision should be made to achieve tension-free flaps.
- Sutures should not be overly tight, and adequate eversion of the flaps is mandatory.
- No compression of any kind should be applied to the surgical area.

Case Reports

Case 1

Vertical ridge augmentation in the posterior mandible (Fig 9-4)
A 55-year-old man presented with bilateral mandibular edentulism. The teeth were lost many years earlier because of periodontal disease. The standard one-stage protocol was applied in this patient because the initial bone height was adequate to allow correct primary implant stability.

The surgery was performed after administration of local anesthetic combined with sedative premedication. A full-thickness incision was made within the keratinized mucosa, starting from the distal aspect of the first premolar. An intrasulcular incision was made buccally around the premolar and lingually extending to the canine. A vertical releasing incision was made at the mesiobuccal angle and at the distal aspect of the crestal incision. Buccal and lingual flaps were reflected with a periosteal elevator.

Once exposed, the cortical bone was curetted with a back-action chisel to remove all residual connective tissue and the periosteum. Cortical perforations were made with a round diamond bur to enhance and stimulate bleeding. Two titanium dental implants were inserted and left to protrude to the appropriate height. Their function was analogous to that of tenting screws, ie, to support the overlying membrane and the particulated graft.

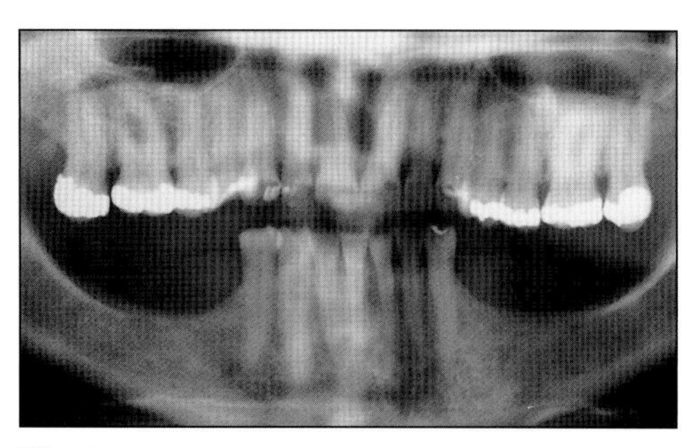

Fig 9-4a A panoramic radiograph indicates that bilateral mandibular atrophy is present. Treatment of the mandibular right side is presented in Figs 9-4b to 9-4h.

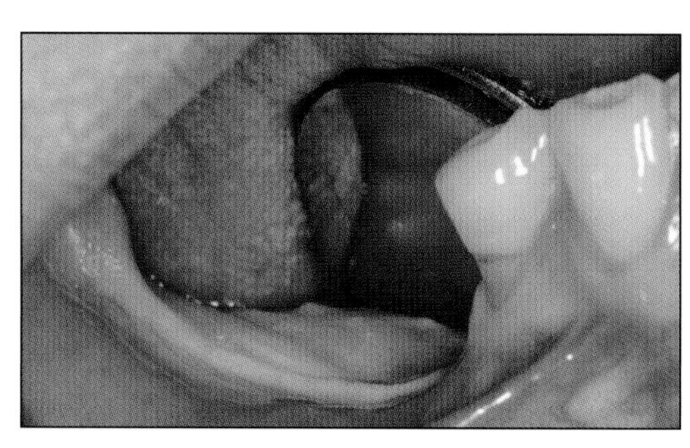

Fig 9-4b The patient's edentulous mandibular right segment exhibits severe atrophy. Minimal keratinized gingiva is present.

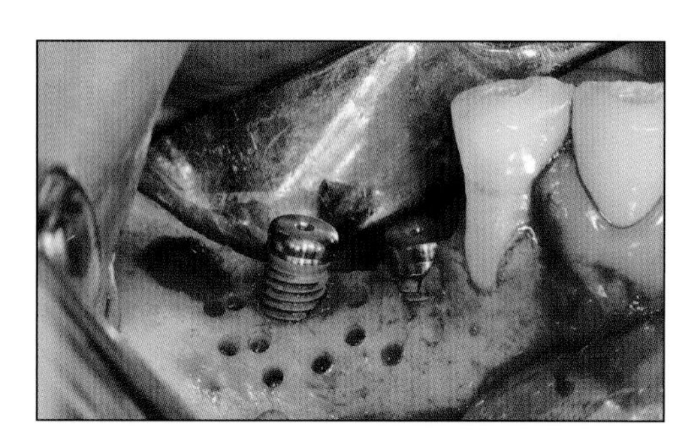

Fig 9-4c Once exposed by flap elevation, the cortical bone is curetted with a back-action chisel to remove all residual connective tissue and the periosteum. Cortical perforations are made with a diamond round bur to increase bleeding. Two titanium dental implants are placed and left to protrude in order to support the overlying membrane and the particulated graft.

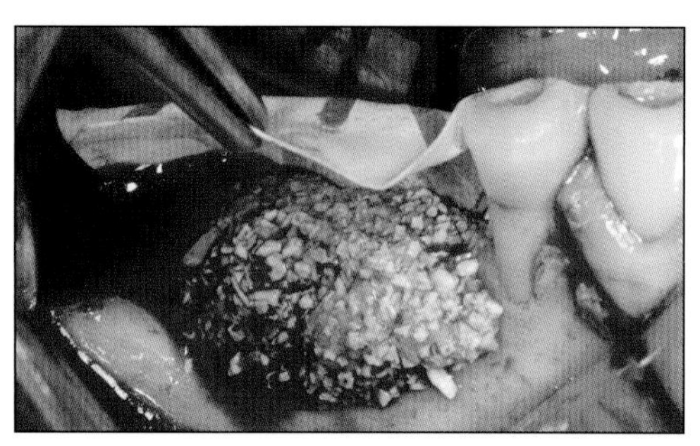

Fig 9-4d Autogenous bone chips are harvested in situ at the distolateral aspect of the mandibular ramus, mixed with DBBM particles, placed around the defect, and protected with a titanium-reinforced ePTFE membrane.

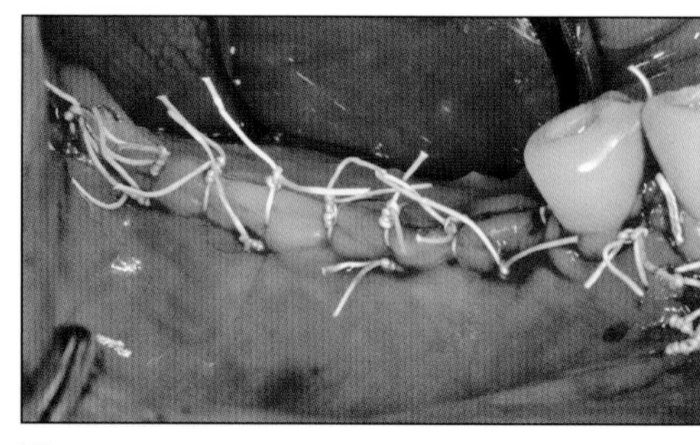

Fig 9-4e Primary wound closure is achieved with alternating nonresorbable horizontal mattress sutures and interrupted sutures.

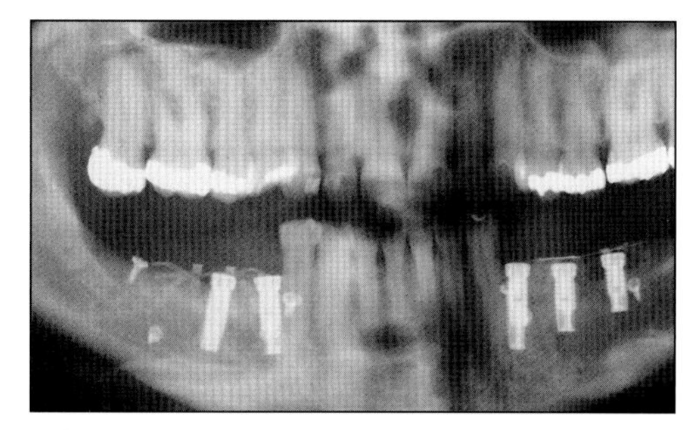

Fig 9-4f Control radiograph with the titanium-reinforced ePTFE membranes and titanium dental implants in place.

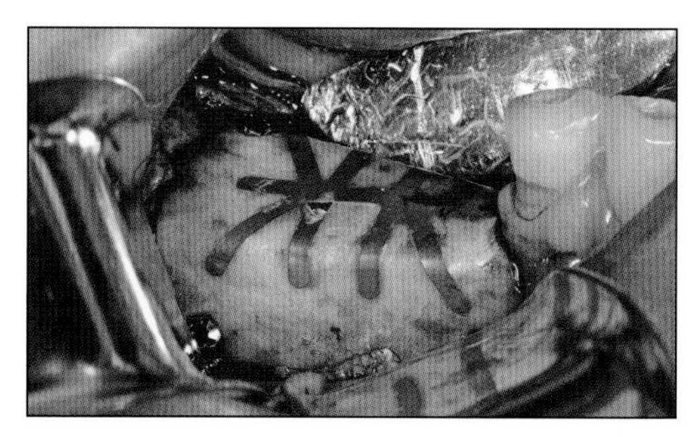

Fig 9-4g At reopening of the site, the titanium-reinforced membrane appears stable with the fixation screws in place.

Fig 9-4h The membrane is carefully removed, and the two dental implants are connected to their healing abutments.

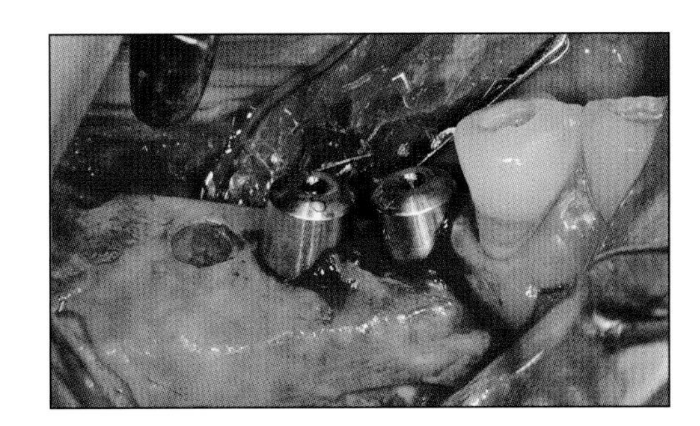

Autogenous bone was harvested in situ at the distolateral aspect of the mandibular ramus and mixed in a 1:1 ratio with DBBM particles. Prior to application of the graft, the ePTFE membrane was secured lingually with mesial and distal screws. The titanium-reinforced ePTFE membrane was then shaped to adapt to the defect without touching the distal margin of the adjacent tooth. The membrane was secured buccally with two fixation screws.

The patient was prescribed prophylactic antibiotics and advised to perform mouthrinses with 0.2 % chlorhexidine gluconate for 15 days. To minimize swelling and pain, the patient received one vial of steroids intramuscularly immediately after surgery and anti-inflammatory agents for 4 days postoperatively. The sutures were removed after 12 days.

Healing was uneventful. The patient was examined weekly during the first 2 months and then once a month until the stage-two surgery. Abutment connection was performed 6 months later.

Case 2

Alveolar bone augmentation in the anterior maxilla (Fig 9-5)

A 26-year-old man sought treatment for his edentulism in the area of the two maxillary central incisors. The incisors were previously lost in a car accident, resulting in inadequate bone volume both vertically and horizontally for traditional implant placement. In addition, there was clinical attachment loss on the adjacent teeth. Examination revealed clinical attachment loss of 4 mm on the mesial aspect of the right lateral incisor and 2 mm on the mesial aspect of the left lateral incisor.

The treatment protocol called for three tenting screws to be inserted to predetermine the height and thickness of the regenerated bone and to support the overlying membrane. A titanium-reinforced ePTFE augmentation membrane supported a mixture of autogenous bone graft and DBBM in a 1:1 ratio. The graft mixture was infused with recombinant human platelet-derived growth factor BB (rhPDGF-BB).

The patient was provided with a provisional fixed partial denture that served only esthetic purposes. No compression was allowed on the surgical site during the healing period. At the time of reopening, 6 months after surgery, the membrane was removed, and two titanium dental implants were placed in the augmented bone. The implants exhibited healthy surrounding soft tissues after stage-two surgery.

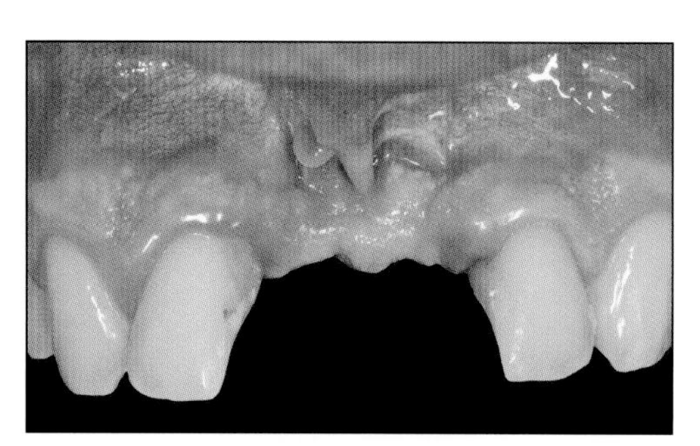

Fig 9-5a A 26-year-old man has lost both maxillary central incisors in an accident.

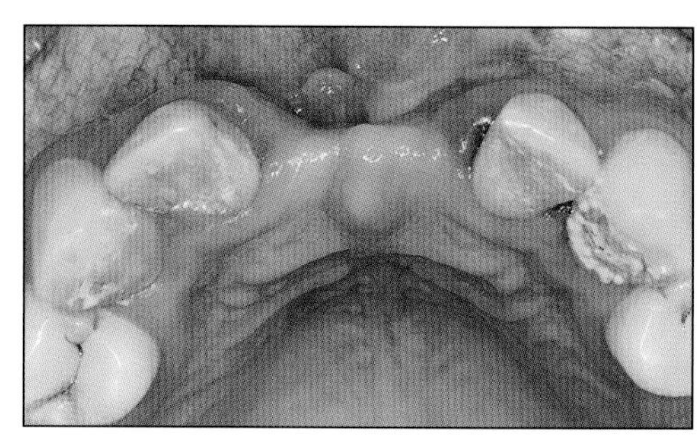

Fig 9-5b The occlusal view reveals the lack of adequate bone volume for traditional implant placement.

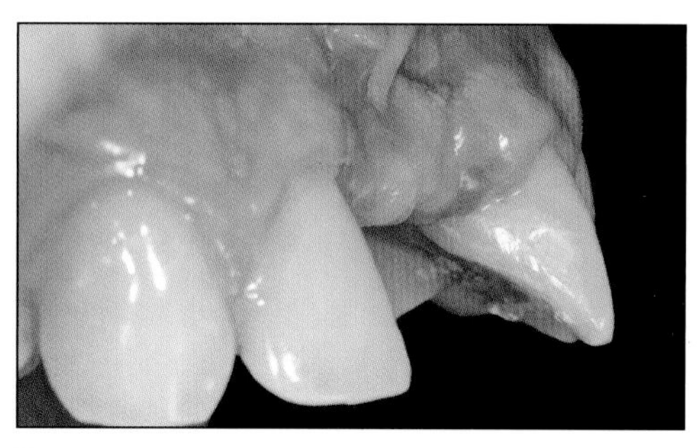

Fig 9-5c Lateral view of the site.

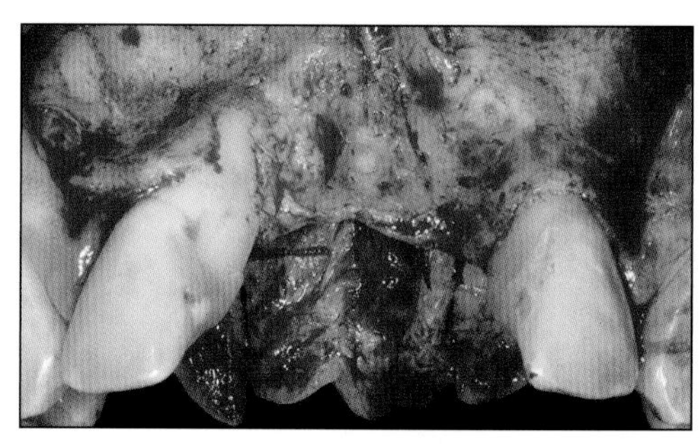

Fig 9-5d Elevation of a full-thickness flap reveals three-dimensional atrophy of the alveolar ridge and clinical attachment loss on the lateral maxillary incisors.

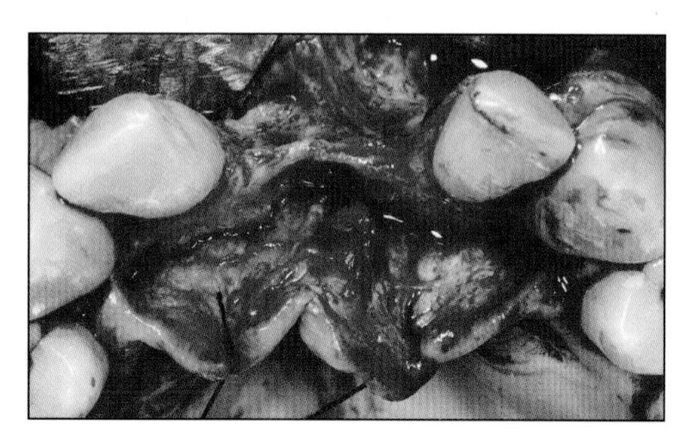

Fig 9-5e The occlusal view of the site after flap elevation reveals a severe bone defect in a horizontal direction.

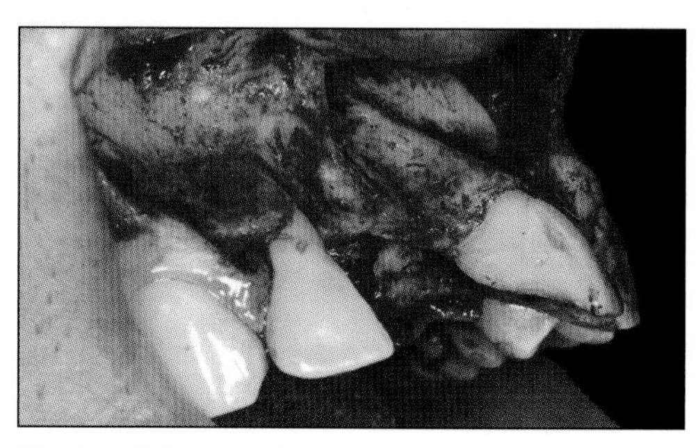

Fig 9-5f Lateral view of the exposed defect.

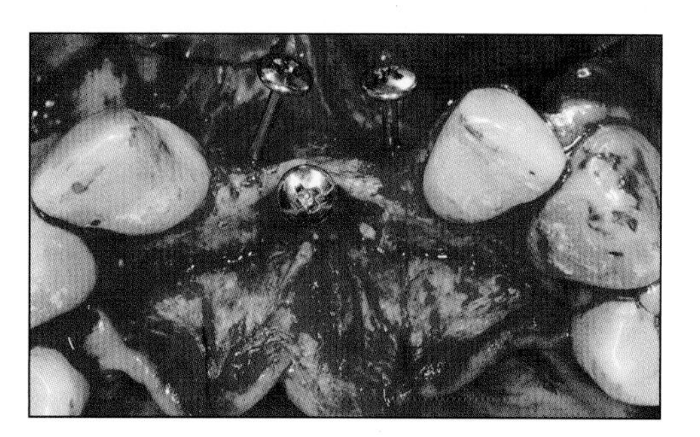

Fig 9-5g Three tenting screws are inserted to predetermine the height and thickness of the regenerated bone and to support the overlying membrane.

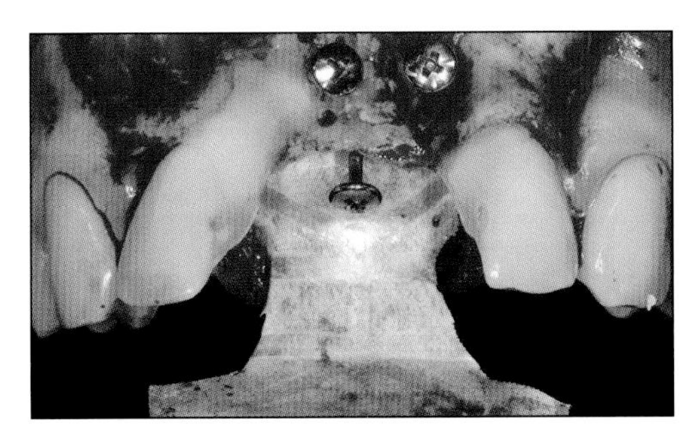

Fig 9-5h A titanium-reinforced ePTFE augmentation membrane is shaped appropriately and fixed to the palate.

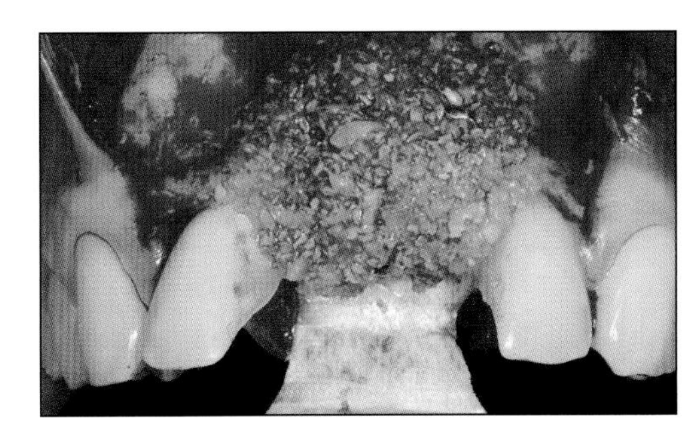

Fig 9-5i The membrane supports a mixture of autogenous bone graft and DBBM in a 1:1 ratio. The graft mixture is infused with rhPDGF-BB.

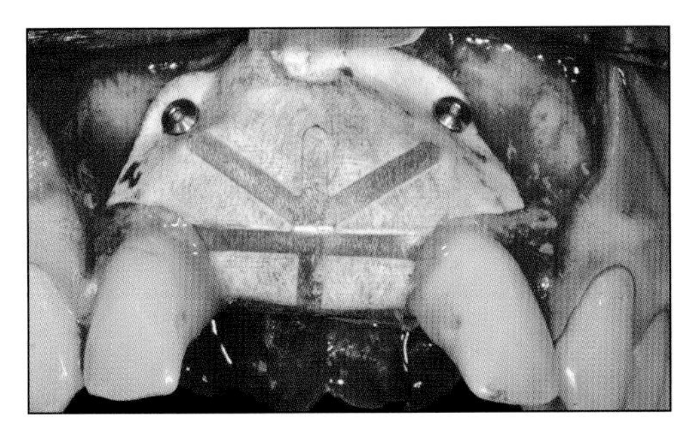

Fig 9-5j The titanium-reinforced ePTFE membrane is secured by four fixation tacks. About 1 mm of crestal bone is left uncovered next to the adjacent teeth so as not to interfere with the healing process of the periodontal tissues.

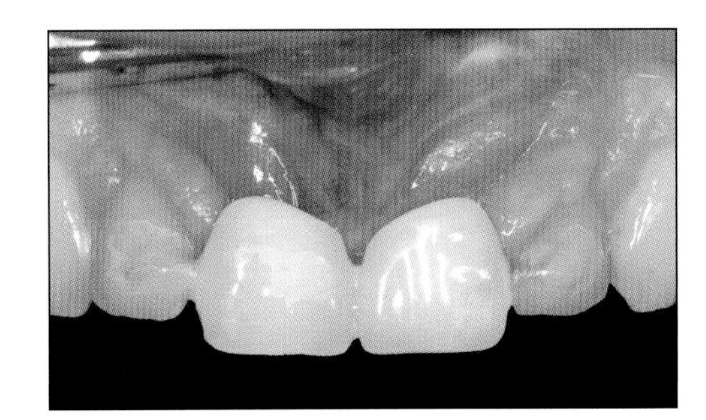

Fig 9-5k Clinical appearance after 6 months of healing. Immediately after surgery, the patient has been provided with a provisional fixed partial denture that served only esthetic purposes. No compression has been allowed on the surgical site during the entire healing period.

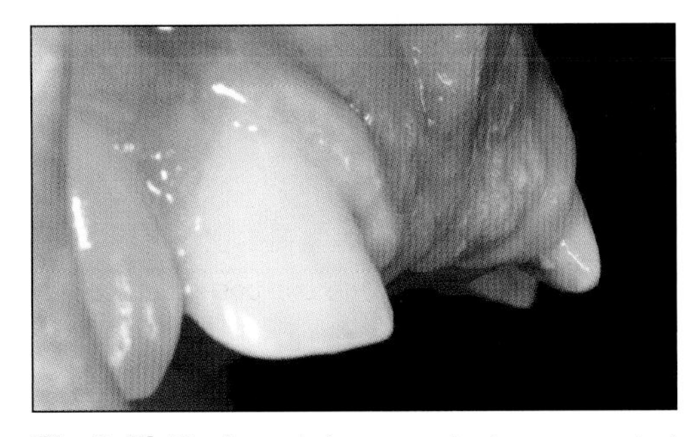

Fig 9-5l The lateral view reveals the augmented bone volume.

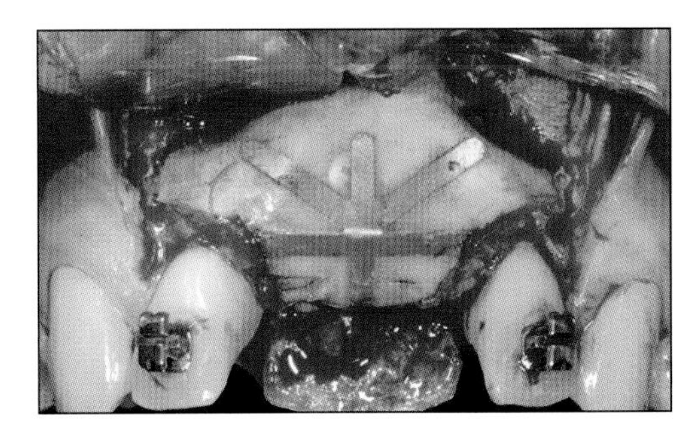

Fig 9-5m The reopening procedure after 6 months reveals the membrane in place and the volume of regenerated hard tissue.

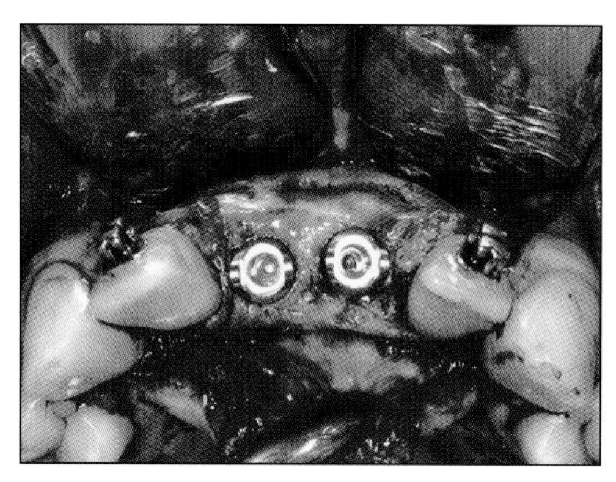

Fig 9-5n At the time of reopening, the membrane is removed, and two titanium dental implants are inserted.

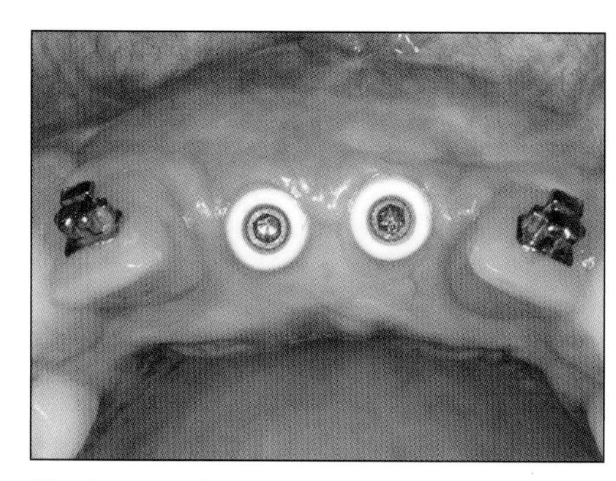

Fig 9-5o A clinical view of the implants in place reveals their healthy surrounding soft tissues after stage-two surgery.

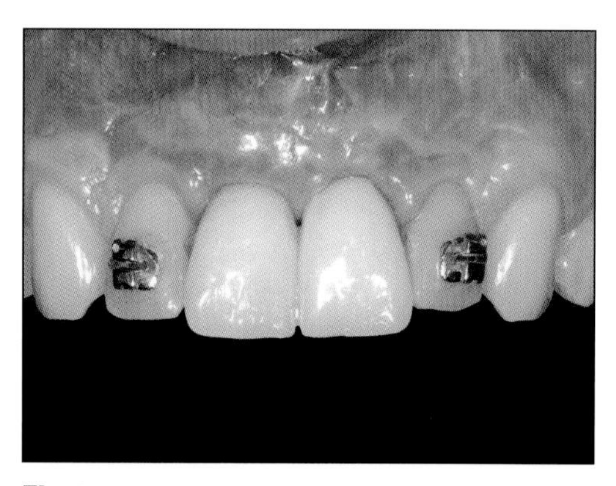

Fig 9-5p The provisional prosthetic restoration is in place. (Courtesy of Dr M. Fradeani, Pesaro, Italy.)

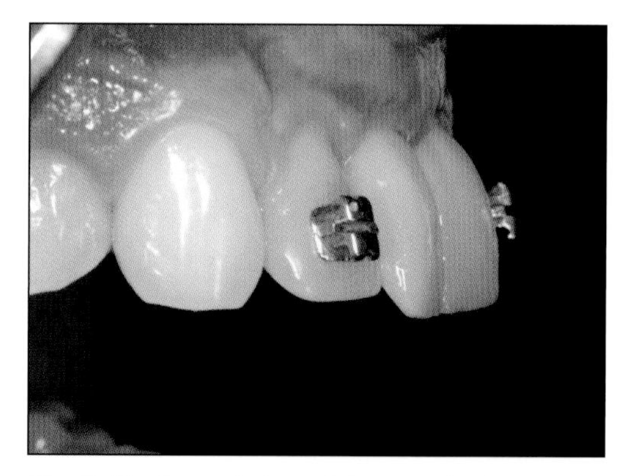

Fig 9-5q Lateral view of the prosthetic restoration. (Courtesy of Dr M. Fradeani, Pesaro, Italy.)

Case 3

Three-dimensional alveolar bone reconstruction (Fig 9-6)
A 34-year-old woman presented with severe disfigurement of the maxillary left lateral incisor and canine area following oncologic surgery. The bone defect extended 20 mm from the cervical margin of the adjacent teeth up to and including the nasal cavity.

The treatment regimen included augmentation with a 1:1 ratio of autogenous bone graft harvested from the retromolar region and DBBM particles. The composite graft was hydrolyzed with rhPDGF-BB and covered by a titanium-reinforced nonresorbable ePTFE membrane. Stage-two surgery was performed at 6 months, when the ePTFE membrane was removed and two titanium dental implants were successfully inserted. The time frame from initial surgery to final prosthesis was 14 months.

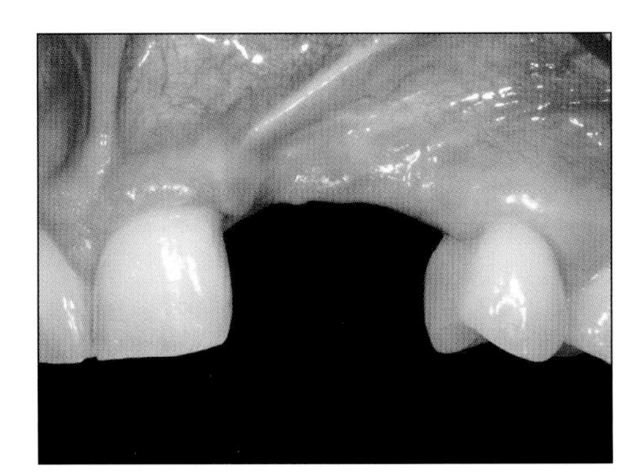

Fig 9-6a Previous oncologic resection resulted in the loss of the left lateral maxillary incisor and the canine and an extensive bone defect in a 34-year-old woman.

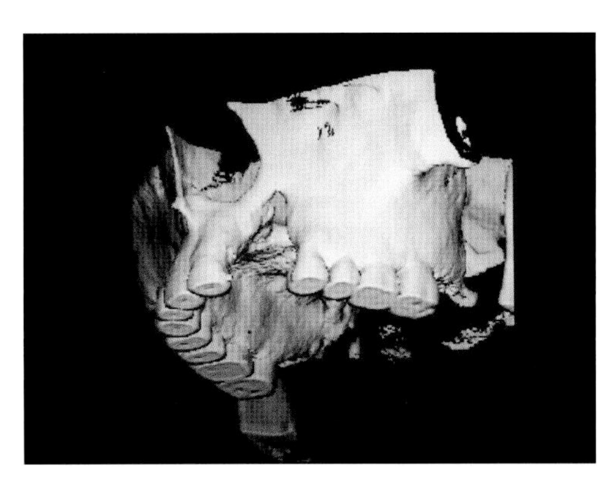

Fig 9-6b Three-dimensional computed tomography reconstruction reveals severe bone loss in direct continuity with the nasal cavity.

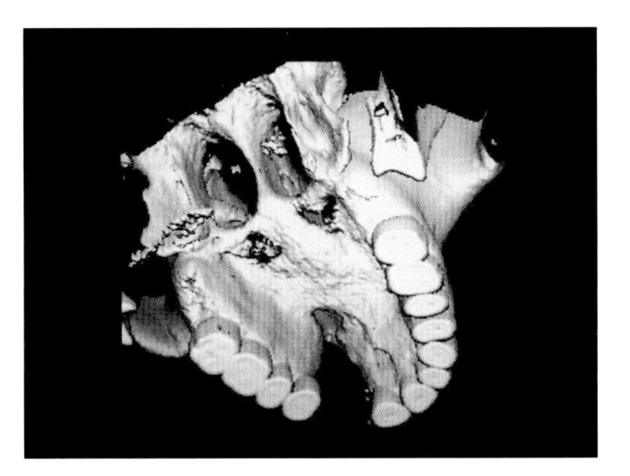

Fig 9-6c Inferoposterior view of the three-dimensional reconstruction shown in Fig 9-6b.

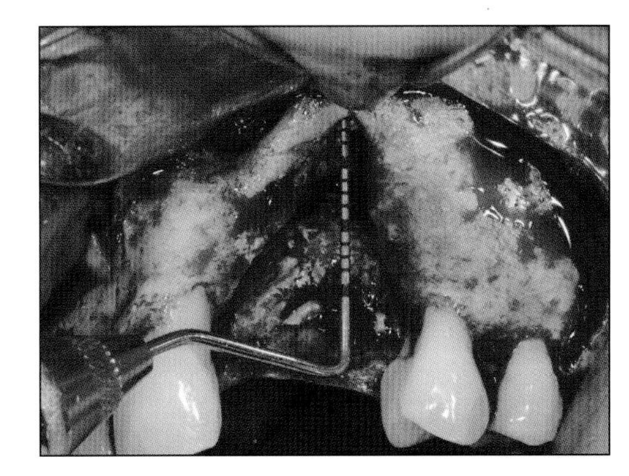

Fig 9-6d Full-thickness flap elevation reveals that the vertical bone loss approaches 20 mm.

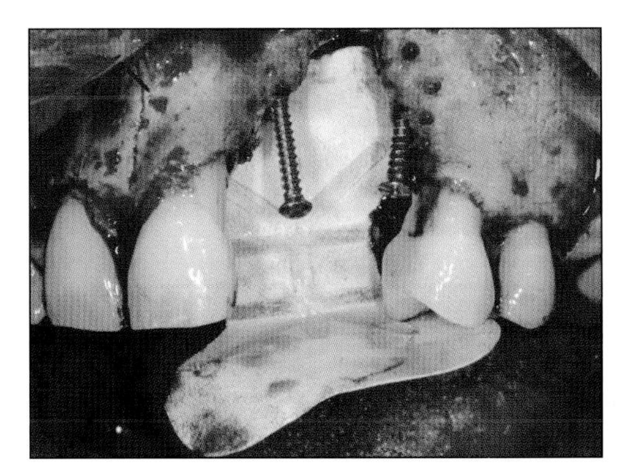

Fig 9-6e Two tenting screws are positioned to support the composite graft and prevent a collapse of the overlying membrane and soft tissues.

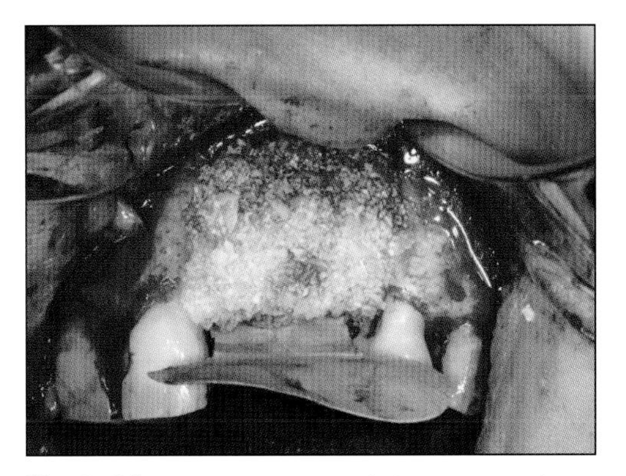

Fig 9-6f The composite graft (autogenous bone and DBBM in a 1:1 ratio) is placed and compacted in the deficient site. The graft had been hydrolyzed by rhPDGF-BB.

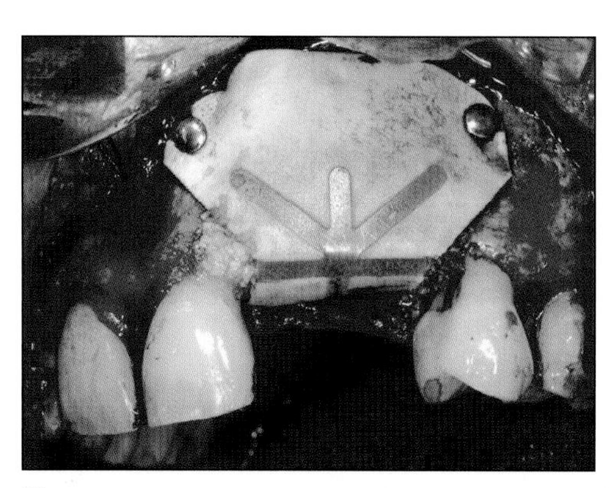

Fig 9-6g The overlying ePTFE membrane is accurately trimmed and secured to the defect area with buccal and palatal tacks.

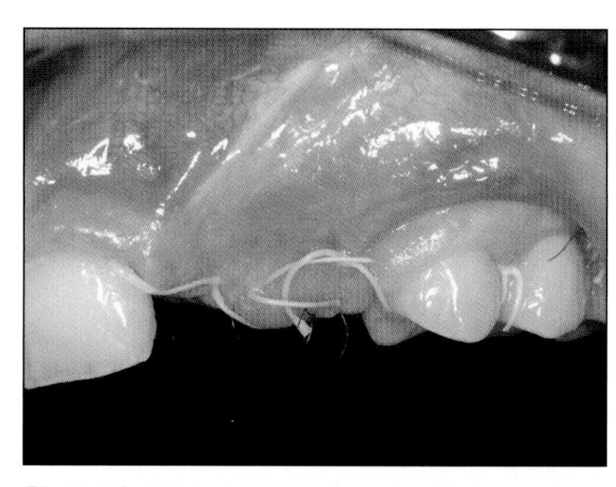

Fig 9-6h Clinical appearance after 12 days, prior to suture removal. Tension-free soft tissue closure was achieved with horizontal and interrupted sutures.

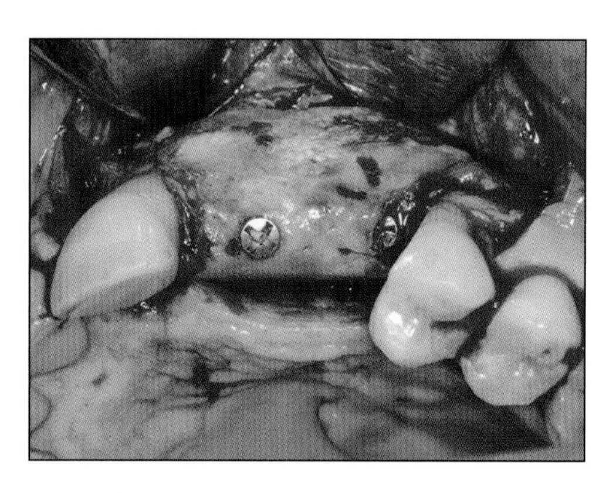

Fig 9-6i The reopening of the site after 6 months reveals substantial bone fill of the defect. The heads of the tenting screws are visible. The ePTFE membrane is removed, and two titanium dental implants are placed.

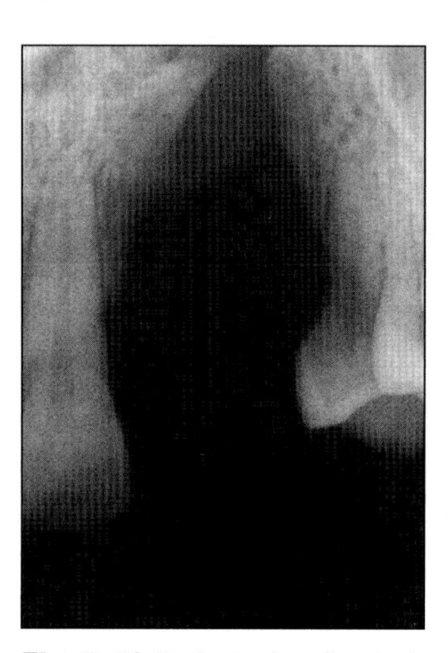

Fig 9-6j Periapical radiograph of the initial defect.

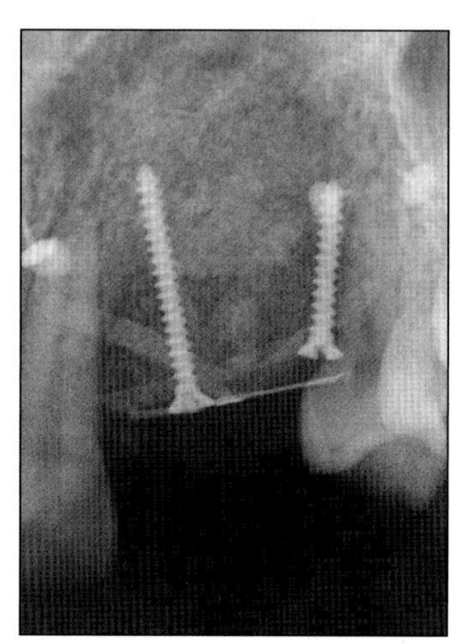

Fig 9-6k The tenting screws are in place with the overlying ePTFE membrane.

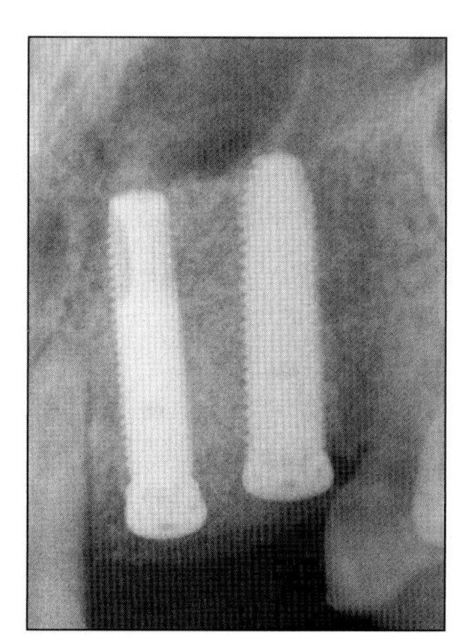

Fig 9-6l The two titanium dental implants are completely surrounded by regenerated bone.

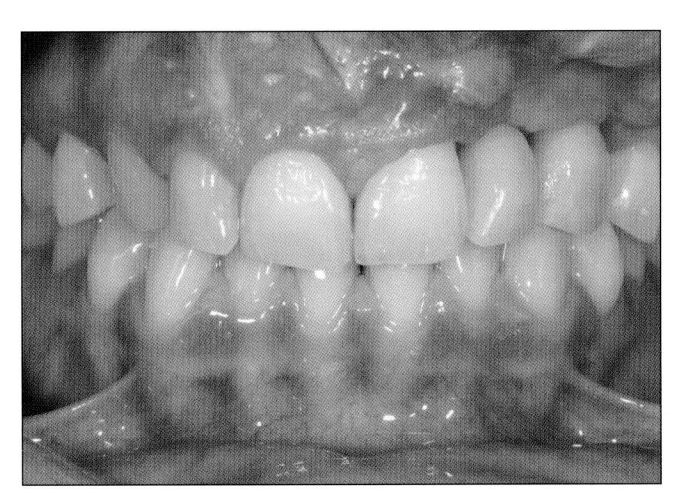

Fig 9-6m Clinical appearance of the final prosthesis in place. (Courtesy of Dr M. Maglione, Milan, Italy.)

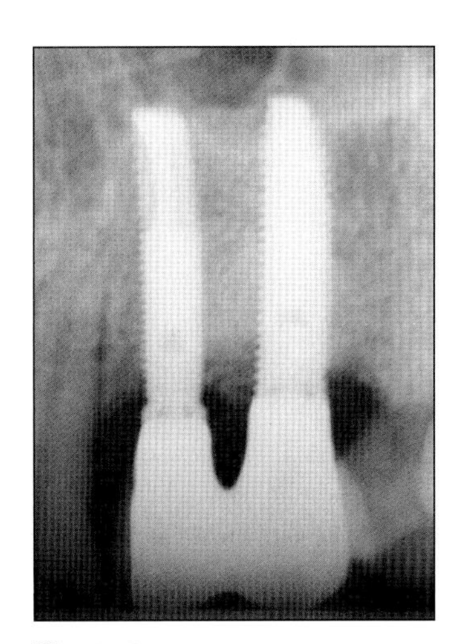

Fig 9-6n Periapical radiograph of the implants and the final prosthesis.

Future Directions: Tissue Engineering

Tissue engineering refers to any attempt to regenerate tissues in the body, whether accomplished in the laboratory or directly in the patient, by the addition of appropriate biologic mediators and matrices. The tissue engineering approach to bone regeneration combines three key elements: *(1)* conductive scaffolds, *(2)* signaling molecules, and *(3)* cells. To regenerate new bone in the treated site more predictably, osteoblasts or bone cell precursors must be encouraged, through cell signaling, to migrate to the engineered graft material, proliferate, and synthesize new bone.

One signaling molecule that has been studied extensively in both animals and humans is platelet-derived growth factor (PDGF), which is found in the granules of blood platelets and bone matrix[44] and is now recombinantly produced. PDGF plays a fundamental role in the wound healing cascade. It is present in high concentrations in platelets and released in the fluids generated during the early stage of wound healing.[45] PDGF is a potent chemotactic and mitogenic factor for cells of mesenchymal origin, including fibroblasts, osteoblasts, and chondrocytes, and is thus believed to be capable of enhancing tissue regeneration and repair.[46] Additionally, PDGF is angiogenic, promoting capillary budding into the graft site.

The use of purified rhPDGF-BB mixed with bone allograft (as described in cases 2 and 3) results in robust periodontal regeneration in both class II furcation invasions and intrabony defects. Histologic evidence has demonstrated that the combination of demineralized freeze-dried bone allograft with 0.5 mg/mL of rhPDGF-BB results in periodontal regeneration.[47–49] In addition, no unfavorable tissue reaction or other safety concern was associated with the treatment throughout the course of the studies. Hence, evidence of periodontal regeneration in humans has been reported with the use of PDGF.

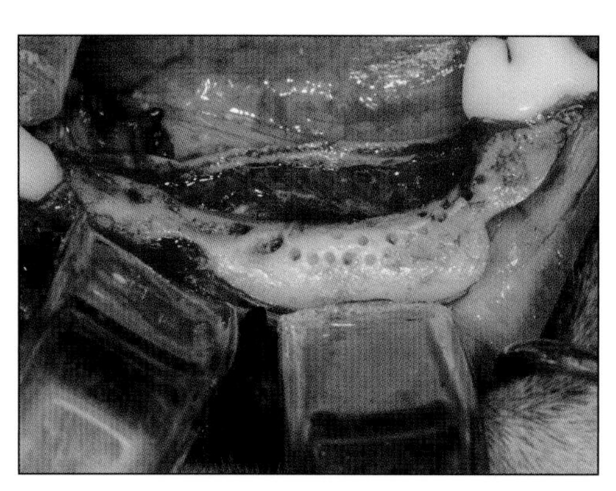

Fig 9-7 A full-thickness mandibular flap is elevated, and cortical perforations are made to encourage bleeding. The measurements of the defect are 3 cm mesiodistally and 1 cm apicocoronally. (Reprinted from Simion and Rocchietta[51] with permission.)

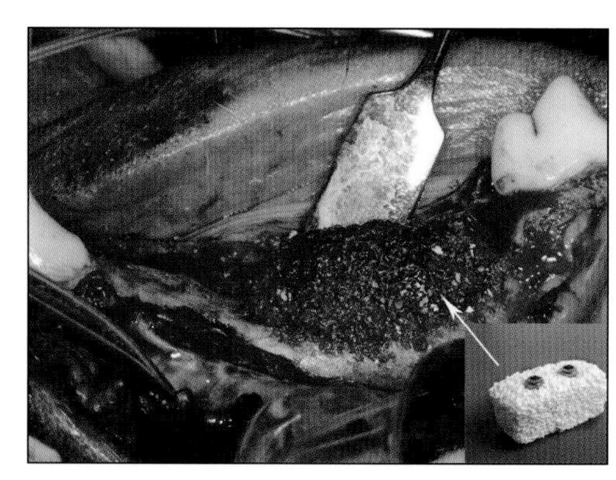

Fig 9-8 A block DBBM graft is placed over the atrophic mandible and secured by means of two titanium dental implants in mesial and distal positions. In eight sites (groups B and C), the block was infused with rhPDGF-BB. (Reprinted from Simion et al[50] with permission.)

The ability to vertically regenerate bone in severe chronic defects was investigated recently.[50] In the study, the effect of PDGF treatment on bone grafts positioned under a full-thickness mucoperiosteal flap was investigated using an established canine model[11] for alveolar ridge defects. Defects were created by bilateral extraction of all four mandibular premolars in six female fox hounds. The edentulous ridge was then surgically reduced, resulting in a flat defect approximately 10 mm deep and 30 mm long (Fig 9-7). The wound was closed and allowed to heal for 3 months. Following healing, full-thickness mucoperiosteal flaps extending the full length of the chronic defect were carefully elevated. The defects remained largely unhealed, verifying their critical-sized nature (ie, inability to heal naturally).

A block DBBM graft (Bio-Oss cancellous block, 20 × 10 × 10 mm, Geistlich) was shaped and placed in the site and stabilized by two titanium dental implants (Fig 9-8). Group A (n = 4) received a graft block in combination with a cell-occlusive bilayer collagen membrane placed between the periosteum and the graft block; group B (n = 4) received a block graft infused with PDGF with no collagen membrane (rhPDGF-BB, BioMimetic Therapeutics); and group C (n = 4) received a block graft infused with PDGF and overlaid with a collagen barrier. Animals were killed 4 months postimplantation. At this time, a specimen from group B was clinically reopened, and extensive hard tissue formation was observed (Fig 9-9).

None of the sites in group A (control) demonstrated regeneration of bone in the entire block graft area (Fig 9-10). Three of four sites in group A exhibited soft tissue healing complications in which the surgical wounds experienced dehiscence.

In contrast, extensive bone formation was observed in all group B sites (block graft and rhPDGF-BB; Fig 9-11). The dense new bone formed in contact with and completely covered the titanium implants. The density was greatest in the regions contacting the periosteum and the residual bone. All transient stages of woven bone to

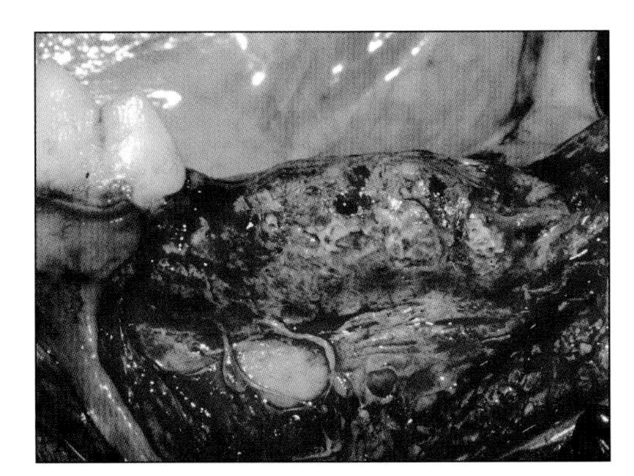

Fig 9-9 At reentry of a block DBBM graft plus rhPDGF-BB site after 4 months of submerged healing, the implants are covered with tissue resembling bone. Note the hard bleeding surface and the volume of regenerated bone. (Reprinted from Simion and Rocchietta[51] with permission.)

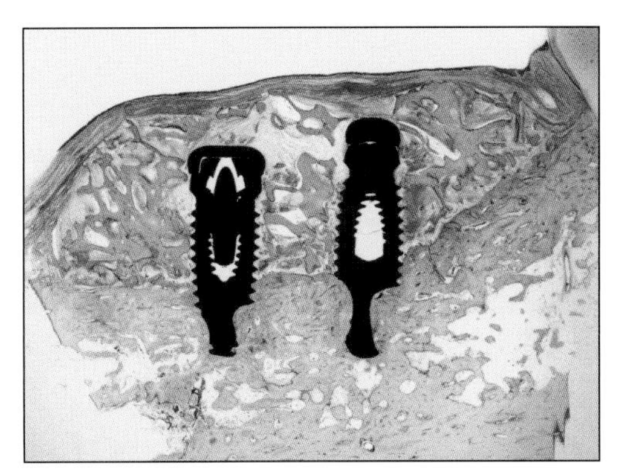

Fig 9-10 Control specimen (block DBBM graft plus membrane). The block is embedded in healthy connective tissue with no bone regeneration (mesiodistal ground section; toluidine blue-pyronine G stain; original magnification ×8). (Reprinted from Simion et al[50] with permission.)

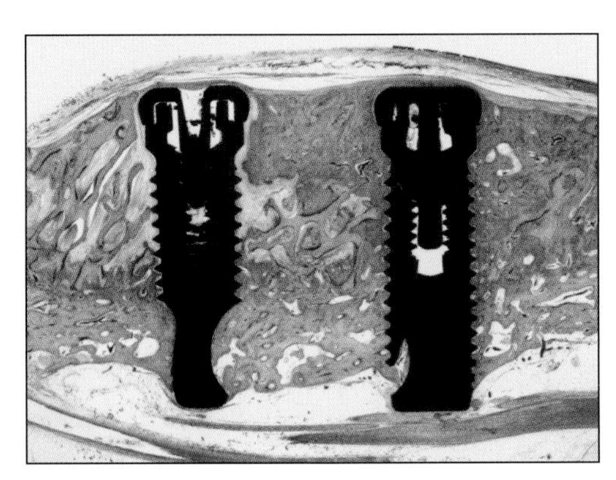

Fig 9-11a Specimen with block DBBM graft plus rhPDGF-BB. Note the formation of new bone around the two implants. The deproteinized bovine block is replaced by new bone. Inflammation-free connective tissue is present in the bovine block areas where bone formation has occurred (mesiodistal ground section; toluidine blue-pyronine G stain; original magnification ×12.5). (Reprinted from Simion et al[50] with permission.)

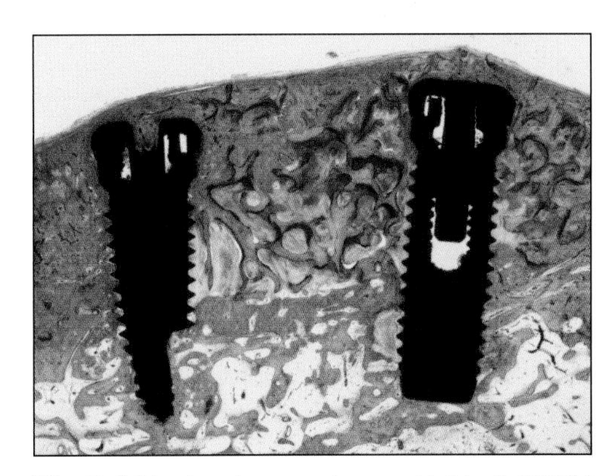

Fig 9-11b Another specimen with block DBBM graft plus rhPDGF-BB, showing similar formation of new bone around the implants (mesiodistal ground section; toluidine blue-pyronine G stain; original magnification ×12.5). (Reprinted from Simion et al[50] with permission.)

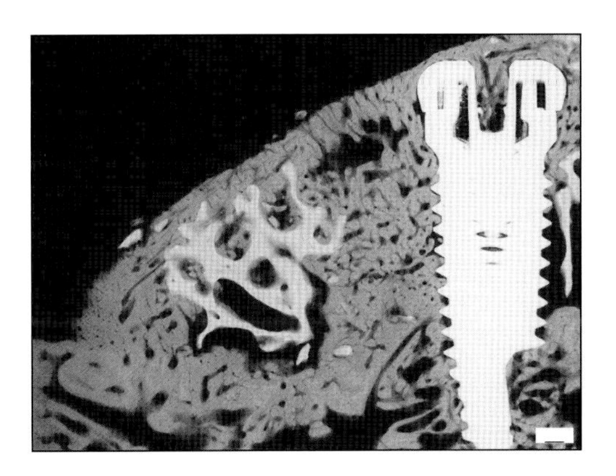

Fig 9-11c Microradiograph of an area of the specimen in Fig 9-11b. (Reprinted from Simion and Rocchietta[51] with permission.)

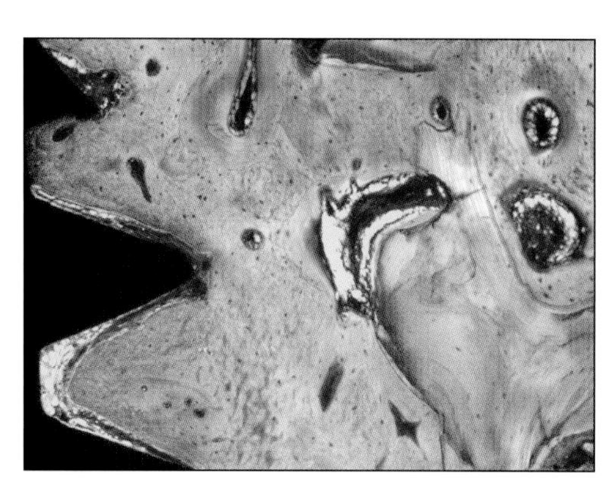

Fig 9-12 Intense osteoblastic activity and remodeling with mature osteons (toluidine blue–pyronine G stain; original magnification ×160). (Reprinted from Simion and Rocchietta[51] with permission.)

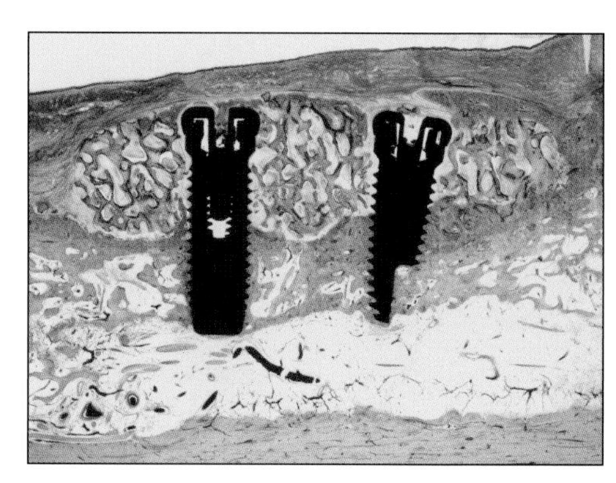

Fig 9-13 Specimen with block DBBM graft plus rhPDGF-BB plus membrane. Only a thin layer of new bone is visible at the coronal aspect of the specimen (mesiodistal ground section; toluidine blue–pyronine G stain; original magnification ×8). (Reprinted from Simion and Rocchietta[51] with permission.)

lamellar bone remodeling were detected in the newly formed bone. Intense osteoblastic activity was apparent, along with an unusually large number of bone remodeling units and well-developed osteons (Fig 9-12). Bone appeared to form from the periphery of the block inward, indicating that cell recruitment occurred from both periosteal and medullary sources. Whereas most of the block graft remained in group A, extensive remodeling of the graft had occurred in group B so that only a small amount of graft remained in the center of the site, embedded within healthy tissue.

Less bone regeneration was observed in group C (block graft, rhPDGF-BB, and barrier membrane) than in group B. New bone was observed growing coronally to the location of the barrier membrane in group C, which has not previously been reported in barrier-protected sites and was not observed in any group A sites. A large remnant of the graft block, surrounded by a thin layer of new bone, was typically present (Fig 9-13).

The infused specimens treated with a barrier membrane demonstrated significantly less bone regeneration, which is consistent with findings found in studies of recombinant bone morphogenetic protein.[52,53] The tissue-occlusive barrier membrane seems not to provide additional value to growth factors; in contrast, it appears that they may complicate wound healing. A possible explanation for this derives from the observation in this study that rhPDGF-BB seems to have strongly stimulated more bone formation from the periosteal surface than did the residual native bone. Therefore, the use of a membrane could have impeded the osteoblastic differentiation stimulated by the periosteum.[54–56]

In this preclinical proof-of-principle canine study, recombinantly produced platelet-derived growth factor (rhPDGF-BB), used in combination with a cancellous block DBBM graft but without a barrier membrane, evidenced significant new bone regeneration with high bone-to-implant contact, accelerated remodeling of the xenograft carrier, and restored the atrophic ridge to its normal anatomical form. Preclinical studies in larger cohorts are ongoing, as are human case reports, to confirm these promising results.[57,58]

Conclusion

Implant placement may not be possible in areas with limited bone height. Guided bone regeneration is one of a number of different techniques developed to reconstruct vertically deficient alveolar ridges. Careful adherence to the outlined surgical principles is mandatory to achieve a successful functional and esthetic outcome.

Clinical researchers continue their efforts to develop new technologies based on the principles of tissue engineering so that a less invasive surgical protocol can be developed for treatment of severe bone defects with decreased postoperative morbidity, faster healing time, improved predictability, and excellent functional and esthetic outcomes. Encouraging results are emerging, but time is still needed to confirm these very promising outcomes.

References

1. Mecall RA, Rosenfield AL. The influence of residual ridge resorption patterns on fixture placement and tooth position. 1. Int J Periodontics Restorative Dent 1991;11:9–23.
2. Nyman S, Karring T, Lindhe J, Planten S. Healing following implantation of periodontitis-affected roots into gingival connective tissue. J Clin Periodontol 1980;7:394–401.
3. Schenk RK, Buser D, Hardwick WR, Dahlin C. Healing pattern of bone regeneration in membrane-protected defects: A histologic study in the canine mandible. Int J Oral Maxillofac Implants 1994;9:13–29.
4. Schmid J, Hämmerle CH, Stich H, Lang NP. Supraplant, a novel implant system based on the principle of guided bone generation. A preliminary study in the rabbit. Clin Oral Implants Res 1991;2:199–202.
5. Linde A, Thorén C, Dahlin C, Sandberg E. Creation of new bone by an osteopromotive membrane technique: An experimental study in rats. J Oral Maxillofac Surg 1993;51:892–897.
6. Jovanovic SA, Schenk RK, Orsini M, Kenney EB. Supracrestal bone formation around dental implants: An experimental dog study. Int J Oral Maxillofac Implants 1995;10:23–31.
7. Jensen OT, Greer RO, Johnson L, Kassebaum D. Vertical guided bone-graft augmentation in a new canine mandibular model. Int J Oral Maxillofac Implants 1995;10:335–344.
8. Renvert S, Claffey N, Orafi H, Albrektsson T. Supracrestal bone growth around partially inserted titanium implants in dogs. A pilot study. Clin Oral Implants Res 1996;7:360–365.
9. Schliephake H, Kracht D. Vertical ridge augmentation using polylactic membranes in conjunction with immediate implants in periodontally compromised extraction sites: An experimental study in dogs. Int J Oral Maxillofac Implants 1997;12:325–334.
10. Schliephake H, Dard M, Planck H, Hierlemann H, Stern U. Alveolar ridge repair using resorbable membranes and autogenous bone particles with simultaneous placement of implants: An experimental pilot study in dogs. Int J Oral Maxillofac Implants 2000;15:364–373.
11. Simion M, Dahlin C, Rocchietta I, Stavropoulos A, Sanchez R, Karring T. Vertical ridge augmentation with guided bone regeneration in association with dental implants: An experimental study in dogs. Clin Oral Implants Res 2007;18:86–94.
12. Simion M, Trisi P, Piattelli A. Vertical ridge augmentation using a membrane technique associated with osseointegrated implants. Int J Periodontics Restorative Dent 1994;14:496–511.
13. Tinti C, Parma-Benfenati S, Polizzi G. Vertical ridge augmentation: What is the limit? Int J Periodontics Restorative Dent 1996;16:220–229.

14. Simion M, Jovanovic SA, Trisi P, Scarano A, Piattelli A. Vertical ridge augmentation around dental implants using a membrane technique and autogenous bone or allografts in humans. Int J Periodontics Restorative Dent 1998;18:8–23.
15. Tinti C, Parma-Benfenati S. Vertical ridge augmentation: Surgical protocol and retrospective evaluation of 48 consecutively inserted implants. Int J Periodontics Restorative Dent 1998;18:434–443.
16. Parma-Benfenati S, Tinti C, Albrektsson T, Johansson C. Histologic evaluation of guided vertical ridge augmentation around implants in humans. Int J Periodontics Restorative Dent 1999;19:424–437.
17. Simion M, Jovanovic SA, Tinti C, Parma-Benfenati S. Long-term evaluation of osseointegrated implants inserted at the time or after vertical ridge augmentation. A retrospective study on 123 implants with 1-5 year follow-up. Clin Oral Implants Res 2001;12:35–45.
18. Dahlin C, Lekholm U, Linde A. Membrane-induced bone augmentation at titanium implants. A report on ten fixtures followed from 1 to 3 years after loading. Int J Periodontics Restorative Dent 1991;11:273–281.
19. Dahlin C, Lekholm U, Becker W, et al. Treatment of fenestration and dehiscence bone defects around oral implants using the guided tissue regeneration technique: A prospective multicenter study. Int J Oral Maxillofac Implants 1995;10:312–318.
20. Fugazzotto PA. Success and failure rates of osseointegrated implants in function in regenerated bone for 6 to 51 months: A preliminary report. Int J Oral Maxillofac Implants 1997;12:17–24.
21. Adell R, Lekholm U, Rockler B, Brånemark PI. A 15-year study of osseointegrated implants in the treatment of the edentulous jaw. Int J Oral Surg 1981;10:387–416.
22. Lekholm U, Adell R, Lindhe J, et al. Marginal tissue reactions at osseointegrated titanium fixtures. 2. A cross-sectional retrospective study. Int J Oral Maxillofac Surg 1986;15:53–61.
23. Nevins M, Langer B. The successful application of osseointegrated implants to the posterior jaw: A long-term retrospective study. Int J Oral Maxillofac Implants 1993;8:428–432.
24. Albrektsson T, Zarb G, Worthington P, Eriksson B. Long-term efficacy of currently used dental implants: A review and proposed criteria of implant success. Int J Oral Maxillofac Implants 1986;1:11–25.
25. Simion M, Fontana F, Rasperini G, Maiorana C. Long-term evaluation of osseointegrated implants placed in sites augmented with sinus floor elevation associated with vertical ridge augmentation: A retrospective study of 38 consecutive implants with 1- to 7-year follow-up. Int J Periodontics Restorative Dent 2004;24:208–221.
26. Szpalski M, Gunzburg R. Recombinant human bone morphogenetic protein-2: A novel osteoinductive alternative to autogenous bone graft? Acta Orthop Belg 2005;71:133–148.
27. Ito K, Yamada Y, Nagasaka T, Baba S, Ueda M. Osteogenic potential of injectable tissue-engineered bone: A comparison among autogenous bone, bone substitute (Bio-Oss), platelet-rich plasma, and tissue-engineered bone with respect to their mechanical properties and histological findings. J Biomed Mater Res A 2005;73:63–72.
28. Kirmeier R, Payer M, Lorenzoni M, Wegscheider WA, Seibert FJ, Jakse N. Harvesting of cancellous bone from the proximal tibia under local anesthesia: Donor site morbidity and patient experience. J Oral Maxillofac Surg 2007;65:2235–2241.
29. Raghoebar GM, Louwerse C, Kalk WW, Vissink A. Morbidity of chin bone harvesting. Clin Oral Implants Res 2001;12:503–507.
30. Clavero J, Lundgren S. Ramus or chin grafts for maxillary sinus inlay and local onlay augmentation: Comparison of donor site morbidity and complications. Clin Implant Dent Relat Res 2003;5:154–160.
31. Raghoebar GM, Meijndert L, Kalk WW, Vissink A. Morbidity of mandibular bone harvesting: A comparative study. Int J Oral Maxillofac Implants 2007; 22:359–365.
32. Valentini P, Abensur D. Maxillary sinus floor elevation for implant placement with demineralized freeze-dried bone and bovine bone (Bio-Oss): A clinical study of 20 patients. Int J Periodontics Restorative Dent 1997;17:232–241.
33. Zitzmann NU, Naef R, Schärer P. Resorbable versus nonresorbable membranes in combination with Bio-Oss for guided bone regeneration. Int J Oral Maxillofac Implants 1997;12:844–852.
34. Zitzmann NU, Schärer P, Marinello CP. Long-term results of implants treated with guided bone regeneration: A 5-year prospective study. Int J Oral Maxillofac Implants 2001;16:355–366.
35. Hammerle CH, Lang NP. Single stage surgery combining transmucosal implant placement with guided bone regeneration and bioresorbable materials. Clin Oral Implants Res 2001;12:9–18.
36. Camelo M, Nevins ML, Schenk RK, et al. Clinical, radiographic, and histologic evaluation of human periodontal defects treated with Bio-Oss and Bio-Gide. Int J Periodontics Restorative Dent 1998;18: 321–331.
37. Hammerle CH, Karring T. Guided bone regeneration at oral implant sites. Periodontol 2000 1998;17:151–175.
38. Peetz M. Characterization of xenogenic bone material. In: Boyne PJ (ed). Osseous Reconstruction of the Maxilla and the Mandible. Chicago: Quintessence, 1997:87–100.
39. Rocchietta I, Dellavia C, Nevins M, Simion M. Bone regenerated via rhPDGF-BB and a deproteinized bovine bone matrix: Backscattered electron microscope element analysis. Int J Periodontics Restorative Dent 2007;27:539–545.
40. Camelo M, Nevins ML, Lynch SE, Schenk RK, Simion M, Nevins M. Periodontal regeneration with an autogenous bone–Bio-Oss composite graft and a Bio-Gide membrane. Int J Periodontics Restorative Dent 2001;21:109–119.
41. Simion M, Fontana F, Raperini G, Maiorana C. Vertical ridge augmentation by expanded-polytetrafluoroethylene membrane and a combination of intraoral autogenous bone graft and deproteinized anorganic bovine bone (Bio-Oss). Clin Oral Implants Res 2007;18:620–629.

42. Simion M, Trisi P, Maglione M, Piattelli A. A preliminary report on a method for studying the permeability of expanded polytetrafluoroethylene membrane to bacteria in vitro: A scanning electron microscopic and histological study. J Periodontol 1994;65:755–761.
43. Simion M, Trisi P, Maglione M, Piattelli A. Bacterial contamination in vitro through GTAM membrane with and without topical chlorhexidine application. A light and scanning electron microscopic study. J Clin Periodontol 1995;22:321–331.
44. Lynch SE. Introduction. In: Lynch SE, Genco RJ, Marx RE (eds). Tissue Engineering Applications in Maxillofacial Surgery and Periodontics. Chicago: Quintessence, 1999: xi–xviii.
45. Spindler KP, Mayes CE, Miller RR, Imro AK, Davidson JM. Regional mitogenic response of the meniscus to platelet-derived growth factor (PDGF-AB). J Orthop Res 1995;13:201–207.
46. Bhargava MM, Attia ET, Murrell GA, Dolan MM, Warren RF, Hannafin JA. The effect of cytokines on the proliferation and migration of bovine meniscal cells. Am J Sports Med 1999;27:636–643.
47. Nevins M, Camelo M, Nevins ML, Schenk RK, Lynch SE. Periodontal regeneration in humans using recombinant human platelet-derived growth factor-BB (rhPDGF-BB) and allogenic bone. J Periodontol 2003;74:1282–1292.
48. Camelo M, Nevins ML, Schenk RK, Lynch SE, Nevins M. Periodontal regeneration in human Class II furcations using purified recombinant human platelet-derived growth factor-BB (rhPDGF-BB) with bone allograft. Int J Periodontics Restorative Dent 2003;23:213–225.
49. Nevins M, Giannobile WV, McGuire MK, et al. Platelet-derived growth factor stimulates bone fill and rate of attachment level gain: Results of a large multicenter randomized controlled trial. J Periodontol 2005;76:2205–2215.
50. Simion M, Rocchietta I, Kim D, Nevins M, Fiorellini J. Vertical ridge augmentation by means of deproteinized bovine bone block and recombinant human platelet-derived growth factor-BB: A histologic study in a dog model. Int J Periodontics Restorative Dent 2006;26:415–423.
51. Simion M, Rocchietta I. Minimally invasive strategies for vertical ridge augmentation. In: Lynch SE, Marx RE, Nevins M, Wisner-Lynch LA (eds). Tissue Engineering: Applications in Oral and Maxillofacial Surgery and Periodontics, ed 2. Chicago: Quintessence, 2008: 145–158.
52. Hunt DR, Jovanovic SA, Wikesjo UME, Wozney JM, Bernard GW. Hyaluronan supports rh-BMP-2 induced bone reconstruction of advanced alveolar defects in dogs. A pilot study. J Periodontol 2001;72: 651–658.
53. Zellin G, Linde A. Importance of delivery systems for growth-stimulatory factors in combination with osteopromotive membranes. An experimental study using rh-BMP-2 in rat mandibular defects. Biomed Materials Res 1997;35:181–190.
54. Weng D, Hurzeler MB, Quinones CR, Ohlms A, Caffesse RG. Contribution of the periosteum to bone formation in guided bone regeneration. A study in monkeys. Clin Oral Implants Res 2000;11: 546–554.
55. Shimizu T, Sasano Y, Nakajo S, Kagayama M, Shimauchi H. Osteoblastic differentiation of periosteum-derived cells is promoted by the physical contact with the bone matrix in vivo. Anat Rec 2001;264:72–81.
56. Li M, Amizuka N, Oda K, et al. Histochemical evidence of the initial chondrogenesis and osteogenesis in the periosteum of a rib fractured model: Implications of osteocyte involvement in periosteal chondrogenesis. Microsc Res Tech 2004;64:330–342.
57. Simion M, Dellavia C. Three-dimensional ridge augmentation with xenograft and recombinant human platelet-derived growth factor-BB in humans: Report of two cases. Int J Periodontics Restorative Dent 2007;27:109–115.
58. Simion M, Rocchietta I, Monforte M, Maschera E. Three-dimensional alveolar bone reconstruction by means of a combination of recombinant human platelet-derived growth factor-BB and guided bone regeneration: A case report. Int J Periodontics Restorative Dent 2008;28:239–245.

Index

Note: Page numbers followed by "f" indicate figures; "t" indicate tables; "b" indicate boxes.

C

D

E

F

G